Lecture Notes of the Institute for Computer Sciences, Social Informatics and Telecommunications Engineering 247

More information about this series at http://www.springer.com/series/8197

Paolo Perego · Amir M. Rahmani
Nima TaheriNejad (Eds.)

Wireless Mobile Communication and Healthcare

7th International Conference, MobiHealth 2017
Vienna, Austria, November 14–15, 2017
Proceedings

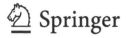 Springer

Editors
Paolo Perego
Polytechnic University of Milan
Milan
Italy

Amir M. Rahmani
University of California
Irvine, CA
USA

Nima TaheriNejad
ICT, Institute of Computer Technology
Vienna University of Technology
Vienna
Austria

ISSN 1867-8211   ISSN 1867-822X (electronic)
Lecture Notes of the Institute for Computer Sciences, Social Informatics
and Telecommunications Engineering
ISBN 978-3-319-98550-3   ISBN 978-3-319-98551-0 (eBook)
https://doi.org/10.1007/978-3-319-98551-0

Library of Congress Control Number: 2018950656

This Springer imprint is published by the registered company Springer Nature Switzerland AG
The registered company address is: Gewerbestrasse 11, 6330 Cham, Switzerland

Preface

The MobiHealth 2017 Conference was the 7th in a series of scientific events bringing together expertise from medical, technological, design, and even from social domains. MobiHealth 2017, which took place in Vienna, Austria, during November 14–15, 2017, focused on wearables, algorithms, virtual reality, and design, with some papers on machine learning in medicine and mobile health. Mobihealth 2017 offered participants a keynote on computer and emotions with Rosallind Picard, founder and director of the Affective Computing Research Group at the MIT Media Lab. The conference had nine sessions and more than 50 authors coming from all over the world.

Mobihealth started in 2010, just at the beginning of the Smartphone revolution, as one of the first conferences on Mobile technology and evolved over the years to an event with an interdisciplinary approach with authors involved from machine learning to service design. The conference also covers technological and biomedical facilities, legal, ethical, social, as well as the necessary basic research for enabling the future of mobile health-care paradigms.

The present volume includes the articles presented during the two-day conference in Vienna. The conference received more than 50 papers, which were accurately checked via a double-blind review process, involving about 20 reviewers: members of the Technical Program Committee and experts from different countries worldwide. The highly selective review process resulted in a full-paper rejection rate of 30%, by that way guaranteeing a high scientific level of the accepted and finally published papers.

The papers were divided into eight sessions:

1. Data Analysis
2. Systems
3. Work in Progress
4. Pervasive and Wearable Health Monitoring
5. Advances in Personalized Health-Care Services
6. Design for Health Care
7. Advances in Soft Wearable Technology for Mobile Health
8. Sensors and Circuits

We are grateful to the Technische Universität Wien and the European Alliance for Innovation for sponsoring this event. Finally, we would like to thank all the participants for the hard work preparing manuscripts and the presentations. The papers included in these proceedings are the end result of a tremendous amount of creative work and a highly selective review process. We hope that they will serve as a valuable source of information on the state of the art of mobile health and technology. Moreover, the editors are indebted to the acknowledged and highly experienced reviewers for having contributed significantly to the quality of the conference and this book. The editors are also grateful to the dedicated efforts of the local Organizing Committee members and their supporters for carefully and smoothly preparing and operating the conference. They especially thank Prof. Nima TaheriNejad from the Institute for Computer Technology (ICT) of the TU Wien and all his team for their dedication to the organization and realization of the conference.

July 2018   Paolo Perego

Organization

Steering Committee

Steering Committee Chair

Imrich Chlamtac   CREATE-NET, EAI

Founding Chair

James C. Lin   University of Illinois at Chicago, USA

Members

Dimitrios Koutsouris	National Technical University of Athens, Greece
Janet Lin	University of Illinois at Chicago, USA
Arye Nehorai	Washington University in St. Louis, USA
Konstantina S. Nikita	National Technical University of Athens, Greece
George Papadopoulos	University of Cyprus, Cyprus
Oscar Mayora	CREATE-NET, Italy

Organizing Committee

General Co-chairs

Nima TaheriNejad	TU Wien, Austria
Giuseppe Andreoni	Polytechnic University of Milan, Italy
Axel Jantsch	TU Wien, Austria

Technical Program Committee Co-chairs

Maria Renata Guarneri	Polytechnic University of Milan, Italy
Nima TaheriNejad	TU Wien, Austria
Akram Alomainy	Queen Mary University of London, UK

Web Chairs

Sai Manoj	TU Wien, Austria
Alessandra Mazzola	Polytechnic University of Milan

Publicity and Social Media Chairs

M. Ali Shami	TU Wien, Austria
Alessandra Mazzola	Polytechnic University of Milan

Workshops Chair

Kalle Tammemäe   Tallinn University of Technology, Estonia

Sponsorship and Exhibits Chair

Marcus Meisel   TU Wien, Austria

Publications Chairs

Paolo Perego   Polytechnic University of Milan, Italy
Amir M. Rahmani   University of California, Irvine, USA

Panels Chairs

Pasi Liljeberg   University of Turku, Finland
Muhammad Shafique   TU Wien, Austria

Tutorials Chair

Amir M. Rahmani   University of California, Irvine, USA

Demos Chair

Albert Treytl   Danube University Krems, Austria

Local Chair

Thilo Sauter   TU Wien, Austria

Conference Manager

Dominika Belisová   EAI

Contents

Data Analysis

Design for Healthcare

Advances in Personalized Healthcare Services

Advances in Soft Wearable Technology for Mobile-Health

Systems

Enhancing the Self-Aware Early Warning Score System Through Fuzzified Data Reliability Assessment

Maximilian Götzinger[1(✉)], Arman Anzanpour[1], Iman Azimi[1], Nima TaheriNejad[2], and Amir M. Rahmani[2,3]

[1] Department of Information Technology, University of Turku, Turku, Finland
{maxgot,armanz,imaazi}@utu.fi
[2] Institute of Computer Technology, TU Wien, Vienna, Austria
nima.taherinejad@tuwien.ac.at
[3] Department of Computer Science, University of California Irvine, Irvine, USA
amirr1@uci.edu

Abstract. Early Warning Score (EWS) systems are a common practice in hospitals. Health-care professionals use them to measure and predict amelioration or deterioration of patients' health status. However, it is desired to monitor EWS of many patients in everyday settings and outside the hospitals as well. For portable EWS devices, which monitor patients outside a hospital, it is important to have an acceptable level of reliability. In an earlier work, we presented a self-aware modified EWS system that adaptively corrects the EWS in the case of faulty or noisy input data. In this paper, we propose an enhancement of such data reliability validation through deploying a hierarchical agent-based system that classifies data reliability but using Fuzzy logic instead of conventional Boolean values. In our experiments, we demonstrate how our reliability enhancement method can offer a more accurate and more robust EWS monitoring system.

Keywords: Early Warning Score · Modified early warning score
Self-awareness · Data reliability · Consistency · Plausibility
Fuzzy logic · Hierarchical agent-based system

1 Introduction

Chronic diseases such as cardiovascular diseases are the leading cause of death in the world [1]. Such diseases put patients at the risk of sudden health deterioration, which is reflected in patient's vital signs up to 24 h in advance. Early enough health deterioration detection effectively increases the chance of patient's survival [2].

In hospitals, particularly in intensive care units, the Early Warning Score (EWS) is a prevalent manual tool, by which patient's vital signs are periodically recorded and the emergency level is interpreted [3]. To this end, a score

© ICST Institute for Computer Sciences, Social Informatics and Telecommunications Engineering 2018
P. Perego et al. (Eds.): MobiHealth 2017, LNICST 247, pp. 3–11, 2018.
https://doi.org/10.1007/978-3-319-98551-0_1

(0 for a perfect condition and 3 for the worst condition) is allocated to each vital sign according to its value and the predefined limits (see Table 1). The summation of the obtained scores indicates the degree of health deterioration of the patient (the higher the EWS, the worse the patient's health condition). However, there are two major restrictions in this manual tool. First, unreliable interpretation might be made due to the presence of inaccuracy and latency in the manual data collection. Secondly, and the more important restriction from a practical point of view, this manual tool is not applicable to out-of-hospital situations where no professional caregiver is available to perform the measurements. Recent advancements in Internet of Things (IoT) technologies can mitigate these restrictions by providing 24/7 remote health monitoring. In EWS systems based on IoT devices, patients' vital signs along with context data are continuously monitored via mobile/wearable sensors, while cloud server performs data analysis and decision making algorithms for the score determination [4,5].

Data reliability of such IoT-based EWS systems in remote health monitoring is of paramount importance. In our previous work [6], we proposed an architecture which exploits self-awareness techniques to adaptively adjust the EWS in the case of faulty readings from the sensor. We indicated a binary decision-making technique to determine whether the sensory data is reliable, and if needed we accordingly adjusted the EWS. However, like many other natural phenomena, data reliability of the sensory data is a continuous value and treating it in a binary manner, although simplifying the analysis, can lead to loss of information. For example, many somewhat reliable sensory data can lead to an unreliable assessment whereas in a binary assessment they may be interpreted as reliable (since they may fall closer to a reliable value in the spectrum) and thus create a wrong assessment.

In this paper, we propose a data reliability validation technique that is based on Fuzzy logic. The usage of Fuzzy logic instead of Boolean logic to classify input data as reliable or faulty covers the unsharp (fuzzy) ranges in which vital signs can indeed be correct or incorrect. In our extensive experiments, we show how our Self-Aware Early Warning Score (SA-EWS) method can be leveraged to enhance the reliability and robustness of health monitoring systems.

Table 1. Score classification table of a set of vital signals

Vital signal score	3	2	1	0	1	2	3
Heart rate (beats/min)	<40	40–51	51–60	60–100	100–110	110–129	>129
Systolic blood pressure (mmHg)	<70	70–81	81–101	101–149	149–169	169–179	>179
Respiratory rate (breaths/min)		<9		9–14	14–20	20–29	>29
Oxygen saturation (%)	<85	85–90	90–95	>95			
Body temperature (°C)	<28	28–32	32–35	35–38		38–39.5	>39.5

2   Data Reliability Concepts

Data reliability is an additional meta-data which describes the quality of the measured data. The reliability consists of accuracy and precision of sensory data [7] and grants a higher level of comprehension on the validity of the input data. If a sensor is broken, the monitored vital sign will be most probably inaccurate and not precise. Whereas the data provided by the sensor can still be accurate and precise when the sensor is detached from the patient's body. However, in both of these cases, an EWS calculated based on their values is invalid and therefore, unreliable in the given context. Hence, determining the reliability of the input data can be very challenging, but there exist potential solutions; consistency and plausibility controls, as well as cross validation are among them [7]. While the calculation of the EWS is based on the absolute values of the vital signs, the reliability of the EWS uses additional information about slopes and inter-correlations of the vital signs.

Consistency: Signals often have some limits such as maximum rate of change, these limits can be exploited to assess the reliability of a signal. Consistency is an aspect that can provide information on whether an observed input signal is reliable or not based on its history. A signal with a physically impossible slope indicates a problem which can be evoked by a sensor failure or a detachment of the sensor from the body. Regardless of the reason, a faulty monitored vital sign affects the calculation of the EWS negatively and should be avoided. For example, a change of the body temperature of several degrees per minute is impossible [8]. Therefore, in such a case the gathered sensory data should be classified as unreliable and treated accordingly.

Plausibility and Correlation: One aspect of plausibility is the absolute value of an input signal. For example, the oxygen saturation can only be between 0% and 100%. An input data that shows values of the oxygen saturation outside of this boundary must be classified as unreliable.

Another aspect of plausibility is the cross-reliability or co-existence plausibility. Various efforts have been conducted to indicate correlations between different vital signs [9–11]. For instance, considering the possible effect of the body temperature on the heart rate value, the probability of an increase in heart rate is high in the case of elevated body temperature [10]. As a second example, we can consider that a body temperature of $-30\,°C$ is implausible in the case of a living patient, although a deceased person lying in a very cold area can have such a low body temperature.

3   Fuzzified Reliability Assessment

In contrast to our previous work [6] where the data reliability validation was based on Boolean logic, we propose here the use of Fuzzy logic. Because of the lack of complete knowledge of all body functions, determining whether a vital sign is monitored correctly is a hard task. Fuzzy logic brings the significant advantage of covering unsharp (fuzzy) ranges in which vital signs cannot be easily tagged as correctly monitored or not. Thus, a vital sign can have a reliability value between 0 and 1 (0% and 100%), instead of just being reliable or unreliable.

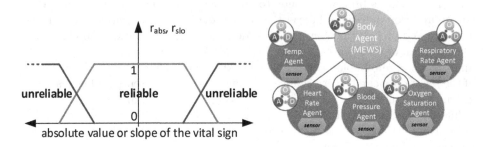

Fig. 1. Example for a fuzzy membership function.

Fig. 2. System architecture.

In the proposed system, the first task of reliability module is to analyze two metrics of a vital sign, the absolute value of the signal and its slope. For this analysis, fuzzy membership functions (shown in Fig. 1) are needed, each of which is configured to match the properties of the assigned signal. The result of this analysis is given by two parameters, the reliability of the absolute value r_{abs} and that of the signal slope r_{slo}. Subsequently, the reliability of an input signal r_{sig} is calculated with

$$r_{sig} = r_{abs} \wedge r_{slo} \tag{1}$$

where the fuzzy "and" ($\wedge$) is equal to a minimum function [12]. The parameter r_{sig} gives information about the reliability of each signal considered separately and omits the correlation of the different vital signs (reviewed in Sect. 2). To consider the correlation, more highly abstracted information is needed on how one vital sign can impact another. The cross-validated reliability, r_{cro}, which exists for each pair of signals is given by

$$r_{cro} = \begin{cases} 1 & \text{if } S_{vs1} = S_{vs2} \\ \frac{1}{p_{cro}|S_{vs1}-S_{vs2}|} & \text{if } S_{vs1} \neq S_{vs2} \end{cases} \tag{2}$$

where $p_{cro} \in (0, \infty)$ denotes a coefficient of the strength of the correlation[1] between vital signs vs_1 and vs_2, and S_{vs1} as well as S_{vs2} are the abstracted scores of these two vital signs.

---

[1] The reliability module in our implementation limits the cross-reliability r_{cro} to a value between 0 to 1, although theoretically, a coefficient less than 1 can lead to a r_{cro} higher that 1.

When all reliability and cross-reliability values are available, the reliability of the calculated EWS is given by

$$r = \left(r_{sig_1} \wedge \cdots \wedge r_{sig_n}\right) \wedge \left(r_{cro_{12}} \wedge r_{cro_{13}} \wedge \cdots \wedge r_{cro_{mn}}\right) \tag{3}$$

where the first term conjugates all reliabilities of the various vital signs, and the second term contains the conjunction of all combinations of cross-reliabilities.

4 Experiments

4.1 Implemented System Architecture

As in our last work [6], a hierarchical agent-based model, implemented in C++, constitutes the base of the SA-EWS system (Fig. 2). Such an agent-based approach combined with the usage of mini ODA loops enable a good modularity and simple implementation. Every agent works according to an ODA loop; which means that every single agent monitors certain inputs, decides what to do, and acts accordingly.

Beside its modularity, such hierarchical agent-based architecture has another essential advantage. The input data with all its semantic content and contextual information can be abstracted in different layers [13]. As shown in Fig. 2, each agent of the lower hierarchical level is connected to a sensor. Due to the agent-based design, the scoring of vital signs and the calculation of the EWS are performed independently in different locations.

4.2 Functional Description of the System

First, each low-level agent reads the actual value of the vital sign the sensor attached to it provides. Subsequently, it abstracts the raw input data to a vital sign score S (Table 1) and validates the reliability of the signal, r_{sig} (Eq. 1). Finally, the low-level agent sends both values (score S and the signal reliability r_{sig}) to the agent of the higher hierarchical level; the "Body Agent".

Similar to the low-level agents, the body agent starts its task with reading the input values, although these are coming from the low-level agents and not from sensors. This high-level agent is responsible for the calculation of the EWS as well as the reliability of the calculated EWS. While the agent's binding module sums up all gathered scores to calculate the EWS, the reliability module calculates the cross-reliability, r_{cro}, for each pair of vital signs (Eq. 2) followed by the reliability, r, of the overall EWS (Eq. 3). As the last step and before the next data sets are read, the calculated EWS and its reliability, r, are outputted.

4.3 Experimental Data

All vital signs are collected from a 36 years old male subject with diastolic hypertension. Several sensors and devices are used for data collection. The Bioharness 3 [14] chest strap with a wearable Bluetooth sensor set is used to record the

heart rate and the respiration rate. Blood pressure and blood Oxygen saturation are recorded using iHealth BP5 [15] arm blood pressure monitor and iHealth
PO3 [16] finger grip pulse oximeter which both of them are Bluetooth-enabled
monitoring devices. Body temperature sensor is a DS18b20 [17] digital temperature sensor connected to ATMEGA328P [18] microcontroller and nRF51822 [19]
Bluetooth low energy module. We used an Android phone to collect data from
all sensors during the experiments with the rate of one sample per second.

We conditioned the data collection phase to emulate certain faults and errors.
These conditions are applied in order to show how the system is able to detect
the changes from normal to the abnormal condition and back from abnormal to
normal condition. To this end, a change has been applied for around 5 min in the
middle of a 15-min data collection. We note that the conducted experiments are
proof-of-concept experiments and more extensive tests with more patients are
planned for the future. The applied abnormal conditions are: (i) The temperature
sensor has been detached from the body and brought to contact with an object
at room temperature, (ii) The temperature sensor has been detached from the
body and brought to contact with a cold object, (iii) The temperature sensor
has been detached from the body and brought to contact with a hot object, (iv)
A biceps contraction has happened during the blood pressure measurements,
and (v) The chest strap for the heart rate and respiration rate monitor has been
loosened.

4.4 Configuration

Several factors influenced the setup of the fuzzy membership functions and the
correlation coefficients. Besides the medical publications [8–11,20], expert's opin-
ions from various physicians, the accuracy of the sensors used, and the medical
condition of the patient were considered in configuring the system. To repeat
the experiments with other sensors or patients, the setup should be reconfigured
again to reflect such personalization. Although reconfiguration of these parameters is easy in our system, finding our the right values is a complex task which
requires further research for enabling its automation.

5 Results

Our experiments show that the SA-EWS system works correctly, and the reliability of the calculated EWS coincides with the condition of the measurement
setup. In other words, erroneous input data leads to a lower reliability. Due to
the space limitation, only two of these cases are shown here in this section.

In the first experiment (shown in Fig. 3(a)) at around 350 s the body temperature sensor is detached and measures the room temperature until it is again
attached (around 700 s). Over this period the reliability value decreases drastically. Whereas the validation of the slope causes the low reliability during
the beginning and the ending phase of the period of detachment, the cross-
plausibility validation does this for the rest of this period. Because of the medical condition (high respiration rate) of the test subject, the correlation between

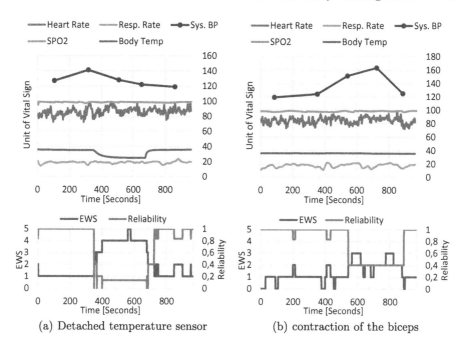

(a) Detached temperature sensor   (b) contraction of the biceps

Fig. 3. The monitored vital signs, the EWS and its reliability. (a) the body temperature sensor is detached from the patient and temporarily measures the room temperature (b) a contraction of the biceps interferes with the blood pressure measurement.

the respiration and the other vital signs was set to weak (decreased from the default value of 1.5 to 0.6). Nevertheless, during the moments when the respiration frequency reaches values greater than or equal to 20 (score 2), reliability level decreases even further.

For the second experiment shown here (Fig. 3(b)), we tampered with the measurement of the blood pressure. The gathered input data shows a high blood pressure value because the patient tensed his biceps during two of the samples (around 550 s and 700 s). Since there is a strong correlation between heart rate and blood pressure [9], the correlation coefficient p_{cro} was increased from 1.5 to 2.5. As the heart rate was more or less constant while the blood pressure was increased, the cross-reliability led to a low reliability. As in the first experiment, the temporary breathing rate with a score of 2 or higher leads to short periods of slightly reduced reliability at around 200 s and 400 s.

6   Conclusion and Future Work

In this paper, we presented an SA-EWS system with a fuzzified reliability validation which recognizes erroneous vital signs caused by various measurement artifacts such as loose sensors, detached sensors or other interferences. In our experiments, the proposed system was successful in detecting such events and decreased the data reliability during such events. This observation shows that self-awareness techniques such as the one proposed and used here can provide more robust EWS calculations. We note that deciding the value of parameters such as possible absolute values, signal slopes, and correlations among various vital signs demands domain knowledge. As the human body is an extremely complex system, not every phenomenon is already known. Therefore, although domain knowledge can be helpful for general cases, it does not replace personalized assessment which experts can provide each patient with. For this reason, we plan to add a learning module to the SA-EWS system which should learn about the patient's body functions and its basic health condition. In addition, more metrics should be generated and used, such as the derivation or the variability of a vital sign.

Acknowledgement. The authors wish to acknowledge the financial support by the Marie Curie Actions of the European Union's H2020 Programme.

References

1. WHO: Chronic diseases and health promotion. http://www.who.int/chp/en/. Accessed June 2017
2. Kyriacos, U.: Monitoring vital signs using early warning scoring systems: a review of the literature. J. Nurs. Manag. **19**(3), 311–330 (2011)
3. Morgan, R.J.M.: An early warning scoring system for detecting developing critical illness. Clin. Intensive Care **8**(2), 100 (1997)
4. Anzanpour, A., et al.: Internet of Things enabled in-home health monitoring system using early warning score. In: Proceedings of MobiHealth (2015)
5. Anzanpour, A., et al.: Self-awareness in remote health monitoring systems using wearable electronics. In: DATE Conference (2017)
6. Götzinger, M., Taherinejad, N., Rahmani, A.M., Liljeberg, P., Jantsch, A., Tenhunen, H.: Enhancing the early warning score system using data confidence. In: Perego, P., Andreoni, G., Rizzo, G. (eds.) MobiHealth 2016. LNICST, vol. 192, pp. 91–99. Springer, Cham (2017). https://doi.org/10.1007/978-3-319-58877-3_12
7. TaheriNejad, N., et al.: Comprehensive observation and its role in self-awareness; an emotion recognition system example. In: Proceedings of FedCSIS (2016)
8. Pasquier, M., et al.: Cooling rate of 9.4 °C in an hour in an avalanche victim. Resuscitation **93**, e17–e18 (2015)
9. Reule, S.: Heart rate and blood pressure: any possible implications for management of hypertension? Curr. Hypertens. Rep. **14**(6), 478–484 (2012)
10. Davies, P.: The relationship between body temperature, heart rate and respiratory rate in children. Emerg. Med. J. **26**(9), 641–643 (2009)
11. Zila, I., Calkovska, A.: Effects of elevated body temperature on control of breathing. Acta Medica Martiniana **2011**(Supp 1), 24–30 (2011)
12. Ross, T.J.: Fuzzy Logic with Engineering Applications. Wiley, New York (2009)
13. Guang, L.: Hierarchical agent monitoring design approach towards self-aware parallel soc. ACM Trans. Embed. Comput. Syst. **9**(3), 25 (2010)
14. Zephyr: Bioharness 3. www.zephyranywhere.com. Accessed June 2017
15. iHealth: iHealth BP5. www.ihealthlabs.com/blood-pressure-monitors/feel/. Accessed June 2017

16. iHealth: iHealth   PO3.   www.ihealthlabs.com/fitness-devices/wireless-pulse-oximeter/. Accessed June 2017
17. Maxim Integrated: DS18b20. www.maximintegrated.com/en/products/analog/sensors-and-sensor-interface/DS18B20.html. Accessed June 2017
18. ATMEL: Atmega328p. www.atmel.com/devices/atmega328p. Accessed June 2017
19. Nordic Semiconductor: nrf51822. www.nordicsemi.com/eng/Products/Bluetooth-low-energy/nRF51822. Accessed June 2017
20. Song, H.S., et al.: The effects of specific respiratory rates on heart rate and heart rate variability. Appl. Psychophysiol. Biofeedback **28**(1), 13–23 (2003)

Large-Scale Continuous Mobility Monitoring of Parkinson's Disease Patients Using Smartphones

Wei-Yi Cheng[1], Florian Lipsmeier[2], Andrew Creigh[2,3], Alf Scotland[2],
Timothy Kilchenmann[2], Liping Jin[1], Jens Schjodt-Eriksen[2], Detlef Wolf[2],
Yan-Ping Zhang-Schaerer[2], Ignacio Fernandez Garcia[2],
Juliane Siebourg-Polster[2], Jay Soto[4], Lynne Verselis[1], Meret Martin Facklam[2],
Frank Boess[2], Martin Koller[4], Machael Grundman[4,5,6], Andreas U. Monsch[7,8],
Ron Postuma[9], Anirvan Ghosh[2], Thomas Kremer[2], Kirsten I. Taylor[2],
Christian Czech[2], Christian Gossens[2(✉)], and Michael Lindemann[2,10]

[1] Roche Innovation Center New York, Roche TCRC Inc., New York, USA
[2] Roche Innovation Center Basel, F. Hoffmann-La Roche Ltd., Basel, Switzerland
christian.gossens@roche.com
[3] University of Oxford, England, UK
[4] Prothena Biosciences Inc., South San Francisco, USA
[5] Global R&D Partners, LLC, San Diego, USA
[6] University of California, San Diego, USA
[7] University Center for Medicine of Aging, Memory Clinic, Felix Platter Hospital,
Basel, Switzerland
[8] University of Basel, Basel, Switzerland
[9] Department of Neurology, McGill University, Montreal General Hospital,
Montreal, Canada
[10] Baden-Wuerttemberg Cooperative State University, Loerrach, Germany

Abstract. Smartphone-based assessments have been considered a potential solution for continuously monitoring gait and mobility in mild to moderate Parkinson's disease (PD) patients. Forty-four PD patients from cohorts 4 to 6 of the Multiple Ascending Dose (MAD) study of PRX002/RG7935 and thirty-five age- and gender-matched healthy individuals (i.e. healthy controls - HC) in a separate study performed smartphone-based assessments for up to 24 weeks and up to 6 weeks, respectively. The assessments included "active gait tests", where all participants were asked to walk for 30 s with at least one 180° turn, and "passive monitoring", in which subjects carried the smartphone in a pocket or fanny pack as part of their daily routine. In total, over 6,600 active gait tests and over 30,000 h of passive monitoring data were collected. A mobility analysis indicates that patients with PD are less mobile than HCs, as manifested in time spent in gait-related activities, number of turns and sit-to-stand transitions, and power per step. It supports the potential use of smartphones for continuous mobility monitoring in future clinical practice and drug development.

© ICST Institute for Computer Sciences, Social Informatics and Telecommunications Engineering 2018
P. Perego et al. (Eds.): MobiHealth 2017, LNICST 247, pp. 12–19, 2018.
https://doi.org/10.1007/978-3-319-98551-0_2

Keywords: Sensors · Activity recognition · Smartphone
Accelerometer · Machine learning · Deep learning
Parkinson's disease · Clinical trial

1   Introduction

Mobility-related symptoms are among the earliest symptoms of Parkinson's disease (PD) and are part of the clinical diagnosis [1]. Functional impact of PD on mobility-related activities such as walking, turning or rising from chair has an impact on patients' quality of life and is also used clinically as an indication for disease progression. In order to provide an objective and quantitative assessment of gait and mobility, many studies have implemented wearable systems or body-fixed sensors in both controlled [2,3] and free-living settings [4,5]. While the on-body sensors are light-weighted and inexpensive, the difficulties of integrating them into daily living pose an extra burden to the subjects and usually limit the length of the study to less than one month [5].

Most smartphones have built-in sensors to provide more environment-aware services and applications utilize these sensors, such as accelerometers, gyroscope and magnetometers. As smartphones have become standard equipment in daily life, they provide a more natural way of performing long-term mobility assessment in a clinical setting. In this paper, we present the results of a large-scale, longitudinal gait and mobility assessment of PD patients in a clinical trial setting using smartphones and compare them with age and gender matched controls.

2   Methods

2.1   Data Collection

Information on the MAD clinical trial of PRX002/RG7935 study can be found online [6]. Our analysis focused on exploring the between-group differences between HC and PD, and did not assess PRX002/RG7935-related effects. PD subjects from cohorts 4 to 6 of the MAD study and all participants from the HC study were provided with a locked-down smartphone only running a dedicated app, which allowed for the execution of active tests and continuous sensor recordings.

Active Gait Tests. Each participant was asked to perform at least one active test in the morning. Participants were requested to walk in a straight line with minimal turns for 30 s. In the trial, 5,107 active gait tests were completed by the PD cohort and 1,589 in the HCs. The sensor readouts of the accelerometer and gyroscopes were measured at 66 Hz. All of the gait and mobility features in the active tests were extracted while excluding the first and last 5 s of the test, as during these time spans often the subjects were putting the smartphones into or removing it from their pockets or fanny packs.

Passive Monitoring. Every day the participants were requested to carry the smartphone in their pocket or in a fanny pack for as long as the battery life allowed (approximately 6 h), while the sensors recorded their movement. In total, 24,104 h of passive monitoring data were recorded for the PD cohort, and 8,614 h for the HCs. In line with a previously published approach [7], we filtered out accelerometer data where the standard deviation of Euclidean norm was less than $0.03 \, \text{m/s}^2$ for more than 30 min, as during these spans smartphones were likely not carried by the subjects. This step removed 24% of the passive monitoring data.

2.2 Human Activity Recognition (HAR)

A diagram of the 9-layer neural network model structure and an example data flow is shown in Fig. 1. Similar structures have been used previously for HAR and have been shown to out-perform the traditional machine learning methods [8]. Our HAR model was trained on two public data sets [9,10] to classify six activities: walking, stairs, jogging, sitting, standing, and lying down. The continuous accelerometer data were down-sampled into 20 Hz and segmented into 4-s windows with 75% overlapping with adjacent ones.

When making predictions, the model classifies the overlapping windows into the six activities. As each second in the trial data was covered by four windows, we determined the final predictions on each second by performing a majority vote using the predicted activities of the four windows. In case of a tie, the predicted activity was determined by the one with highest summed predicted probability.

For sit-to-stand and stand-to-sit (STS) detection, we counted the number of occurrence of sit or lying down spans preceded by or followed by stand, walk, stairs, or jog spans. The STS extraction algorithm would only accept the event as a true STS event if and only if during the span transition the phone orientation has changed, or step detection algorithm has detected steps in the gait spans.

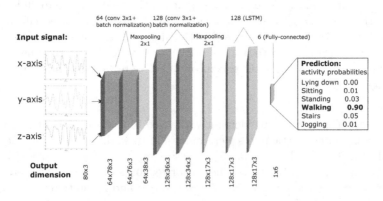

Fig. 1. Example dataflow from raw signal to activity classification

2.3   Gait and Mobility Feature Extraction

The mobility features we extracted from gaits and turns are all based on previously investigated features [5, 11–13].

We applied the adaptive step detection algorithm proposed by Lee *et al.* [14] to determine the time points of step initiation. After steps were identified in the gait spans, we calculated average step frequencies (number of steps divided by time) per subject. For the passive monitoring data we only performed the step detection and feature extraction algorithm in gait-related activities (walking, stairs, jogging) that were longer than five seconds. To infer the power invested during walk, we calculated the integral of the variance of the Euclidean norm of the acceleration signal, divided by the number of steps as the per-step power coefficient. This metric is a surrogate coefficient for power given that we do not have mass of the subject.

For turn detection, we followed a three-step process. First, we used a minimization method to identify the optimal rotation matrix $R^* = R_x(pitch)R_y(roll)$ such that the average of the acceleration signal on the z-axis follows gravity. That is, $\text{argmin}_{pitch,roll}(\int_t R_x(pitch)R_y(roll)a_z g\, dt)$, where $pitch$ and $roll$ are the pitch angle and roll angel, g is the gravity, and a_z is the z-axis component of the acceleration signal. In the second step we applied the rotation matrix R^* on the gyroscope signal. To detect turns around the z-axis, we integrated the angular velocity on a 1.5 s rolling window to obtain the yaw angles: $\int_t (R^* \text{gyro})_z\, dt$ where $()_z$ takes the z-axis component of the rotated signal. We then detect peaks in yaw angles that are higher than 1.5 rad ($\sim$86°) as one turn event. Our method is comparable to similar methods described in [12, 15], but uses a more stringent turn criterion in terms of degrees and speed of turns. For computational reasons we only estimated turns for gait spans longer than 18 s. This leaves about 57,000 walking spans collected during passive monitoring.

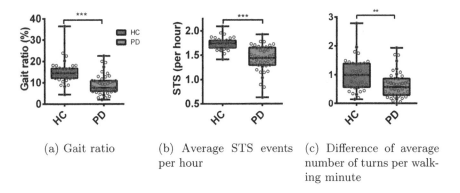

(a) Gait ratio   (b) Average STS events per hour   (c) Difference of average number of turns per walking minute

Fig. 2. Associations between HAR-profiled mobility measurements and clinical features. *Statistical significance:* **P value < 0.01; ***P value < 0.001

3 Results

3.1 Human Activity Recognition Performance Validation

Before applied on the passive monitoring data, the HAR model was validated on two data sets. The first was the held-out test set from the same sources of training data. The HAR model was able to correctly distinguish gait activities (walking, stairs, jogging) from stationary activities (sitting, standing, lying down) with more than 98% of accuracy. In addition, we also performed validation using the labeled daily active test. The active gait test sensor data was used as the positive control for gait detection, while the balance test, during which the subjects stand still for 30 s, was used as negative control. We defined a correct prediction as more than 50% of the span was labeled with the correct activity. The HAR model was also able to successfully profile the gait segments with 96.9% of accuracy, and balance segments with 99.5% accuracy.

3.2 Activity Profiles and Mobility Features Comparison in Passive Monitoring

The mobility of each subject was quantified by gait ratio, defined as the proportion of time the subject engaged in gait activities over the total passive monitoring coverage. Figure 2a shows the between-group difference in gait ratios. In the PD cohort we detected a median of 9.7% of gait spans over all coverage spans as supposed to HC cohort's 15.1%, indicating that the HC cohort had a significantly higher per-subject gait activity level than PD cohort ($P < 0.001$, Mann-Whitney test).

From the activity profile, we calculated the coverage-normalized STS events for each subject. Concordant with the results previously presented [11], the median number of STS per hour in PD patients was 17% lower than in HC subjects, as shown in Fig. 2b ($P < 0.001$, Mann-Whitney test).

Difficulties while turning is a regular symptom of PD [16] and may influence the way PD patients walk during their regular daily life. From our turn detection we calculated the average number of turns per hour per subject. We observed a 38% median reduction in the PD cohort versus HCs ($P < 0.01$, Mann-Whitney test), as shown in Fig. 2c. This result differs from a similar albeit smaller and shorter study by others [13], where no significant difference could be observed. One possible reason for this could be our focus on turns with higher degree change that pose a much higher difficulty for gait impaired PD patients.

3.3 Comparison of Gait Features Between Active Tests and Passive Monitoring

Active tests, such as our Gait Test, constitute an artificial situation and one open question is how much they reflect the subjects' behavior during their regular daily life. We compared three important and typical gait features: step frequency, step power and turning speed, between active test and passive monitoring for HC and

PD patients. Additionally, we also compared group differences between HC and PD cohorts. For the comparison we only used the subset of passive monitoring spans, which the HAR labeled as walking, and span length between 20 to 40 s.

Figure 3a shows that there is a significant mean reduction of 0.05 steps per second between active test and passive monitoring in the PD patient data ($P < 0.01$, paired t-test), whereas the difference in HCs is not significant ($P > 0.1$, paired t-test). However, we observed that during passive monitoring the HCs has much less variability in step frequency than that of PD. This low variability in HCs and the decrease in step frequency for PD patients may help explain the significant difference between HC and PD in passive monitoring ($P < 0.01$, Mann-Whitney test).

For turning speed, as depicted in Fig. 3b, we observed statistically significant difference between active and passive in both groups ($P < 0.001$, paired t-test). While the reduction in turning speed in PD is much more pronounced in the active tests, the differences in both active test and passive monitoring are statistically significant ($P < 0.001$, Mann-Whitney test). Similar to the case of step frequency, the HC cohort harbors much less variability than the PD cohort in passive monitoring.

Finally, Fig. 3c shows the power invested while walking in the active tests versus during passive monitoring. For both active and passive monitoring we observed significant lower power in PD versus HCs ($P < 0.001$, Mann-Whitney test). Both the PD cohort and HCs show significantly higher per-step power in passive monitoring then in the active gait tests ($P < 0.01$, paired t-test). The significance levels of comparisons between various groups are summarized in Table 1.

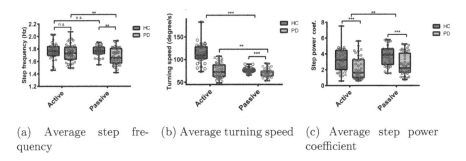

(a) Average step frequency

(b) Average turning speed

(c) Average step power coefficient

Fig. 3. Comparison of active vs. passive in HC and PD as well as between group comparison of HC vs. PD. *Statistical significance:* $^{**}P$ value < 0.01; $^{***}P$ value < 0.001

Table 1. Significance level for active test and passive monitoring comparison.

Test difference in % (P value)	Step frequency	Tuning speed	Step power coefficient
PD vs HC in active test	−2.0% (n.s.)	−33.6% (<0.001)	−50.0% (<0.001)
PD vs HC in passive monitoring	−6.1% (<0.01)	−6.4% (<0.001)	−40.0% (<0.001)
Active vs passive in PD	−4.3% (n.s.)	−2.1% (<0.001)	70.7% (<0.01)
Active vs passive in HC	−0.0% (<0.01)	−30.2% (<0.01)	42.4% (<0.01)

4   Discussions

As mobility reflects a very important aspect in the quality of life while being a diagnostic indication for PD, continuous long-term monitoring can provide valuable insight for treatment strategy development. Our study shows that such monitoring on mild to moderate PD patients is feasible using smartphones. Sensor data collected from both active and passive monitoring provide previously inaccessible information regarding patients' daily behavior and functioning. Specifically we demonstrated that patients with PD in our study were less mobile than healthy controls, as manifested in time spent in gait-related activities, number of turns and sit-to-stand transitions, and power per step. For further understanding on whether these features reflect disease severity as measured by physician rated assessment, we are performing ongoing analyses which include correlating the Movement Disorder Society unified Parkinson's disease rating scale (MDS-UPDRS), that is used in clinic to evaluate PD severity, with the smartphone data. Another important issue is how robust these measurements are across different mobile devices. In this study, all the subjects were using the same smartphone model. In the future, if similar study is to be performed using subjects' own devices, as different commercial smartphone models have different built-in inertial measurement unit (IMU), the acceleration and angular speed readings will require more comprehensive benchmarking so the derived features are comparable across devices.

The comparison of step features between active and passive monitoring provides valuable insight for future practice of remote monitoring programs. While for most step features we observed no significant difference in active test and passive monitoring, larger spread of step frequencies and turning speed in HC during active tests were clearly observed. We also observed that the step power is positively correlated with span length: both PD patients and HCs tended to invest more power in longer walking spans (data not shown). This agrees with the previously published result [5]. These pose interesting questions on human behavior and trial design for future studies.

Finally, the information from this study may be applicable to other motor function-related diseases to further understand disease progression or treatment effects, and eventually provides new perspectives in healthcare practices.

Acknowledgements. We thank Max A. Little for his technical input at the early stages of this research project.

References

1. Ramaker, C., Marinus, J., Stiggelbout, A.M., van Hilten, B.J.: Systematic evaluation of rating scales for impairment and disability in Parkinson's disease. Mov. Disord. **17**(5), 867–876 (2002)
2. González, R.C., López, A.M., Rodriguez-Uría, J., Álvarez, D., Alvarez, J.C.: Real-time gait event detection for normal subjects from lower trunk accelerations. Gait Posture **31**, 322–325 (2010)

3. Zijlstra, A., Zijlstra, W.: Trunk-acceleration based assessment of gait parameters in older persons: a comparison of reliability and validity of four inverted pendulum based estimations. Gait Posture **38**(4), 940–944 (2013)
4. Godfrey, A., Lord, S., Galna, B., Mathers, J.C., Burn, D.J., Rochester, L.: The association between retirement and age on physical activity in older adults. Age Ageing **43**, 386–393 (2014)
5. Del Din, S., Godfrey, A., Galna, B., Lord, S., Rochester, L.: Free-living gait characteristics in ageing and Parkinson's disease: impact of environment and ambulatory bout length. J. NeuroEng. Rehabil. **13**, 46 (2016)
6. ClinicalTrials.gov. https://clinicaltrials.gov
7. Rai, A., Chintalapudi, K.K., Padmanabhan, V.N., Sen R.: Zee: zero-effort crowd-sourcing for indoor localization. In: MobiCom (2012)
8. Ordóñez, F.J., Roggen, D.: Deep convolutional and LSTM recurrent neural networks for multimodal wearable activity recognition. Sensors **16**, 115 (2016)
9. Weiss, G.M., Lockhart J.W.: The impact of personalization on smartphone-based activity recognition. In: Proceedings of the AAAI-12 Workshop on Activity Context Representation: Techniques and Languages, Toronto, Canada (2012)
10. Stisen, A., et al.: Smart devices are different: assessing and mitigating mobile sensing heterogeneities for activity recognition. In: 13th ACM Conference on Embedded Networked Sensor Systems, Seoul, Korea (2015)
11. Zijlstra, A., Mancini, M., Lindermann, U., Chiari, L., Zijlstra, W.: Sit-stand and stand-sit transitions in older adults and patients with Parkinson's disease: event detection based on motion sensors versus force plates. J. NeuroEng. Rehabil. **9**, 75 (2012)
12. El-Gohary, M., et al.: Continuous monitoring of turning in patients with movement disability. Sensors **14**, 356–369 (2014)
13. Mancini, M., et al.: Continuous monitoring of turning in Parkinson's disease: rehabilitation potential. NeuroRehabilitation **37**(1), 3–10 (2015)
14. Lee, H.H., Choi, S., Lee, M.J.: Step detection robust against the dynamics of smartphones. Sensors **15**(10), 27230–27250 (2015)
15. Pham, M.H.: Algorithm for turning detection and analysis validated under home-like conditions in patients with Parkinson's disease and older adults using a 6 degree-of-freedom inertial measurement unit at the lower back. Front. Neurol. **8**, 135 (2017)
16. Stack, E., Ashburn, A.: Dyscuntional turning in Parkinson's disease. Disabil. Rehabil. **30**(16), 1222–1229 (2008)

Design and Development of the MedFit App: A Mobile Application for Cardiovascular Disease Rehabilitation

Ghanashyama Prabhu[1]([✉]), Jogile Kuklyte[1], Leonardo Gualano[1],
Kaushik Venkataraman[1], Amin Ahmadi[1], Orlaith Duff[1], Deirdre Walsh[1],
Catherine Woods[3], Noel E. O'Connor[1], and Kieran Moran[1,2]

[1] Insight Centre for Data Analytics, Dublin City University, Dublin, Ireland
ghanashyama.prabhu@insight-centre.org
[2] Department of Health and Human Performance, Dublin City University,
Dublin, Ireland
[3] Physical Education and Sport Sciences Department, University of Limerick,
Limerick, Ireland

Abstract. Rehabilitation from cardiovascular disease (CVD) usually requires lifestyle changes, especially an increase in exercise and physical activity. However, uptake and adherence to exercise is low for community-based programmes. We propose a mobile application that allows users to choose the type of exercise and compete it at a convenient time in the comfort of their own home. Grounded in a behaviour change framework, the application provides feedback and encouragement to continue exercising and to improve on previous results. The application also utilizes wearable wireless technologies in order to provide highly personalized feedback. The application can accurately detect if a specific exercise is being done, and count the associated number of repetitions utilizing accelerometer or gyroscope signals Machine learning models are employed to recognize individual local muscular endurance (LME) exercises, achieving overall accuracy of more than 98%. This technology allows providing a near real-time personalized feedback which mimics the feedback that the user might expect from an instructor. This is provided to motivate users to continue the recovery process.

Keywords: Cardiovascular disease · Mobile application
Support vector machine · Wearable sensors · Repetition counting

1 Introduction

Cardiovascular disease (CVD) is the leading cause of premature death and disability in Europe and worldwide [1]. While mortality and morbidity rates are improved with effective cardiac rehabilitation (CR) [2], uptake and adherence of community-based CR are very low [3]. Key reasons for this include: lack of disease-specific programmes, travel time to such programmes, scheduling issues,

© ICST Institute for Computer Sciences, Social Informatics and Telecommunications Engineering 2018
P. Perego et al. (Eds.): MobiHealth 2017, LNICST 247, pp. 20–28, 2018.
https://doi.org/10.1007/978-3-319-98551-0_3

and low self-efficacy associated with a perception of poor 'body image' or poor exercise technique [4]. Ideally, a personal instructor could visit the patient's home, provide a tailored programme and monitor the exercise quality and give personalized feedback. Unfortunately, this is not feasible in practice for a variety of reasons, including financial.

The mobile application described in this paper provides a solution to the problem: it allows tailored exercise classes to be completed at any time in a patient's home by offering personalized video exercise classes and feedback during exercise based on the data from wearable sensors (i.e. whether the exercise was completed and, if so, the number of repetitions). It also provides summary feedback and statistics on the completion and overall performance for specified periods of time (day, week, month, etc.). Finally, while the main focus of cardiac rehabilitation is exercise, it is also important to provide the patient with expert information in order to change their behaviour towards a more healthy lifestyle relating to the targeted areas of: smoking cessation, stress management, alcohol use, diet and medication adherence. The overall system is designed to be patient-centric with all technology and functionality choices informed by behaviour theory. The behavioral change techniques and social cognitive theory have been used in conjunction with the focus group feedback to develop and design the content of the application. The mHealth development and evaluation framework have been used to provide a best practice framework for the MedFit app development [5]. The selected behaviour change strategies are being delivered within the intervention through the various app components such as push notifications, testing, feedback, and videos.

The application has three main functionalities provided to the user: (1) A list of personalized exercise classes that guide users through different exercises using video and audio modalities; (2) Feedback provision to the user on the different aspects of activity measurements; (3) Capability to supervise a patient if wearable sensors are worn whilst exercising. The contributions of the work can be divided into two groups: design choices for the application, including wearable sensors that are utilized, and the feedback provisions to the user. Three feedback techniques were selected based on the health behaviour change models and implemented in the application. The experiment results are reported on separate integral parts of the application, while the clinical trial with the medical patients using the complete application is scheduled in the near future.

2 Mobile Application Design

An android application is developed as a prototype of the front-end of the proposed system. The application is aimed at the patients who suffered a cardiac event and are in Phase III of the recovery process[1]. The design of the graphical interface is carefully considered to make sure that patients can easily use the application. The mobile application development framework [5] used follows an iterative process for developing technology-based interventions, by facilitating

---

[1] http://www.uofmhealth.org/health-library/ty6411abc.

and encouraging end-user engagement. Focus groups with cardiac rehabilitation participants (n = 26; 65% male; mean age 64 ± 18.2 years) were undertaken to get feedback on the first prototype of the application. This feedback was then translated into feasible technical improvements.

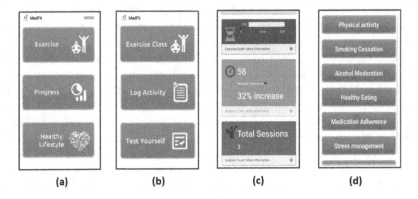

Fig. 1. Graphical user interface (GUI) of the application

As can be seen in Fig. 1(a), the main menu has three options: *Exercise*, *Progress*, and *Healthy Lifestyle*. There are three options related to the *Exercise*, as can be seen in Fig. 1(b). *Exercise Class* brings the user to the list of guided exercise classes that are personalized based on the evaluation of the classes performed earlier. The *Log Activity* section allows the user to manually log any exercise or physical activity that has been done outside of the application (e.g. swimming). The *Test Yourself* option allows the user to evaluate their progress using internationally accepted standard physical activity health tests [6]. The *Progress* option provides the users with the statistical representation of the activities performed so far (see Fig. 1(c)). The *Healthy Lifestyle* option brings the user to the key rehabilitation lifestyle topics picked by experts, as shown in Fig. 1(d). Apart from the design of the application, a lot of considerations went into the selection of wearable sensors that would allow the users to get the best possible feedback about their performance.

2.1   Multi-sensor Connectivity

Wearable sensors became ubiquitous and are now available off-the-shelf to use with an impressive list of sensing modalities made available. After an in-depth analysis of the suitability of the available sensors, an off-the-shelf wearable fitness tracker was utilized to retrieved step count and heart rate measure (Fitbit Charge2[2]). These two measures, in combination with the statistical information related to the exercise provided by the application, are sufficient to provide in-depth and meaningful information to the user about their progress.

---

[2] https://www.fitbit.com/ie/charge2.

Additional, more in-depth analysis of the actual performed exercises is made available to the user using the Shimmer3 inertial sensor[3]. The Shimmer is a small wireless sensor platform with integrated accelerometer and gyroscope sensors, large storage and low-power standards-based communication capabilities. The Shimmer sensor data is used to detect whether a particular LME exercise is being completed (activity recognition) and count the associated number of repetitions. It enables the near real-time feedback to the user during the performance of the exercises. Fitbit measurements are used to give an insight on the heart-rate and step counts to the user. The performance measures are carried out with shimmer sensor data.

3 Motivational Feedback

It is well accepted that motivation to continue and progress on any activity, including rehabilitation program, is closely related to the performance feedback available [7]. In this work, three main feedback delivery methods are employed, namely self monitoring, message notifications and near-real-time feedback.

3.1 Self Monitoring

In a review of applications to promote physical activity among adults, providing feedback and self-monitoring were the most frequently used techniques [7]. The application provides a feedback on four main statistical measures of user performance. The number of exercise minutes completed, the number of exercises classes completed, the daily step count and the average heart-rate captured during exercises.

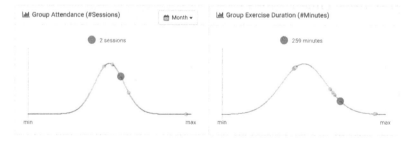

Fig. 2. Patient performance compared to other group members (Color figure online)

In addition to personal statistics, the user can also compare his/her performance with that of other group members (Fig. 2). In this Figure, the user status is highlighted in red on the Gaussian curve. The left and right graphs

---

[3] https://www.shimmersensing.com.

represent the number of classes (sessions) completed and the number of minutes spent exercising, respectively. The progress of the other users is marked, but anonymised, using yellow dots. This graphical visualization is created in order to notify the user that there are other people who are carrying out the same exercises. It allows the user to feel more part of a community of rehabilitators and increase the chance of adhering to the rehabilitation program. Furthermore, it allows the user to determine where he/she is standing in comparison to other group members (in an anonymized manner) and as a result become more motivated and engaged with the entire program to enhance his/her performance level. Users have the option of creating and opting in/out of these groups.

3.2   Message Notifications

Previous research, has shown that most interventions provided personally tailored SMS messages [8]. This application provides a tailored feedback to be delivered to end users based on health behaviour change theory, as well as a delivery schedule based on the 'six A' programme of changing behaviour [9]. Messaging is provided to remind users to exercise, to give encouragement or just to give feedback on their progress. Text messages are sent three times a week in the morning and at the end of the week; the user receives a summary of their performance for the entire week. An example of a personalized message sent on Sunday to a user called Mike, who has completed more than half of his target goal by the end of the week, would look like this:

"Hi Mike, your physical activity goal for this week was at least 150 minutes. You fell short of your goal by 75 minutes this week. Think positively next week and keep your mind set on reaching your goal. You can do it!".

3.3   Near Real-Time Feedback

At the end of each exercise, the repetition count report acts as an important feedback mechanism for the patient. The 3D accelerometer and 3D gyroscope, from the Shimmer sensor unit, can provide accurate translational and rotational data [10]. Fourteen LME exercises associated with cardiac rehabilitation are used for evaluating activity detection and repetition counting (Table 1) [11].

Data Capture and Pre-processing: Shimmer3 unit is calibrated in order to obtain accurate and consistent data and is configured with a sampling rate of 512 Hz for data capturing. The calibrated sensor unit is worn on the right wrist by each participant. For each LME exercise listed in Table 1 data is captured and a 30 s data segment is used, which corresponds to the length of the exercise. To introduce variability to the data, each exercise is performed by six participants (Age group between 20–40, 2 males and 4 females). A 30 s segment of the accelerometer sensor data in the 3D space for Bicep Curl is shown in Fig. 3. The classification model is trained to identify whether the person is performing

Table 1. Local muscular endurance (LME) exercises for cardiac rehabilitation

Exercise	Type of LME	Exercise	Type of LME
Upper body LME exercises			
Ex 1	Bicep Curls	Ex 6	Pec Dec
Ex 2	Triceps extension (right)	Ex 7	Trunk twist
Ex 3	Upright row	Ex 8	Side Bends - alternating sides
Ex 4	Lateral raise (arms up)	Ex 9	Bent Over Row (right arm)
Ex 5	Frontal raise (arms up)	Ex 10	Press up against wall
Lower body LME exercises			
Ex 11	Squats	Ex 13	Standing bicycle
Ex 12	Lunges-alternating sides	Ex 14	Leg lateral raise (right)

an exercise, therefore, random movements are also captured and added to the dataset. Random movements are 'standing relatively still' or 'shuffling around' to represent non-performing of an exercise. The data segments are grouped into two balanced classes: Class 1 for exercise data and Class 0 for random movements data. 80% of the data collected was used to train and validate the generated models utilizing 10-fold cross validation technique. The remaining 20% of the data was used for testing.

A total of 24 time and frequency statistical measurements from all 3 axes of the accelerometer data is used as a feature vector. The features include the mean, standard deviation, correlation coefficients, FFT coefficients, minimum and maximum values, RMS values, and entropy. The features are computed from the concatenated segmented data using a sliding window of 4 s. A window length of 4 s with 2 s of overlap is chosen as it is sufficient time for each repetition of the selected LME exercises to be completed.

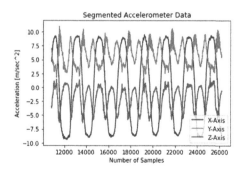

Fig. 3. Segmented Bicep Curls data for 30 s

Classification: There are a number of machine learning algorithms that could be used for classification. Since the dataset consists of two classes, an optimized support vector machine (SVM) classifier is chosen for this binary classification task [14]. One SVM model is created for each exercise with optimum hyper parameters. The models are used for recognition of each LME exercise from the random movement [12]. Ten-fold cross-validation as well as a regularization technique is used to avoid overfitting. A grid search for SVM hyper parameter optimization technique is implemented to improve the performance of the designed models by finding the optimal combination of hyper parameter values, including the regularization parameters and kernel options [13].

Classification results are measure using f-score, precision, and recall for each LME exercise recognition and are listed in Table 2. Individual accuracies of no lower that $\geq 96\%$ are found using a single wrist-worn 3D wearable sensor, with an overall accuracy of $\geq 98\%$. The accuracy of the lower body exercises does not suffer form the sensor placement on the right wrist due to wrist movements that are also associated with these exercises.

Repetition Counting: Data from the best suitable axis, either from the accelerometer or from the gyroscope sensor is used to count the repetitions. The best axis data from the sensor is filtered using a Savitzky-Golay filter [15] of order 4 and a repetition counting algorithm (peak-to-peak detection (PP) or threshold crossing (ThC)) is used to count the repetition.

Repetition counting results for each exercise are accurate to 100% with repetition rate of a repetition per one, two and four seconds.

Table 2. Performance measures associated with each LME exercise

Exercise	Precision	Recall	F1-score	Exercise	Precision	Recall	F1-score
Upper body LME exercises							
Ex 1	1.000	1.000	1.000	Ex 6	1.000	1.000	1.000
Ex 2	1.000	1.000	1.000	Ex 7	1.000	1.000	1.000
Ex 3	1.000	1.000	1.000	Ex 8	1.000	0.963	0.981
Ex 4	1.000	1.000	1.000	Ex 9	1.000	1.000	1.000
Ex 5	1.000	1.000	1.000	Ex 10	1.000	1.000	1.000
Lower body LME exercises							
Ex 11	1.000	1.000	1.000	Ex 13	1.000	1.000	1.000
Ex 12	0.963	0.963	0.963	Ex 14	1.000	0.963	0.963

4 Conclusion

Physical activity, as part of cardiac rehabilitation, is crucial to reducing the likelihood of premature death and increasing the quality of life following CVD. While patients are encouraged to join community-based programmes, uptake and adherence are very low. Our mobile application is created to be a personal trainer/rehabilitator to the patient and to provide live and summary feedback in order to increase the motivation to continue exercising. The proposed system, whose design was driven by behavioural change theory in combination with patient feedback, is a starting point of the independent recovery plan for the patient and aims to motivate the user to uptake and adhere long term to a personalized programme. The application is currently undergoing extensive user/patient testing as part of a clinical trial with results to be reported in the future.

Acknowledgements. We acknowledge financial support from SFI under the Insight Centre award, Grant Number SFI/12/RC/2289, and ACQUIS BI, an industrial partner of Insight Centre for Data Analytics, Dublin City University, Ireland.

References

1. Perk, J., et al.: European Guidelines on cardiovascular disease prevention in clinical practice (version 2012). Europ. Heart J. **33**(13), 1635–1701 (2012)
2. Balady, G.J., Williams, M.A., Ades, P.A., Bittner, V., Comoss, P., Foody, J.M., et al.: Core components of cardiac rehabilitation/secondary prevention programs: 2007 update. Circulation **115**(20), 2675–2682 (2007)
3. Dalal, H.M., Zawada, A., Jolly, K., Moxham, T., Taylor, R.S.: Home based versus centre based cardiac rehabilitation: Cochrane systematic review and meta-analysis. BMJ (Clin. Res. Ed.) **340**, b5631 (2010)
4. Jackson, L., Leclerc, J., Erskine, Y., Linden, W.: Getting the most out of cardiac rehabilitation: a review of referral and adherence predictors. Heart **91**(1), 10–14 (2005)
5. Whittaker, R., Merry, S., Dorey, E., Maddison, R.: A development and evaluation process for mHealth interventions: examples from new zealand. J. Health Commun. **17**(suppl. 1), 11–21 (2012)
6. American Thoracic Society: ATS statement: guidelines for the six-minute walk test. Am. J. Respir. Crit. Care Med. **166**, 111–117 (2002)
7. Middelweerd, A., Mollee, J.S., van der Wal, C.N., Brug, J., te Velde, S.J.: Apps to promote physical activity among adults: a review and content analysis. Int. J. Behav. Nutr. Phys. Act. **11**(1), 97 (2014)
8. Fjeldsoe, B.S., Marshall, A.L., Miller, Y.D.: Behavior change interventions delivered by mobile telephone short-message service. Am. J. Prev. Med. **36**(2), 165–173 (2009)
9. Person-Centred Care Resource Centre, NHC: 6 'A's-Tip Sheet For Self-Management Support (2016). http://personcentredcare.health.org.uk/sites/default/files/resources/a_a_cliniciantipsip
10. Ahmadi, A.: 3D human gait reconstruction and monitoring using body-worn inertial sensors and kinematic modeling. IEEE Sens. J. **16**(24), 8823–8831 (2016)

11. Prabhu, G., Ahmadi, A., O'Connor, N.E., Moran, K.: Activity recognition of local muscular endurance (LME) exercises using an inertial sensor. In: Lames, M., Saupe, D., Wiemeyer, J. (eds.) IACSS 2017. AISC, vol. 663, pp. 35–47. Springer, Cham (2018). https://doi.org/10.1007/978-3-319-67846-7_4

12. Bulling, A.: A tutorial on human activity recognition using body-worn inertial sensors. ACM Comput. Surv. (CSUR) **46**(3), 33 (2014)

13. Ahmadi, A.: Toward automatic activity classification and movement assessment during a sports training session. IEEE Internet Things J. **2**(1), 23–32 (2015)

14. Vapnik, V.: The Nature of Statistical Learning Theory. Springer, New York (2013)

15. Savitzky, A., Golay, M.J.: Smoothing and differentiation of data by simplified least squares procedures. Anal. Chem. **36**(8), 1627–1639 (1964)

16. Buys, R., Claes, J., Walsh, D., Cornelis, N., Moran, K., Budts, W.: Cardiac patients show high interest in technology enabled cardiovascular rehabilitation. BMC Med. Inform. Decis. Making **16**(1), 95 (2016)

17. Adams, J., Cline, M., Reed, M., Masters, A., Ehlke, K., Hartman, J.: Importance of resistance training for patients after a cardiac event. Proc. (Bayl. Univ. Med. Cent.) **19**(3), 246–248 (2006)

Adoption of Mobile Apps for Mental Health: Socio-psychological and Technological Factors

Soontae An[(⊠)] and Hannah Lee

Division of Communication and Media, College of Social Sciences,
Ewha Womans University, Seoul, Korea
soontae@ewha.ac.kr, hoyl222@naver.com

Abstract. The purpose of this research is to explore the factors affecting intention to use a mobile application for mental health in South Korea. Based on the Health Belief Model and Extended Technology Acceptance Model, this research aims to advance our understanding of mobile app adoption for mental health. A total of 218 men and women participated in an online survey. Results showed that perceived usefulness and perceived ease of use had significant effects on all stages of behavioral intention: app subscription, information seeking, information sharing, and following recommendations. Subjective norm and output quality were also significant predictors for intention to use a mobile app. Results provide useful insights for utilization of mobile apps to address mental health issues in Korean society.

Keywords: Mental health · Mental health app · Mobile app
Extended Technology Acceptance Model

1 Introduction

1.1 Purpose of Research

The purpose of this research is to explore the factors affecting intention to use a mobile application for mental health in South Korea. Despite the high suicide rates and increasing mental health illness [1], little attention has been paid to mobile applications as a tool to help people receive appropriate help and treatment. Given the high penetration of smartphones among Koreans [2], mobile applications are a promising venue for prevention and treatment of mental illnesses in Korean society. Based on the Health Belief Model and Extended Technology Acceptance Model, we explored socio-psychological and technological factors in determining people's intention to use a mobile application for mental health.

1.2 Research Model

As shown in Fig. 1, perceived *Ease of Use* and perceived *Usefulness* are two primary factors influencing adoption of mobile applications for mental health. Extended Technology Acceptance Model (TAM2) posits that *Subjective Norm*, *Image* and *Output Quality* influence people's perceived *Usefulness* which, in turn, leads to *Intention to*

© ICST Institute for Computer Sciences, Social Informatics and Telecommunications Engineering 2018
P. Perego et al. (Eds.): MobiHealth 2017, LNICST 247, pp. 29–37, 2018.
https://doi.org/10.1007/978-3-319-98551-0_4

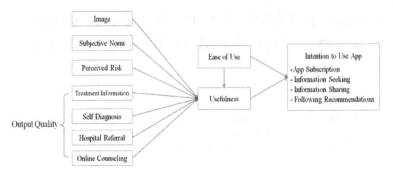

Fig. 1. Proposed research model

Use, along with perceived *Ease of Use* [3]. *Perceived Risk* is one of the key constructs in Health Belief Model (HBM), a widely used theoretical framework to understand health behaviors [4]. By integrating HBM and TAM2, this research aims to advance our understanding of mobile app adoption for mental health.

Subjective Norm was defined as "A person's perception that most people who are important to him/her think he/she should or should not perform the behavior in questions" (p. 302) [5]. *Image* was operationalized as "the degree to which use of an innovation perceived to enhance one's status in one's social system" (p. 195) [6]. *Perceive risk* was operationally defined as "one's subjective perception of the risk of contracting a health condition and feelings concerning the seriousness of contracting an ailment or of leaving it untreated" [7]. *Output Quality* was defined as users' perceptions of "how well the system performs the tasks that match their job relevance" (p. 985) [8]. *Output Quality* was measured by four dimensions in the current study: treatment information, self-diagnosis, hospital referral, and online counseling.

Perceived *Ease of Use* was defined as "the degree to which a person believes that using a particular system would be free of effort" [9]. Perceived *Usefulness* referred to "the degree to which a person believes that using a particular system would enhance his or her job performance (p. 320) [9]. Finally, *Intention to Use* was measured by four outcome variables: subscription of the mobile app, information seeking, information sharing, and following recommendations [10].

2   Methods

A total of 228 people participated in the online survey. Among the participants, 51.3% were males while 48.7% were females. Their average age was 39.16 years (Min = 20.00, Max = 58.00, SD = 10.45). Table 1 shows basic characteristics of the sample.

The online survey was conducted by a professional research firm. Screen shots of a mobile app were shown with explanations of its key features. The mobile app is currently provided by the Ministry of Patriots and Veterans Affairs in South Korea. After showing features of the mobile app, participants' intention to use the app as well as other factors were measured.

Table 1. Sample characteristics

Variables	N (%)	Variables	N (%)
Gender		**Income**	
Male	117 (51.3%)	Less than $1,000	14 (6.1%)
Female	111 (48.7%)	$1,000~$2,000	19 (8.3%)
Age		$2,000~$3,000	52 (32.8%)
20~30 years	58 (25.4%)	$3,000~$4,000	46 (20.2%)
30~40 years	60 (26.3%)	$4,000~$5,000	72 (31.5%)
40~50 years	59 (25.9%)	More than $5,000	25 (11.0%)
50~60 years	51 (22.4%)		
		Experience of Psychotherapy	
Education		Yes	29 (12.7%)
Lower than high school degree	6 (2.6%)	No	199 (87.3%)
High school graduate	34 (14.9%)		
College graduate	171 (75.0%)		
Graduate student	17 (7.5%)		

Key descriptive statistics are as follows: *Usefulness* (Four items, M = 3.6, SD = .66, Cronbach's α = .81), *Ease of Use* (Three items, M = 3.62, SD = .70, Cronbach's α = .79), *Subjective Norms* (Two items, M = 2.87, SD = .89, Cronbach's α = .77), *Image* (Two items, M = 2.80, SD = .81, Cronbach's α = .73), *Perceived Risk* (Six items, M = 3.61, SD = .68, Cronbach's α = .83), *Output Quality* (Twelve items, M = 3.60, SD = .65, Cronbach's α = .94), and *Intention to Use the Mental Health App* (Seven items, M = 3.47, SD = .66, Cronbach's α = .87). Scales for measuring all variables were adopted and modified based on Venkatesh and Davis [3]'s and Lin [11]'s items. Each statement was measured on a 5-point Likert scale from 1 (strongly disagree) to 5 (strongly agree).

3 Results

3.1 Attitudes Toward Mental Health Services

First, we examined barriers deterring use of mental health services. About half of participants (47.8%) mentioned social stigma as a barrier. Table 2 shows a list of barriers including lack of information (17%) and shame (9.6%).

Table 2. Barriers of mental health care use

	Lack of information	Medical mistrust	Treatment cost	Shame	Stigma	Total
N (%)	40 (17.5%)	30 (13.2%)	27 (11.8%)	22 (9.6%)	109 (47.8%)	228 (100%)

Next, participants were asked: "If you are suffering from mental health problems, who would be the first to ask for help?" As shown in Table 3, most participants responded that they would look for mental health information via the Internet (40.8%), followed by family (25.4%) and doctor (11.8%).

Table 3. The first help-seeking for mental health crisis

	Most likely	Second most likely	Third most likely	Total index
Friends	17 (7.5%)	27 (11.8%)	39 (17.1%)	14400
Family	58 (25.4%)	**55 (24.1%)**	36 (15.8%)	**32000**
Doctor	27 (11.8%)	48 (21.1%)	35 (15.4%)	**21200**
For myself	26 (11.4%)	39 (17.7%)	**45 (19.7%)**	20100
Internet	**93 (40.8%)**	41 (18.0%)	43 (18.9%)	**40400**
Religion	6 (2.6%)	13 (5.7%)	12 (5.3%)	5600

3.2 Correlations Among Variables

Table 4 displays Pearson Correlations among variables.

Table 4. Correlations between variables

	1	2	3	4	5	6	7	8	9	10	11	12	13
1.Subject Norm	1												
2.Image	.71**	1											
3.Treatment Information	-.49**	-.58**	1										
4.Self Diagnosis	-.47**	-.54**	.79**	1									
5.Hospital Referral	-.49**	-.59**	.76**	.75**	1								
6.Online Counseling	-.51**	-.63**	.80**	.79**	.79**	1							
7.Risk Perception	-.21**	-.24**	.37**	.38**	.37**	.39**	1						
8.Usefulness	-.55**	-.62**	.79**	.74**	.72**	.79**	.39**	1					
9.Ease to Use	-.32**	-.44**	.53**	.50**	.49**	.51**	.33**	.58**	1				
10.Subscription	-.52**	-.57**	.70**	.68**	.64**	.69**	.40**	.69**	.51**	1			
11.Information Seeking	-.53**	-.56**	.70**	.61**	.64**	.69**	.42**	.67**	.54**	.70**	1		
12.Information Sharing	-.57**	-.63**	.60**	.54**	.60**	.59**	.33**	.60**	.46**	.61**	.64**	1	
13.Following Recommendations	-.42**	-.47**	.62**	.56**	.57**	.60**	.38**	.60**	.40**	.61**	.58**	.51**	1

*p<.05, **p<.01

3.3 Tests of the Proposed Model

Structural equation models were run to test the proposed research model with four different outcome variables (app subscription, information seeking, information sharing, and following recommendations). In this study, AMOS was used and the estimation procedure was maximum likelihood estimation. Table 5 provides information on the fit indices of the four models, indicating acceptable fits.

Three endogenous variables were tested in model 1. Perceived usefulness was found to be significantly determined by subjective norm, treatment information, self diagnosis, online counseling and perceived ease of use, resulting in an R^2 of .74. The dependent variable, subscription app, was significantly determined by perceived usefulness and perceived ease of use, resulting in R^2 of .49.

Table 5. Fit Indices of proposed research models

Fit index	χ^2	Df	GFI	NFI	CFI	RMSEA	SRMR
Level of acceptable fit			>.90	>.90	>.90	<.06	<.05
Proposed research model 1	57.96	6	.95	.97	.97	.18	.02
Proposed research model 2	63.68	6	.95	.96	.97	.19	.02
Proposed research model 3	61.61	6	.96	.96	.97	.19	.03
Proposed research model 4	34.23	6	.97	.98	.98	.13	.03

In model 2, perceived usefulness was significantly determined by subjective norm, treatment information, self diagnosis, online counseling and perceived ease of use at R^2 of .74, indicating that the variables explained 74% of the variance in perceived usefulness. The dependent variable, information seeking, was significantly determined by perceived usefulness and perceived ease of use, resulting in R^2 of .49.

In model 3, perceived usefulness was found to be significantly determined by subjective norm, treatment information, self diagnosis, online counseling and perceived ease of use, resulting in an R^2 of .74. Information sharing was significantly determined by perceived usefulness and perceived ease of use, resulting in R^2 of .38.

In model 4, the combined effects of subjective norm, treatment information, self diagnosis, online counseling and perceived ease of use explained 73.7% of the variance in perceived usefulness. Perceived usefulness, easy to use explained 36% ($R^2 = .36$) of the variance in the dependent variable, following recommendations.

Figure 2 shows the resulting path coefficients of the proposed research model 1. The results showed that subject norm ($\beta = -.12$, $p < .05$), treatment information ($\beta = .28$, $p < .01$), self diagnosis ($\beta = .12$, $p < .05$), and online counseling ($\beta = .25$, $p < .01$) significantly influenced perceived usefulness. Perceived ease of use was found to be significant in influencing both perceived usefulness ($\beta = .15$, $p < .01$) and intention to subscribe the app ($\beta = .16$, $p < .01$). We also found a significant indirect path between perceived ease of use and intention to use app, mediated by perceived usefulness ($\beta = .09$, $p < .05$). We noted that perceived usefulness not only played a key role in its direct effect on intention to use the app ($\beta = .59$, $p < .01$), but also as a mediator variable (Fig. 2).

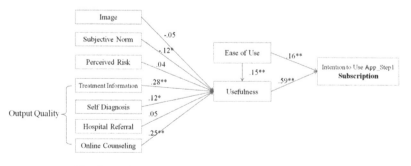

Fig. 2. Path model 1 (Mental health app subscription)

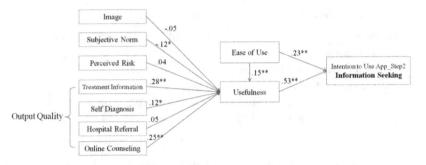

Fig. 3. Path model 2 (Information seeking)

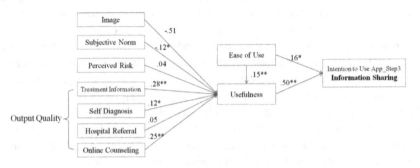

Fig. 4. Path model 3 (Information sharing)

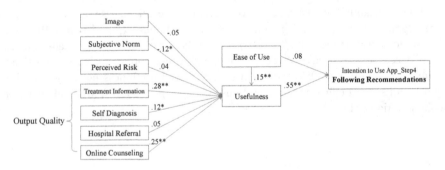

Fig. 5. Path model 4 (Following recommendations)

In model 2 (see Fig. 3) and model 3 (see Fig. 4), the same results were obtained as in model 1. In model 4 (see Fig. 5), on the other hand, perceived ease of use had no significant effect on intention to follow recommendations ($\beta = .08$, $p > .05$) (Tables 6 and 7).

Table 6. Results of path model 1 and path model 2

Path	Research model 1 subscription			Research model 2 information seeking		
	β	S.E	C.R.	β	S.E	C.R.
Direct effect						
Subject Norm → Usefulness	−.12	.04	−2.37*	−.12	.04	−2.37*
Image → Usefulness	−.05	.05	−0.93	−.05	.05	−0.93
Risk Perception → Usefulness	.04	.04	0.99	.04	.04	0.99
Treatment Information → Usefulness	.28	.06	4.21**	.28	.06	4.21**
Self Diagnosis → Usefulness	.12	.06	1.91*	.12	.06	1.91*
Hospital Referral → Usefulness	.05	.06	0.74	.05	.06	0.74
Online Counseling → Usefulness	.25	.06	3.62**	.25	.06	3.62**
Easy to Use → Usefulness	.15	.04	3.59**	.15	.04	3.59**
Usefulness → Intention to Use	.59	.07	10.2**	.53	.07	9.12**
Easy to Use → Intention to Use	.16	.06	2.76**	.23	.06	3.99**
Indirect effect						
Easy to Use → Usefulness → Intention to Use	.09*	.04	–	.08*	.03	–
Subject Norm → Usefulness → Intention to Use	−.07	.04	–	−.06	.03	–
Image → Usefulness → Intention to Use	−.03	.03	–	−.03	.03	–
Risk Perception → Usefulness → Intention to Use	.02	.02	–	.02	.02	–
Treatment Information → Usefulness → Intention to Use	.16**	.05	–	.15**	.05	–
Self Diagnosis → Usefulness → Intention to Use	.07	.05	–	.06	.04	–
Hospital Referral → Usefulness → Intention to Use	.03	.04	–	.02	.03	–
Online Counseling → Usefulness → Intention to Use	.15**	.04	–	.14**	.04	–

*$p < .05$, **$p < .01$

Table 7. Results of path model 3 and path model 4

Path	Research model 3 information sharing			Research model 4 following recommendations		
	β	S.E	C.R.	β	S.E	C.R.
Direct effect						
Subject Norm → Usefulness	−0.12	0.04	−2.37*	−0.12	0.04	−2.30*
Image → Usefulness	−0.05	0.05	−0.93	−0.05	0.05	−0.93
Risk Perception → Usefulness	0.04	0.04	0.99	0.04	0.04	0.99

(continued)

Table 7. (*continued*)

Path	Research model 3 information sharing			Research model 4 following recommendations		
	β	S.E	C.R.	β	S.E	C.R.
Treatment Information → Usefulness	0.28	0.06	4.21**	0.28	0.06	4.21**
Self Diagnosis → Usefulness	0.12	0.06	1.91*	0.12	0.06	1.91*
Hospital Referral → Usefulness	0.05	0.06	0.74	0.05	0.06	0.74
Online Counseling → Usefulness	0.25	0.06	3.62**	0.25	0.06	3.62**
Easy to Use → Usefulness	0.15	0.04	3.59**	0.15	0.04	3.59**
Usefulness → Intention to Use	0.50	0.08	7.81**	0.55	0.08	8.52**
Easy to Use → Intention to Use	0.16	0.07	2.55**	0.08	0.08	1.21
Indirect effect						
Easy to Use → Usefulness → Intention to Use	.08*	.03	–	.08*	.03	–
Subject Norm → Usefulness → Intention to Use	–.06	.03	–	–.06*	.03	–
Image → Usefulness → Intention to Use	–.03	.03	–	–.03	.03	–
Risk Perception → Usefulness → Intention to Use	.02	.02	–	.02	.02	–
Treatment Information → Usefulness → Intention to Use	.14**	.05	–	.15**	.05	–
Self Diagnosis → Usefulness → Intention to Use	.06	.04	–	.07	.04	–
Hospital Referral → Usefulness → Intention to Use	.02	.03	–	.03	.04	–
Online Counseling → Usefulness → Intention to Use	.13**	.04	–	.14**	.04	–

$*p < .05, **p < .01$

4 Discussions

The main aims of this study were to identify key determinants of intention to use a mental health app. The results of path analysis showed that perceived usefulness and perceived ease of use had significant effects on all stages of behavior intention (app subscription, information seeking, information sharing, and following recommendations). In addition, the two external factors, subjective norm and output quality, were also significant in predicting intention to use app. Among sub factors of output quality, treatment information, self-diagnosis and online counseling were significantly associated with increased perceived usefulness. Hospital referral, on the other hand, had no significant effect on perceived usefulness.

Previous studies [12] have shown that social factors (subjective norm and image) influenced acceptance of new technologies. Similarly, this study confirmed the significant relationships between subjective norm and perceived usefulness. However, unlike previous studies [12], subjective norm was negatively associated with perceived usefulness. These results are likely due to the high level of mental health stigma in South Korea. This study also found online counseling to be a strong influential factor of perceived usefulness of mental health app. However, no significant relationship was found between hospital referral and perceived usefulness. The results supported current stigma researches [13] in that stigma attached to mental illnesses discourages people to help-seeking. Berger et al. [14] proved that people with stigmatized illnesses were more likely to use online health information than people with non-stigmatized conditions. Given the increasing mental health problems and the widespread use of smartphones in South Korea, mobile apps for mental health provide a great potential to aid those with symptoms receive appropriate and timely treatment and care.

References

1. World Health Organization: World Health Statistics 2016: Monitoring health for the SDGs. http://www.who.int/gho/publications/world_health_statistics/2016/en/
2. Statista: Share of population in South Korea that use a smartphone from 2015 to 2021. https://www.statista.com/statistics/321408/smartphone-user-penetration-in-south-korea/
3. Venkatesh, V., Davis, F.D.: A theoretical extension of the technology acceptance model: four longitudinal field studies. Manag. Sci. **46**, 186–204 (2000)
4. Carpenter, C.J.: A meta-analysis of the effectiveness of health belief model variables in predicting behavior. Health Commun. **25**, 661–669 (2010)
5. Fishbein, M., Ajzen, I.: Belief, Attitude, Intention, and Behavior. Addison-Wesley, Reading (1975)
6. Moore, G.C., Benbasat, I.: Development of an instrument to measure the perceptions of adopting an information technology innovation. Inf. Syst. Res. **2**, 192–222 (1991)
7. Rosenstock, I.M.: The health belief model and preventive health behavior. Health Educ. Monogr. **2**, 354–386 (1974)
8. Davis, F.D., Bagozzi, R.P., Warshaw, P.R.: Extrinsic and intrinsic motivation to use computers in the workplace1. JASP **22**, 1111–1132 (1992)
9. Davis, F.D.: Perceived usefulness, perceived ease of use, and user acceptance of information technology. MIS Q. **13**(3), 319–340 (1989)
10. Park, Y., Chen, J.V.: Acceptance and adoption of the innovative use of smartphone. IMDS **107**, 1349–1365 (2007)
11. Lin, S.P.: Determinants of adoption of mobile healthcare service. IJMC **9**(3), 298–315 (2011)
12. Schepers, J., Wetzels, M.: A meta-analysis of the technology acceptance model: investigating subjective norm and moderation effects. Inf. Manag. **44**(1), 90–103 (2007)
13. Cukrowicz, K.C., Duberstein, P.R., Vannoy, S.D., Lin, E.H., Unützer, J.: What factors determine disclosure of suicide ideation in adults 60 and older to a treatment provider? Suicide Life Threat. Behav. **44**(3), 331–337 (2014)
14. Berger, M., Wagner, T.H., Baker, L.C.: Internet use and stigmatized illness. Soc. Sci. Med. **61**(8), 1821–1827 (2005)

Sensors and Circuits

Ultra Low Power Programmable Wireless ExG SoC Design for IoT Healthcare System

Mahesh Kumar Adimulam$^{(\boxtimes)}$ and M. B. Srinivas

EE Department, Birla Institute of Technology and Science – Pilani,
Hyderabad Campus, Hyderabad 500078, India
mahesh.kumar@ieee.org

Abstract. An 8-channel ultra low power programmable wireless ExG (ECG, EMG and EEG) system-on-chip (SoC) design for bio-signal processing applications is presented in this paper. The proposed design consists of a capacitive coupled programmable gain instrumentation amplifier (CC-PGIA) with an improved transconductance of amplifier. A 12-bit programmable hybrid SAR-Cyclic analog-to-digital converter (ADC) is introduced for improved performance and low power consumption that consists of a 6-bit SAR ADC (SADC) followed by a 6-bit cyclic ADC (CADC). The remaining blocks implemented in the SoC are programmable low pass filter (PLPF), programmable wireless transmitter (PWT), power management unit (PMU) and a digital block. The proposed programmable wireless ExG (PW-ExG) design is implemented in 180 nm standard CMOS process with a core area of 4 mm^2. The performance parameters are found to be, power consumption of 286 µW @ 0.6 V supply voltage, input referred noise voltage of 0.96 µV$_{rms}$ over 0.5 Hz–1 kHz range, gain of 30–65 dB and signal-to-noise-and-distortion ratio (SNDR) of 69.2 dB.

Keywords: PW-ExG (ECG, EMG and EEG) SoC · CC-PGIA
Cyclic-SAR ADC · Programmable wireless transmitter · Ultra low power
IoT healthcare system

1 Introduction

Technologies related to IoT have been developed recently to improve the interface between healthcare architectures and portable bio-medical systems [1]. The main advantage of IoT technology is that it enables real time monitoring of the patient's health by integrating wireless transmitting systems with, let us say, ExG signal processing circuits. In bio-medical signal processing applications, remote monitoring of signals such as electrocardiography (ECG), electromyography (EMG) & electroencephalography (EEG) through wireless is difficult due to challenges such as signal radius coverage meeting clinical requirements and designs that consume ultra low power, low cost and higher efficiency [2, 3].

In last two decades, significant amount of research has been carried out both at architectural level and circuit implementation for analog front end (AFE) and wireless transmitters [1–4] to improve the performance and power efficiency. The AFE consists of instrumentation amplifier (IA), PLPF and ADC. The operational transconductance

© ICST Institute for Computer Sciences, Social Informatics and Telecommunications Engineering 2018
P. Perego et al. (Eds.): MobiHealth 2017, LNICST 247, pp. 41–49, 2018.
https://doi.org/10.1007/978-3-319-98551-0_5

amplifier (OTA) is the fundamental building block for IA design; different topologies of OTA such as folded cascode, recycling structure, and improved recycling structure [5] have been implemented to improve the ratio of transconductance. In this paper an improved transconductance amplifier with DC offset adjustment circuit is used in CC-PGIA to improve the performance such as common mode rejection ratio (CMRR), power supply rejection ratio (PSRR) and input referred noise without increasing the power consumption and area.

The performance and power consumption of AFE also depend up on ADC sub-block while the ADC performance and power consumption are very critical in processing the bio-signals. Successive approximation register (SAR) ADC is most commonly used for bio-potential signal processing applications [6, 7] which at higher resolutions ($\geq$ 10-bits) has performance degradation due to capacitive mis-matches also power consumption increases significantly due to dynamic switching of the digital-to-analog converter (DAC). In this paper, authors introduce a hybrid SAR-Cyclic ADC for 12-bit operation with low power consumption and improved performance. The proposed SAR-Cyclic ADC overcomes the limitations of the conventional SAR ADC.

Apart from AFE, power consumption by the wireless transmitter is also significant in overall ExG SoC design. In this work, a low power wireless transmitter, operating in the unlicensed 2.4 GHz ISM band, has been designed following IEEE 802.15.4 specifications [8]. The power consumption of this transmitter is reduced by operating at lower supply voltage ($\sim$0.4 V) generated from the internal low power regulator and the power efficiency is improved by calibration.

The organization of this paper is as follows: Sect. 2 describes the architecture of the proposed PW-ExG SoC, Sect. 3 describes the circuit implementation, Sect. 4 presents the simulation results and finally Sect. 5 presents the conclusion.

2 Architecture of the Proposed PW-ExG SoC Design

Figure 1 shows the architecture of the proposed 8-channel PW-ExG SoC design. The operation of the single channel signal path from input electrodes to wireless transmitter output can be described as follows: the differential analog inputs $V_{INP, INM}$ are applied to CC-PGIA block through electrodes, the CC-PGIA circuit can be programmed for a gain of 30–65 dB with digital control bits based upon ExG input signal amplitude levels and the differential outputs of the CC-PGIA are given as inputs to PLPF which is a second order filter. The bandwidth of the PLPF can be programmed from 500 Hz–4 kHz with digital control bits based upon ExG signals operating frequency bands and the filtered outputs are given to the proposed 12-bit hybrid SAR-Cyclic ADC through 8 × 1 ADC MUX. The proposed SAR-Cyclic ADC can be programmed for 10-bit or 12-bit resolutions based on ExG signal amplitude level, the SAR-Cyclic ADC consists of 6-bit SAR ADC followed by 6-bit Cyclic ADC for 12-bit operation. The 12-bit SAR-Cyclic ADC converts analog input provided from PLPF to digital format. The digital data from ADC is post processed through digital block and transmitted over wireless transmitter, while the post processed digital data can also be displayed on display system for monitoring. The performance and power efficiency of the proposed PW-ExG SoC are

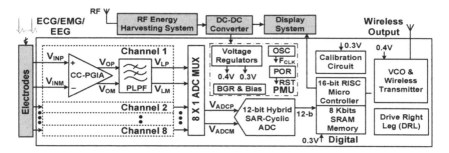

Fig. 1. Architecture of the proposed PW-ExG SoC design

improved by implementing an improved transconductance amplifier with DC offset cancellation and with proposed 12-bit SAR-Cyclic ADC.

The timing operation of the PW-ExG SoC design can be described as follows: the power-on-reset (POR) circuit generates RST signal with 10 mS delay after power supply ramp up while the PMU sub blocks settle within 50 mS time. The calibration circuit provides codes for signal processing path circuits within 15 mS. The analog front end (AFE) channel processes input signal in 12 mS while 12-bit hybrid SAR-Cyclic ADC converts analog input to digital format in 50 uS and the digital block performs post processing in 5 mS. Finally, the data is transmitted by the wireless transmitter which has a settling time of less than 0.5 ns.

3   Circuit Implementation of the PW-ExG SoC Design

3.1   CC-PGIA Design

Figure 2(a) shows the block diagram of the CC-PGIA design. The differential analog inputs $V_{EIP, EIM}$ are applied to CC-PGIA and the differential outputs $V_{OM, OP}$ are captured. The gain of the CC-PGIA design is given as $\Delta V = C_{IN}/C_F$, where C_{IN} is digitally programmable for the gain range of 30–65 dB based upon ExG signals amplitude levels and the ADC input dynamic range.

The improved transconductance amplifier with DC input common adjustment circuit is shown in Fig. 2(b). The transistors M_{1P}–M_{6P} & M_{3N}–M_{8N} form fully differential amplifier while the transistor M_{1N}–M_{2N} are implemented to improve the transconductance. These transistors are biased by M_{5R}. The transistors M_{1R}–M_{5R} adjust the input common mode voltage to V_R and this reduces the DC offset voltage due to electrodes. The transistors M_{1C}–M_{8C} forms the static CMFB circuit to adjust the output common mode voltage. The improved transconductance amplifier increases the DC gain, CMRR, PSRR and reduces the input referred noise voltage.

Table 1 shows the performance of CC-PGIA and a comparison with recent designs. Performance parameters are found to be CMRR of 122 dB, PSRR of 124 dB, input referred noise of 0.96 μV_{rms} and SNDR of 75.8 dB @ 500 Hz input frequency. Power spectrum analysis has been carried out to capture SNDR and Fig. 3 shows the SNDR to be 75.8 dB @ 500 Hz input frequency. The results demonstrate that most of the

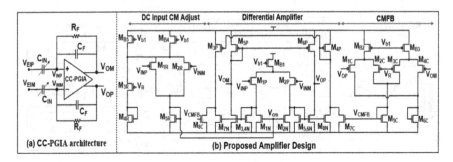

Fig. 2. Block diagram of CC-PGIA and proposed amplifier design

Table 1. Performance   parameters comparison

	[9] 2012	[10] 2016	This work
Technology (nm)	180	180	180
Supply voltage (V)	0.6	0.5	0.6
Supply current (µA)	1.0	1.1	0.48
CMRR (dB)	>120	102	122
PSRR (dB)	>120	104	124
Input referred noise (μV_{rms})	5.41	1.32	0.96
SNDR (dB)	63.0	N/A	75.8

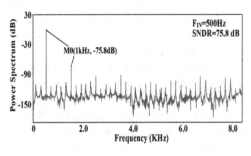

Fig. 3. CC-PGIA SNDR vs frequency

performance parameters are better than those of recent designs and highly suitable for bio-medical applications.

3.2   SAR-Cyclic ADC Design

In the proposed PW-ExG SoC design authors introduced a fully differential hybrid 12-bit SAR-Cyclic ADC to improve the performance and power efficiency. Figure 4 shows the architecture block diagram of the SAR-Cyclic ADC. The coarse ADC is implemented with 6-bit SAR architecture [6, 7] while the fine ADC is implemented

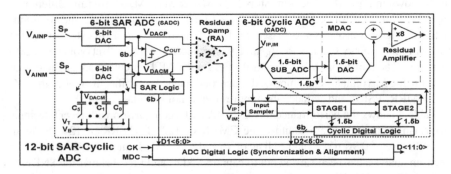

Fig. 4. Architecture of the proposed SAR-Cyclic ADC

with 6-bit cyclic architecture [11] and the integration of the both ADCs is carried out using residual amplifier [12]. The advantage of this architecture is that it reduces the capacitor mis-matches for improving performance and reduces the DAC switching logic for improving power efficiency in conventional SAR ADC at higher resolutions. The selection of Cyclic ADC for fine resolution is due to the requirements of lower sampling speeds, high performance and lower power consumption.

The functional description of the SAR-Cyclic ADC is provided as follows: the differential analog inputs $V_{AINP, AINM}$ are applied to coarse SADC which performs 6-bit operation and provides coarse digital output D1<5:0> to ADC digital logic. The error voltage from the SADC is amplified by a gain of 16 using residual amplifier (RA) which improves voltage dynamic range and provides output to fine 6-bit CADC. The CADC performs 6-bit operation and provides fine digital output D2<5:0> to ADC digital logic. The ADC digital logic performs data synchronization, error correction and combines D1<5:0> & D2<5:0> bits to provide a 12-bit D<11:0> digital output.

The circuit implementation of the 6-bit SADC is adopted from [6] and its performance is improved by reducing the capacitor mis-matches. The cyclic ADC architecture is adopted taken from [11] and designed at 0.6 V supply voltage while the RA circuit is fully differential-bias based inverter with common mode feedback (CMFB). The proposed ADC is programmable to 10-b mode (i.e., 5-b SADC and 5-bit CADC) using MDC control bit.

The performance parameters of the SAR-Cyclic ADC for both 10-b/12-b operation and comparison with recent designs are provided in Table 2. The design has a differential non-linearity (DNL) of ±0.4 LSB and integral non-linearity (INL) of ±0.51 LSB while among dynamic parameters, ENOB is found to be 11.24. Power spectrum analysis was carried out to capture SNDR, Fig. 5 shows an SNDR of 69.4 dB @ 500 Hz input frequency. Thus, it can be safely said that most of the performance parameters of the proposed ADC are better than those of recent designs and the ADC is highly suitable for bio-medical applications.

Table 2 Performance parameters comparison of the proposed ADC with recent designs

	[6] 2014	[7] 2015	[11] 2016	This work	
Technology (nm)	180	180	180	180	
Supply voltage (V)	0.6	0.6	0.9	0.6	
Architecture	SAR	SAR	Cyclic	SAR-Cyclic	
Sampling rate (KHz)	100	20	500	100	
Resolution (bits)	10	10	12	10	12
DNL (LSB)	0.5	0.46	±0.5	±0.34	±0.4
INL (LSB)	0.89	0.44	+3.2/−2	±0.42	±0.51
SNDR (dB)	57.14	58.34	62.68	58.7	69.4
ENOB (bits)	9.2	9.4	10.1	9.46	11.24
Power (W)	390n	38n	120μ	124n	308n
FOM (fJ/conv-step)	6.7	2.8	241	1.76	1.27

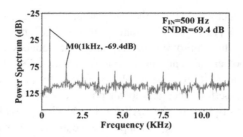

Fig. 5. ADC SNDR vs frequency

3.3 Low Power and Programmable Wireless Transmitter

In design of the wireless transmitter, the super-regenerative OOK transmitter architecture is used [3] following the IEEE 802.15.4 specifications. Figure 6(a) shows the programmable wireless transmitter block diagram where the voltage controlled oscillator (VCO) is designed with complementary cross coupled NMOS/PMOS structure and RF varactor capacitor is used for frequency tuning. Calibration is done to improve performance by controlling V_C voltage and aspect ratios of P[1–4] and N[1–4] devices. The power consumption of the circuit is reduced by operating on 0.4 V internal supply voltage. Figure 6(b) shows the TX output power spectrum at 2.4 GHz tuning frequency and output power is found to be −27.89 dBm compared to −16.36 dB in [3]. Power consumption of transmitter is 276.5 μW @ 0.4 V supply voltage.

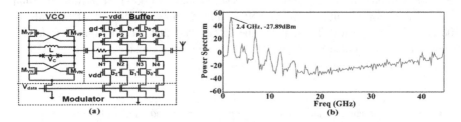

Fig. 6. (a) Block diagram of programmable wireless transmitter (b) Transmitter output spectrum

The PLPF block is designed with improved transconductance amplifier to improve the performance and remaining sub-blocks PMU [6], calibration & digital [3] are designed considering PW-ExG performance and power efficiency.

4   Simulation Results

In this section simulation results of the proposed PW-ExG SoC design are discussed. The proposed design is implemented in 180 nm standard CMOS process with a core area of 2 mm × 2 mm. The worst-case RC post layout simulations are carried out to capture the performance parameters at block level and PW-ExG top level. Figure 7(a) and (b) shows the ±3σ Montecarlo offset voltages for SAR ADC comparator and

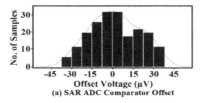 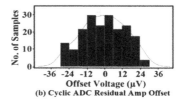

(a) SAR ADC Comparator Offset   (b) Cyclic ADC Residual Amp Offset

Fig. 7. (a) SAR ADC comparator offset voltage (b) Cyclic ADC residual amplifier offset voltage

Cyclic ADC residual amplifier. The SAR ADC comparator offset voltage is ± 36 μV and the same for Cyclic ADC residual amplifier is ± 30 μV. The variation of the offset voltages is reduced by one time calibration. Results show that the comparator and residual amplifier designs meet 12-bit accuracy.

Figure 8(a) shows the simulation setup to validate the results at receive end and Fig. 8(b) shows the data transmission bits at the input of the transmitter, output of the transmitter and output of the receiver model. Data from the PW-ExG SoC design is transmitted over antenna with 2.4 GHz carrier frequency. The Verilog-a model of receiver is built to capture the digital data, de-modulate and analog output is captured for performance analysis after filtering through programmable 12-bit ideal DAC. Results show that there are no data errors, meaning the transmitted data is recovered fully at the receiving end.

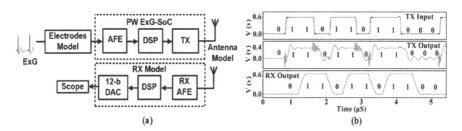

(a)   (b)

Fig. 8. (a) PW-ExG SoC simulation setup (b) Transmitter and receiver data pattern

The ExG signals are taken from [14, 15] and given as inputs to the 8-channel PW-ExG SoC and the results are captured at the output of the ideal 12-bit DAC. Results show SNDR @ 100 Hz input signal as 69.9 dB for ECG signals and at 500 Hz input signal is 69.2 dB for EMG signals. Figure 9(a) and (b) shows the ECG and EMG

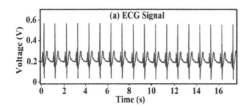 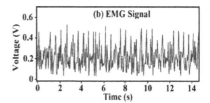

Fig. 9. ECG and EMG signals captured at the output of the Ideal DAC

Table 3. Performance parameters comparison with recent state of art designs

	[13] 2013	[4] 2015	[3] 2015	[2] 2016	This work
Technology (nm)	130	130	180	180	180
Supply voltage (V)	1.0	1.0	1.2	0.95	0.6
Sensor type	Neural, ExG	ExG	ECG	ECG	ExG
Number of channel (s)	1	4	1	1	8
AFE gain (dB)	42–78	40–78	20–28	34	30–65
Input ref noise (μV_{rms})	–	<2	–	16	0.96
ADC arch	8-bit SAR	8-bit SAR	12-bit SDM	8-b LC ADC	12-b SAR-Cyclic
TX data rate	100 kb/s	200 kb/s	5 Mb/s	90 kb/s	5 Mb/s
TX band (GHz)	0.433	0.433	2.4	0.402	2.4
TX O/P power (dBm)	−16.0	−18.5	−16.36	−16.0	−27.89
Power consumption (μW)	500 @ (100% duty cycled)	19 @ (0.013% duty cycled)	606 @ (50% duty cycled)	9.72 (-)	286 @ (50% duty cycled)
Area (mm)	2.5 × 3.3	3.3 × 2.5	1.52 × 1.55	1.9 × 2.0	2.0 × 2.0

signals captured at the output of the Ideal DAC. Table 3 shows the performance parameters of the proposed design and a comparison with recent state of art designs.

5   Conclusion

In this paper, a design of ultra-low power PW-ExG SoC for IoT healthcare system has been presented. It has 8-channels supporting various ExG signal amplitudes and frequency bands. Its performance is improved by CC-PGIA design, hybrid SAR-Cyclic ADC, PWT and calibration technique while the power consumption is reduced by operating on a 0.6 V supply voltage and sub-threshold region. The results in Table 3 show that most of the performance parameters are better than that of recent designs making the design suitable for bio-medical and IoT healthcare applications.

References

1. Redondi, A., et al.: An integrated system based on wireless sensor networks for patient monitoring, localization and tracking. Ad Hoc Netw. **11**(1), 39–53 (2013)
2. Mansano, A.L., et al.: An autonomous wireless sensor node with asynchronous ECG monitoring in 0.18 μm CMOS. IEEE Trans. Biomed. Circ. Syst. **10**(3), 602–611 (2016)

3. Lee, S.-Y., et al.: Low-power wireless ECG acquisition and classification system for body sensor networks. IEEE J. Biomed. Health Inform. **19**(1), 236–246 (2015)
4. Rai, S., et al.: A 500 μW neural tag with 2 μV$_{rms}$ AFE and frequency-multiplying MICS/ISM FSK transmitter. In: IEEE International Solid-State Circuits Conference-Digest of Technical Papers, ISSCC 2009. IEEE (2009)
5. Li, Y.L., et al.: Transconductance enhancement method for operational transconductance amplifiers. Electron. Lett. **46**(19), 1321–1323 (2010)
6. Zhu, Z., Liang, Y.: A 0.6-V 38-nW 9.4-ENOB 20-kS/s SAR ADC in 0.18-μm CMOS for medical implant devices. IEEE Trans. Circ. Syst. I Regul. Pap. **62**(9), 2167–2176 (2015)
7. Jin, J., Gao, Y., Sanchez-Sinencio, E.: An energy-efficient time-domain asynchronous 2 b/step SAR ADC with a hybrid R-2R/C-3C DAC structure. IEEE J. Solid State Circ. **49**(6), 1383–1396 (2014)
8. IEEE Standard Part 15.4: Wireless Medium Access Control (MAC) and Physical Layer (PHY) Specification for Wireless Personal Area Networks (WPANs). IEEE Standard 802.15.4-2003 (2003)
9. Tseng, Y., et al.: A 0.09 μW low power front-end biopotential amplifier for biosignal recording. IEEE Trans. Biomed. Circ. Syst. **6**(5), 508–516 (2012)
10. Zhu, Z., Bai, W.: A 0.5-V 1.3-μW analog front-end CMOS circuit. IEEE Trans. Circ. Syst. II Express Briefs **63**(6), 523–527 (2016)
11. Tang, F., et al.: A column-parallel inverter-based cyclic ADC for CMOS image sensor with capacitance and clock scaling. IEEE Trans. Electron Devices **63**(1), 162–167 (2016)
12. Lim, Y., Flynn, M.P.: A 1 mW 71.5 dB SNDR 50 MS/s 13 bit fully differential ring amplifier based SAR-assisted pipeline ADC. IEEE J. Solid State Circ. **50**(12), 2901–2911 (2015)
13. Zhang, Y., et al.: A batteryless 19 μW MICS/ISM-band energy harvesting body sensor node SoC for ExG applications. IEEE J. Solid State Circ. **48**(1), 199–213 (2013)
14. Databases Webpage on Physionet (2012). http://www.physionet.org/physiobank/database/#ecg
15. iRhythm (2013). http://www.irhythmtech.com

Channel Modeling of In-Vivo THz Nanonetworks: State-of-the-Art and Research Challenges

Vasilis K. Papanikolaou$^{(\boxtimes)}$ and George K. Karagiannidis

Department of Electrical and Computer Engineering,
Aristotle University of Thessaloniki, 54124 Thessaloniki, Greece
{vpapanikk,geokarag}@auth.gr

Abstract. Recently, it has been proposed, that nanodevices can be injected in the human body and perform non-invasive medical diagnostics. However, due to their small size, a plethora of such nanodevices need to be used in practical applications, thus, creating a nanonetwork, which collects the information and communicates with out-of-body nodes. For these networks, several models have been proposed for the THz channel in the in-vivo scenario. Most of them are based on well-defined theories and physical laws, while some of them are based on experiments. In this paper, we review the state-of-the-art of channel modeling of in-vivo communications in the THz band and discuss future trends and research challenges.

Keywords: Terahertz nanonetworks · In-vivo communication
Nanotechnology · Channel modeling

1 Introduction

In recent years, advancements in nanotechnology allowed to envision the use of nanomachines in everyday human life. Nanodevices can be utilised for a plethora of different applications, ranging from flexible electronics to medical technologies [1]. Coordinating and information sharing among them can lead to the creation of nanonetworks that cover different areas simultaneously and can perform several tasks in a non-invasive way [2]. As a result, nanosensing has emerged as a very promising field. Nanosensors are not just tiny sensors, but complete nanomachines that can identify and measure events in the nanoscale. Especially for medical applications, it provides a novel way of diagnosis, since the nanosensors can –for example– detect chemical compounds in concentrations as low as one part per billion [3]. However, in order to achieve such sensing accuracy, the range of sensing must be limited to the nano-environment –just a few micrometers in most cases– of the nanomachine. Also, the need of a mechanism to transmit the collected information outside the body is a challenging task of the nanonetworks scientific field.

© ICST Institute for Computer Sciences, Social Informatics and Telecommunications Engineering 2018
P. Perego et al. (Eds.): MobiHealth 2017, LNICST 247, pp. 50–57, 2018.
https://doi.org/10.1007/978-3-319-98551-0_6

As mentioned above, nanonetworks can cover an area of interest in the human body and perform nanosensing to detect irregularities in the tissues or even perform standard medical exams, in a non-invasive way. It must be noted, that nanonetworks can also be used as drug delivery systems. With the use, recently, of nanomaterials, such as graphene and its derivatives, communication in a nanonetwork can be made feasible. It has been found that the operational frequency of nanoantennas, constructed from such materials, belongs in the band of THz (0.1 THz–10 THz), otherwise known as the *terahertz gap*. Note that THz radiation is non-ionizing and, as such, it is thought to be safe for the human body.

In this paper, we review the state-of-the-art of channel modeling of in-vivo communications in the THz band and discuss future trends and research challenges.

2   Noise Models

Noise in THz systems can originate from multiple sources. The main contribution comes from the *molecular absorption noise*, which is generated during the transmission process. Other sources include the noise created by surrounding nanomachines or the same device, termed as *background noise*. However, while there is no accurate noise model for graphene-based electronic devices, the electronic noise temperature is considered to be very low [4]. As such, the research mostly focuses on the molecular absorption noise.

2.1   Background Noise

Kokkoniemi *et al.* [5] described the background noise with the help of the *sky noise* model. Sky noise is created by the temperature of the absorbing medium, causing the medium to be an effective black body radiator and, as such, it is independent of the transmitted signals. Sky noise is producing a noise temperature T_{mol}, which can be evaluated as

$$T_{mol}(r, f) = T_0 \left(1 - e^{-a(f)r} \right), \tag{1}$$

where T_0 is the reference temperature and $a(f)$ is the absorption coefficient of the medium in terms of frequency f.

In the past, this model was used to describe the atmosphere as a medium for transmission [4]. In [6] it was proposed that this model is not sufficient to describe the *body radiation* noise, since it is not reliable to use the molecular temperature as a parameter in order to evaluate the radiation from the absorbing medium in human tissues. Kokkoniemi *et al.* [5] and Zhang *et al.* [6] used Planck's law to evaluate the background radiation noise as

$$B(T_0, f) = \frac{2h\pi(nf)^3}{c^2} \left(\exp\left(\frac{hf}{k_B T_0} \right) - 1 \right)^{-1}, \tag{2}$$

where k_B is the Boltzmann and h is the Planck constants, correspondingly. Planck's function is multiplied with π to transform the unit from $W/Hz/cm^2/sr$ to $W/Hz/cm^2$.

Assuming that the human tissue can be approximated as an isothermal and homogeneous layer with thickness r and that this radiation is created only from the original energy state of the molecules (black body radiation) the noise power can be evaluated as

$$N_b(r, f) = \lim_{r \to \infty} \int_0^r B(T_0, f) a(f) e^{-a(f)s} ds =$$

$$= \lim_{r \to \infty} B(T_0, f) \left(1 - e^{-a(f)r} \right) = B(T_0, f). \tag{3}$$

Taking into account the antenna aperture term, due to the isotropic radiation at the receiver, the power spectral density (psd) of the body radiation noise with the unit W/Hz is given by

$$N_b(f) = B(T_0, f) \frac{c^2}{4\pi(n_0 f_0)^2}. \tag{4}$$

2.2 Molecular Absorption Noise

This subsection is devoted to the molecular absorption noise, which contributes the most in the noise of the THz channel. What makes this noise different than usual is that it is *self-induced*, which means that it is induced by the transmissions of the users sharing the medium. A part of the radiation that is transmitted is absorbed by the molecules of the medium and becomes kinetic energy, i.e. heat. The other part is re-emitted back in random directions and, as such, it is considered as noise to the receiver. In the pioneering work of Jornet et al. [3], they derived a model for the psd of the molecular absorption noise for the atmosphere. The parameter that describes this phenomenon is the *emissivity* of the channel, ϵ, which is defined as

$$\epsilon(f, r) = 1 - \tau(f, r), \tag{5}$$

where f is the frequency of the electromagnetic propagating wave, r stands for the total path length and τ is the transmissivity of the medium given by the Beer-Lambert Law

$$\tau(f, r) = \frac{P_0}{P_i} = e^{-a(f)r}, \tag{6}$$

with P_i and P_0 being the incident and radiated power, respectively, and $a(f)$ is the absorption coefficient of the medium. Then, the equivalent noise temperature due to molecular absorption can be written as

$$T_{mol}(f, r) = T_0 \epsilon(f, r), \tag{7}$$

where T_0 is the reference temperature and ϵ is given by (5). For a given bandwidth, B, the molecular absorption noise power at the receiver can be evaluated as

$$P_n(f,r) = \int_B N_m(f,r)df = k_B \int_B T_{mol}(f,r)df. \tag{8}$$

This model can be adjusted to fit a different medium. As such, Yang et al. [1] and Piro et al. [7] proposed the use of the same model for in-vivo communications. The only difference is that they use the extinction coefficient, κ, instead of the absorption coefficient. The noise power spectral density is, then, given by

$$N_m(f,r) = k_B T_{mol} = k_B T_0 \left(1 - e^{-4\pi f \kappa(f)r/c}\right) \tag{9}$$

and the absorption coefficient is derived from the extinction coefficient by using the following formula

$$a(f) = \frac{4\pi f}{c}\kappa(f). \tag{10}$$

Kokkoniemi et al. [5] considered that, since it is a *self-induced* noise, the source term (Planck's function) in the sky noise model should be replaced by an appropriate transmit energy function. Furthermore, they noticed that the molecular absorption noise energy at point r depends on the derivative of the complement of the transmittance. Then, accounting for the spreading loss, $1/(4\pi r^2)$, as well, as the transmit signal psd, $S_{Tx}(f)$, they get the existing molecular absorption noise model for the receiver at distance r from the transmitter as

$$N_m(r,f) = \frac{S_{Tx}(f)}{4\pi r^2}\left(1 - e^{-a(f)r}\right). \tag{11}$$

Based on [5], Zhang et al. [6] proposed the following formula

$$N_m(r,f) = S_{Tx}(f)\left(\frac{c}{4\pi n f r}\right)^2\left(1 - e^{-a(f)r}\right), \tag{12}$$

where $S_{Tx}(f)$ is the transmitted signal psd and the term $(c/(4\pi n f r))^2$ accounts for the spreading loss and the antenna aperture.

It is worth mentioning here, that this formula was derived with the assumption that all the absorbed energy from the transmitted signal received at the receiver would turn into molecular absorption noise psd at point r.

2.3   Total Noise

In the previous subsections, we have presented the main noise sources for the THz in-vivo channel. The total channel noise psd for the in-vivo nanonetwork can, then, be derived as the sum of the two

$$N(r,f) = N_b(f) + N_m(r,f). \tag{13}$$

It was shown [4], that the molecular absorption noise tends to be significantly higher than the background radiation noise. As such, in many cases it is considered the dominant noise source in THz in-vivo nanonetworks, Fig. 1.

It is worth noting here that these results are based on graphene-based receivers, which have yet to be developed. The available nanodevices today, are not based on these new materials and thus, the Johnson-Nyquist thermal noise should be taken into account. In Sect. 4, we discuss in more detail the use of new materials and the future challenges on this field.

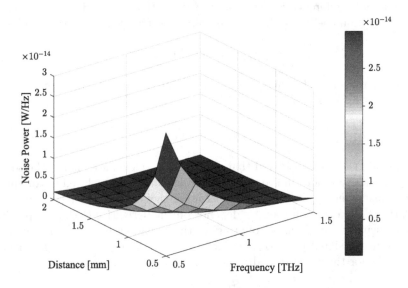

Fig. 1. Total noise for a transmitted signal with flat psd

3   Path Loss Models

As discussed in the previous section, in THz nanonetworks the molecular absorption of the medium deteriorates the propagation of the EM waves. Also, path loss is present, due to the spreading of the signal [8]. Most of the research focuses on spread and absorption losses for the in-vivo THz channel.

3.1   Spreading Loss

Spreading loss is a well known power attenuation contributor in wireless communications. The proposed model, even for in-vivo THz communications, assumes an isotropic radiation and as such, the spreading loss can be defined in dB as

$$PL_{spr}(r)[dB] = 20\log\frac{4\pi r}{\lambda_g}, \tag{14}$$

where r is the propagation distance of the wave and λ_g is the wavelength in the medium.

3.2   Absorption Loss

We have pointed out in Sect. 2, that part of the transmitted energy is absorbed by the medium. Details on the absorption coefficient, $a(f)$, of human tissues was provided in [1] and is frequency dependent. The main issue with the molecular absorption is that there are not any analytic functions of the absorption coefficient and, the numerical data are limited to frequencies in the range of 1 THz or frequencies closer to the optical spectrum.

The behavior of the absorption of each tissue varies with the kind of tissue; more specifically, it seems to depend on the percentage of water, since water molecules create peaks in the absorption-frequency relation, due to resonance phenomena. The transmittance of the medium, τ, can be evaluated using the Beer-Lambert Law, as in (6), which is the fraction of incident EM radiation at a given frequency, that is able to pass through the medium [3]. Obviously, since we need the fraction of the radiation that is absorbed by the medium we need the inverse of τ.

$$PL_{abs}(f,r) = \frac{1}{\tau(f,r)} = e^{a(f)r}, \tag{15}$$

or in dB

$$PL_{abs}(f,r)[dB] = 10a(f)r\log_{10}e. \tag{16}$$

3.3   Total Path Loss

In order to evaluate the total path loss, it is evident that both the spreading path loss and the molecular absorption path loss must be taken into account.

$$PL(f,r)[dB] = PL_{spr}(r)[dB] + PL_{abs}(f,r)[dB] \tag{17}$$

$$= 20\log_{10}\frac{4\pi r}{\lambda_g} + 10a(f)r\log_{10}e. \tag{18}$$

Recently, some research was devoted to obtain alternative, simpler and more accurate formulas, by using experimental data. More specifically, Javed *et al.* [9] proposed an approximation to the analytical path loss model, named *Simple-Nano*, that is described by the following equation,

$$PL(f,r)[dB] = 10\log_{10}K_0 + 10n\log_{10}\left(\frac{r}{r_0}\right) + X_\sigma, \tag{19}$$

where K_0 is the path-loss at a reference distance r_0, which is chosen to be 0.01 m, n is the path loss exponent and X_σ is a log-normal random variable that takes into account the shadowing. In another work of Abbasi *et al.* [10], they used an artificially synthesized collagen layer from QMUL, which was used to model the human skin layer, so that they could perform actual measurements for the path loss in THz frequencies. After intensive experiments they proposed the model

$$PL(f,r)[dB] = A(N) + B(N)r^{0.65} + C(N)f^{4.07}, \tag{20}$$

where the regression technique is used to find the functions $A(N)$, $B(N)$, $C(N)$, which represent the constant offset and the coefficients for distance and frequency respectively, as a function of the number of sweat ducts. The reason that sweat ducts play such an important role is because they are approximately consisted of 99% water and as we mentioned above, water molecules appear to be highly absorbent in THz frequencies. So, variations in the number of sweat ducts can drastically change the channel.

In Fig. 2 we compare the above models through (17) and (20). The equation we used is [10, Eq. 16]

$$PL(f,r)[dB] = -0.2N + 3.98 + (0.44N + 98.48)r^{0.65} + (0.068N + 2.4)f^{4.07}, \tag{21}$$

where r is expressed in mm, and f is expressed in THz. The two models do not match, although in both cases, path loss seems to increase with the frequency. We can justify the difference in the fact that in [10] a synthesized skin model was used out of collagen. However, by tuning the parameters of (20), it is possible to get a variety of results that accommodate the difference between the models.

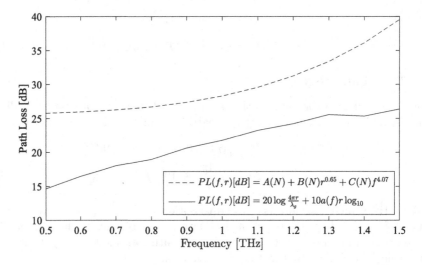

Fig. 2. Comparison of path loss models at $r = 0.1\,\text{mm}$

4   Research Challenges

It is evident from the previous sections, that there is space for research both for noise and path loss models. Some research challenges are as follow:

– In-vivo electromagnetic propagation is a critical topic in nanonetworks. Reflection, diffraction and scattering need to be modeled properly for highly dispersive mediums, such as the blood.

In addition to that, the channel characteristics changes from person to person, depending on health conditions. A complete model needs to capture that behavior and be robust enough to adjust to all scenarios, regarding the human body condition.

- The biggest research challenge is the development of nanodevices, based on new materials. The development of graphene-based nanodevices will provide the opportunity to validate the theoretical models. Furthermore, it important to note here that these nanomachines allow only low complexity coding schemes, due to their limited processing capacity.
- Medical research challenges are also present. The THz band is a part of the EM spectrum, between far infrared light and microwaves, and, as such, it is a non-ionizing radiation that is considered safe for the human body. Despite that, there is still a need to investigate the way that THz radiation interacts with human cells.
- Finally, the effects of the use of carbon in these nanodevices, that are injected into the human body, specifically graphene, need to be investigated.

References

1. Yang, K., Pellegrini, A., Munoz, M.O., Brizzi, A., Alomainy, A., Hao, Y.: Numerical analysis and characterization of Thz propagation channel for body-centric nano-communications. IEEE Trans. Terahertz Sci. Technol. **5**, 419–426 (2015)
2. Akyildiz, I.F., Jornet, J.M.: The Internet of nano-things. IEEE Wirel. Commun. **17**, 58–63 (2010)
3. Jornet, J.M., Akyildiz, I.F.: Channel modeling and capacity analysis for electromagnetic wireless nanonetworks in the terahertz band. IEEE Trans. Wirel. Commun. **10**, 3211–3221 (2011)
4. Jornet, J.M.: Fundamentals of electromagnetic nanonetworks in the terahertz band. Ph.D. thesis, School of Electrical and Computer Engineering, Georgia Institute of Technology (2013)
5. Kokkoniemi, J., Lehtomäki, J., Juntti, M.: A discussion on molecular absorption noise in the terahertz band. Nano Commun. Netw. **8**, 35–45 (2016)
6. Zhang, R., Yang, K., Alomainy, A., Abbasi, Q.H., Qaraqe, K., Shubair, R.M.: Modelling of the terahertz communication channel for in-vivo nano-networks in the presence of noise. In: 2016 16th Mediterranean Microwave Symposium (MMS), pp. 1–4. IEEE (2016)
7. Piro, G., Yang, K., Boggia, G., Chopra, N., Grieco, L.A., Alomainy, A.: Terahertz communications in human tissues at the nanoscale for healthcare applications. IEEE Trans. Nanotechnol. **14**, 404–406 (2015)
8. Zogas, D.A., Karagiannidis, G.K.: Infinite-series representations associated with the bivariate rician distribution and their applications. IEEE Trans. Commun. **53**, 1790–1794 (2005)
9. Javed, I.T., Naqvi, I.H.: Frequency band selection and channel modeling for WNSN applications using simplenano. In: Proceedings of IEEE International Conference on Communications, ICC 2013, Budapest, Hungary, 9–13 June 2013, pp. 5732–5736. IEEE (2013)
10. Abbasi, Q.H., El Sallabi, H., Chopra, N., Yang, K., Qaraqe, K.A., Alomainy, A.: Terahertz channel characterization inside the human skin for nano-scale body-centric networks. IEEE Trans. Terahertz Sci. Technol. **6**, 427–434 (2016)

Designing and Evaluating a Vibrotactile Language for Sensory Substitution Systems

Majid Janidarmian[✉], Atena Roshan Fekr, Katarzyna Radecka, and Zeljko Zilic

Electrical and Computer Engineering Department, McGill University, Montréal, QC, Canada
{majid.janidarmian,atena.roshanfekr}@mail.mcgill.ca,
{katarzyna.radecka,zeljko.zilic}@mcgill.ca

Abstract. The sense of touch can be used for sensory substitution, i.e., to represent visual or auditory cues to impaired users. Sensory substitution often requires the extensive training of subjects, leading to exhaustion and frustration over time. The goal of this paper is to investigate the ability of the subjects to recognize alphanumeric letters on 3×3 vibration array, where the subjects can fully personalize the variables including spatial location, vibratory rhythm, burst duration and intensity. We present a vibrotactile device for delivering the spatiotemporal letter patterns while maintaining the high level of expressiveness. The results prove that this system is an effective solution with a low cognitive load for visually/auditory impaired people and for any context that would benefit from leaving the eyes/ears free for other tasks.

Keywords: Vibrotactile display · Sensory substitution · Wearables · Haptics

1 Background

The skin has been considered as a conduit for information [1, 2], where a vibrotactile display can be added by an array of vibration actuators, with the resolution varying from 2×2 to 64×64 [3] and mostly applied to the skin on the back, abdomen, forehead, thigh, or the fingers. In [4], a camera image is transformed into vibrotactile stimuli using a dynamic tactile coding scheme. The resolution of the image needs to be reduced to fit the low resolution of the *tactor array* as their system consists of 48 (6×8) vibrating motors. The authors also compared their method (M1) in tactilely displaying of the letter with two other typical continuous vibration modes [5, 6]. The first one is an improved handwriting pattern, and the actuation order is similar to handwriting. The vibrating duration time is overlapped between the adjacent motors (M2). In another approach, called scanning mode (M3), the motors are triggered in the lines from top to bottom. As an initial study in pattern identification task, the capital letters were displayed to experienced and inexperienced subjects, using a 20×20 matrix of vibratory tactors placed against the back [6]. Authors reported the results of four modes of stimulus presentation, each letter being presented 42 times under each mode. They found that the sequential tracing by a single moving point leads to the highest recognition accuracy. A tactile stimulator (M8) mounted on a wheelchair is presented in [7], to convert the capital letters into tactile letters using 17×17 Tactile Vision Substitution Systems (TVSS). The dark

© ICST Institute for Computer Sciences, Social Informatics and Telecommunications Engineering 2018
P. Perego et al. (Eds.): MobiHealth 2017, LNICST 247, pp. 58–66, 2018.
https://doi.org/10.1007/978-3-319-98551-0_7

region of the visual display captured by a stationary camera activated the tactors in the corresponding areas of the tactile matrix. Each black line of a letter drawn on a white cardboard activated a line of two tactors wide in the tactile matrix. The experiments demonstrate that at least three independent basic letter features i.e. enclosing shapes, vertical parallel lines, and angle of lines play important parts in tactile letter recognition.

The possibility of differentiating letters by using only a 3×3 array of vibrating motors on the back of a chair has been examined in [8], by providing a sequential pattern for each letter with a "tracing mode." This work (M9) could obtain high recognition rate in reading tactile alphanumeric characters. Recently, a system of spatiotemporal vibration patterns called EdgeVib, for delivering both alphabet (M10) and digits (M11) on wrist-worn vibro-tactile display was presented in [9]. Each unistroke pattern longer than four vibrations is split into multiple 2/3-vibration patterns. The new patterns are consecutively displayed to assist the recognition of the alphanumerical patterns. The study revealed that the recognition rate is significantly improved by modifying the unistroke patterns in both alphabet and digits. Factors such as familiarity with the displayed character set, stimulus duration, inter-stimulus onset interval, type of vibration motors, number of trials, number of letters, and cognition load affect the quality of recognition. Therefore, different studies cannot be directly compared. The results along with some details are brought in Table 1. The discrepancy between studies is due to the differences in equipment, procedure, and style of letters. As summarized in Table 1, the subjects had no time limits for letter perception. Moreover, most of the previous studies only focused on a subset of alphanumerics, and the participants

Table 1. Previous published results.

Vibration modes	Average recognition rate	Cognition load (average repeated times)	Number of letters
M1	82.0% ± 23.3%	2.05	10
M2	76.8% ± 23.5%	2.1	10
M3	47.5% ± 27.5%	2.6	10
M4	34%	$1-2^{\alpha, \beta}$	26
M5	41%	$1-2^{\alpha, \beta}$	26
M6	47%	$1-2^{\alpha, \beta}$	26
M7	51%	$1-2^{\alpha, \beta}$	26
M8	67.53% ± 20%	$1^{\alpha, \gamma}$	26
M9	86% ± 9.7%	1^{α}	34
M10	85.9% ± 6.3%	NA^{δ}	26
M11	88.6% ± 10.4%	NA^{δ}	10

α: The subjects had no time limits for letter perception and they were given as much time to respond as they needed.

β: If the first response was incorrect, they responded with the second guess, after which they were informed of the correct response.

γ: The subjects were trained until they had acquired an identification accuracy of over 80% in each subset of alphabet. The error correction was given when the subjects misidentified. The number of trials per subject was not the same.

δ: After training session, a brief test was performed to ensure that each participant memorizes the patterns correctly. The participants could ask to repeat the questions if they were not confident of their answers. After they gave their answer, the screen prompted the actual answer.

were informed of the correct response. To overcome these limitations, we develop a customizable vibrotactile system to deliver any patterns including all alphanumerics under time constraints for letters perception.

2   The Proposed System

Our tactile display is implemented on an adjustable belt attached on the back of a human. The system comprises nine cylindrical Eccentric Rotating Mass (ERM) motors (8.7 mm in diameter and 25.1 mm in length), Fig. 1(a). The motors are glued to the belt with a spacing of 5 cm (see Fig. 1(c)). This gap between tactors is necessary to perform vibration localization robustly. The motors control the intensity and have fine temporal haptic characteristics (8 ms from off to a perceivable intensity, 21 ms from fully on to off using active breaking with H-bridges). The intensity of the tactors is controlled by Pulse Width Modulation (PWM) signals. The vibration intensity is set to 10 levels from very low to very high. To fully control each motor individually, we used Adafruit 16-Channel 12-bit PWM Driver Shield that can drive up to 16 motors over I2C with only two pins (see Fig. 1(b)). The on-board PWM controller will simultaneously drive all 16 channels with no extra processing overhead. Therefore, the system can incorporate the control of a vast number of different feedback devices into a single and unified interface. The shield plugs in directly into an Arduino device, which also provides the 5 V power to power and control the PWM signal.

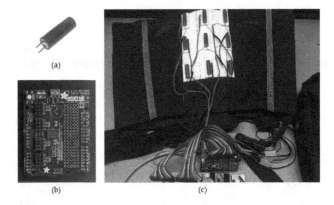

Fig. 1. (a) 9 mm vibration motor from Precision Microdrive, model: 307-103, (b) 16-Channel 12-bit PWM Driver Shield, (c) Back belt with 3 × 3 tactor array

In the proposed platform, the users have full control on the motors variables including spatial location, vibratory rhythm, burst duration, and intensity to generate vibratory patterns. For this purpose, a Graphical User Interface (GUI) is developed to create or revise the patterns and to optimize the temporal-spatial tactile coding according to human tactile perception. Two experiments are conducted with the 3 × 3 tactors array to evaluate the customizable tactile display perception. We report the recognition rate of letters with both default and personalized vibratory patterns.

Algorithm 1 describes the test cases, where each session contains a number of trials with randomly selected characters. Algorithm 2 extracts changes in the motors (events) from the input pattern (line 2). The events stored in an array control the motor operations and 10 intensity levels, defined in line 9. Tactors are activated based on the vibrating order, spatial and temporal properties in lines 10–12.

Algorithm 1. Test_Cases

```
Input: testCase, defaultPatterns, customizedPatterns; output: recognitionRate
1. alphaNumerics ← 'ABCDEFGHIJKLMNOPQRSTUVWXYZ0123456789';
2. numberOfRounds ← 3;
3. switch testCase {
4.      case: 'alphaNumericsRecognition_def' {
5.           targets ← randomPermutation (alphaNumerics(1:end));
             % Make a random order of alphanumeric
6.           hapticPatterns ← extractPatterns (targets, defaultPatterns); }
             % Extract the haptic patterns for the targets according to the default pattern
7.      case: 'alphaNumericsRecognition_per' {
8.           targets ← randomPermutation (alphaNumerics (1:end));
9.           hapticPatterns ← extractPatterns (targets, customizedPatterns); }
             % Extract the haptic patterns for the targets according to the personalized
             pattern through GUI
10.     for i = 1:1: numberOfRounds
11.          for j ← 1:1: length (hapticPatterns)
12.               runHaptic (hapticPatterns (j));
                  % Generate each pattern on the vibration motors
13.     recognitionRate ←accuracy (confMat (targets, userResponses));
14. return recognitionRate;
```

Algorithm 2. runHaptic

```
Input: hapticPattern;
1. resetVibMotors (1:9); % Turn off all 9 motors
2. [events, intensities] = FetchEvents (hapticPattern);
   % Extract the events from the pattern (i.e. default pattern or customized pattern). Events is a
   time-sorted array. events(i): is 1 if a motor should be turned on at this time, events(i): is 0
if
   a motor should be turned off at this time. intensities(i): intensity of the vibration motor
which
   is turned on at this time.
3. i = 0;
4. while (1) {
5.      i = i + 1;
6.      wait (tᵢ); % Wait till it is time for next event.
7.      selectedMotor = events (i).motor;
8.      if (events (i)) { % If at this time a vibration motor should be turned on
9.           intensity = (((maxPW – minPW) × (intensities (i)) / 10) + minPW;
10.          setPWM (selectedMotor, intensity); }
             % Turn on a vibration motor with the determined intensity
11.     else  { % If at this time a vibration motor should be turned off
12.          setPWM (selectedMotor, 0); } % Turn off a vibration motor
13.     if (i == length (events))
14.          break; }
```

3   Experiment Setup

We first conduct an experiment consisted of two sessions of vibrotactile pattern identification tasks, before and the other after the development of each subject's personalized letters. The experiment is carried out with ten healthy volunteers (five males, five females) aged 18 to 46 with (Mean $\pm$ SD) 30.70 ± 8.87. The ethical approval was received from McGill Ethics Committee. The participants had no experience of vibro-tactile display devices, were asked to wear the belt in upright sitting position and to match felt sensations with the alphabets or digits. They had a time limit of 2 s for letter perception, and no chance to repeat the presented tactile stimuli. To have a more realistic scenario, they were not allowed to use any headset to block out the sound caused by the vibrators and environment. We wanted to analyze the results with a minimum cognitive load that is calculated by the average repeated time for the subject to conduct the letter's identification [4]. In the training phase, the subjects knew the characters they perceived through 3×3 tactile grid display. The training and testing phases are composed of 108 (3×36) trials with 3 sets of randomly selected characters. Figure 2 illustrates the sequence of tactors activated in the default patterns setting designed by a left-handed supervisor. There is no time interval between the onsets of stimuli, and the stimulus duration is set to 200 ms.

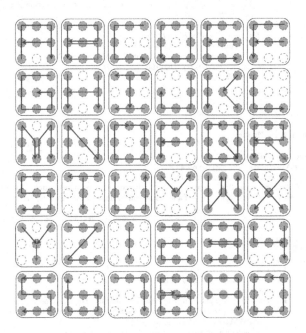

Fig. 2. The sequence of tactors to be activated 36 different alphabets and digits in the default version - The arrows orders: red, green, and blue. (Color figure online)

The default settings help the participants to perceive the letter as a continuous stroke. In the second session, the subjects could revise the default patterns through the GUI. Indeed, each subject can turn the motors on and off in succession and therefore they could customize the tactors' vibration patterns with any preferences such as following their own writing habit. Personalizing the spatiotemporal vibration patterns could deliver more information with easier interpretation and memorizing. Therefore, this property greatly facilitates the users to distinguish the letters.

4   Experimental Results

Figure 3(a) shows the participants' confusions between stimuli with the default patterns. Each cell value of the matrix C (i, j) shows the total number of trials that the response 'j' occurred upon the presentation of stimulus 'i'. The results show that the subjects readily recognize the patterns under mean identification rate of 70.83% ± 24.65%, with a low cognitive load. The subjects reflected that sometimes they had difficulty in distinguishing the patterns different from their own writing habit such as letter 'E'. The patterns 'E' and '7' presented to the participants tended to get highly confused with letters 'G' and '1', respectively. The letter 'O' and number '0' activated the same dot matrix patterns, but they can be discriminated by the direction of the activated tactors. Most participants reported that sometimes they judged a pattern according to their own writing habits. We expect they may be less likely to be confused by revising the spatial locations, stimulus duration and directions, etc. The subjects had a time limit of 2 s and no chance to repeat the stimuli. These constraints are beneficial for the multi-character words. In the second session, where each subject was allowed to make modifications to the default patterns, there is a more uniform confusion matrix (see Fig. 3(b)). For instance, letters 'X' and 'Y' have similar patterns directions, and subjects can apply an alternative writing sequence to create more differentiable patterns. Figure 4 shows some more effective alternative patterns for letters, where the participant used higher level of intensities for letters 'A' and '7' (tick arrows). As seen in Fig. 5, customizing the vibrotactile patterns improved the recognition accuracy by 22.49%. A student's t-test revealed that the customized patterns achieved significantly higher recognition rates than the default patterns (86.76% ± 9.44% vs. 70.83% ± 24.65%, p-value ≪ 0.01). Among the numbers, the number '2' yielded the best accuracy (96.67%) and '5' was the worst (56.67%). For letters, 'I' and 'J' yielded the best accuracy (100%) and the lowest letter accuracies are: 'V' (70%), 'Y' (70%) and 'G' (73.33%). As seen in the confusion matrix, still some letters ('Q' and 'G') exhibited asymmetries. Although the updated patterns increase the total vibratory delivery time, they resolve the confusion between letters and reduce the misrecognition rates. The misidentifications are more likely due to time constraints for letters' perception. Contrary to other studies, the participants could not repeat the questions and the error correction was not given when the subjects misidentified. These constraints are beneficial for the multi-character words. Another observation worth highlighting is the reduction of 'Missed' answers (57.85%) after revising the letters. The subjects could judge the pattern in the first two seconds, and their performance would be improved by tuning the vibratory variables again and practicing them for a couple of more trials.

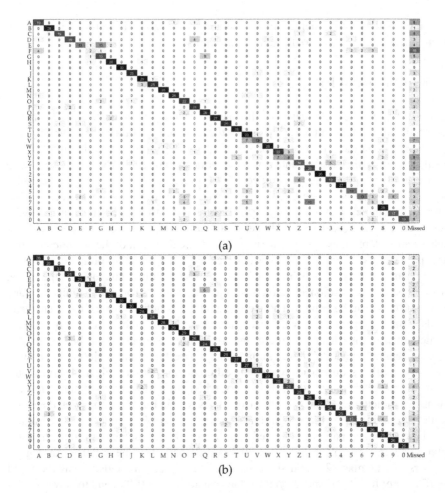

Fig. 3. Confusion matrices for the recognition of (a) default patterns, (b) customized patterns

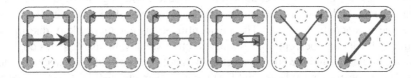

Fig. 4. Examples of customized patterns by one of the participants

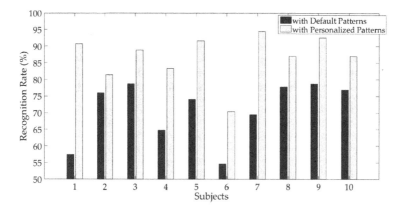

Fig. 5. Recognition rates with default and personalized patterns for each subject

5 Conclusion

We presented a tactile display and the experiments conducted to investigate its effectiveness. The results reveal that the customizable low-resolution vibrotactile display alleviates the perceptional and memory loadings of the users to recognize new patterns with no extensive training sessions. Personalized tactile instructions can be a major component of an assistive wearable device for people with hearing and visual impairments. The applicability and usability can be extended to color and multi-character messages identification tasks.

References

1. Janidarmian, M., Fekr, A.R., Radecka, K., Zilic, Z.: Haptic feedback and human performance in a wearable sensor system. In: 2016 IEEE-EMBS International Conference on Biomedical and Health Informatics (BHI), Las Vegas, NV, pp. 620–624 (2016)
2. Novich, S.D., Eagleman, D.M.: Using space and time to encode vibrotactile information: toward an estimate of the skin's achievable throughput. Exp. Brain Res. **10**, 2777–2788 (2015)
3. Visell, Y.: Tactile sensory substitution: models for enaction in HCI. Interact. Comput. **21**(1–2), 38–53 (2009)
4. Wu, J., Zhang, J., Yan, J., Liu, W., Song, G.: Design of a vibrotactile vest for contour perception. Int. J. Adv. Rob. Syst. **9**, 166 (2012)
5. Kim, H., Seo, C., Lee, J., Ryu, J., Yu, S., Lee, S.: Vibrotactile display for driving safety information. In: IEEE Intelligent Transportation Systems Conference, pp. 573–577 (2006)
6. Loomis, J.M.: Tactile letter recognition under different modes of stimulus presentation. Percept. Psychophysics **16**(2), 401–408 (1974)
7. Kikuchi, T., Yamashita, Y., Sagawa, K., Wake, T.: An analysis of tactile letter confusions. Percept. Psychophysics **26**(4), 295–301 (1979)

8. Yanagida, Y., Kakita, M., Lindeman, R.W., Kume, Y., Tetsutani, N.: Vibrotactile letter reading using a low-resolution tactor array. In: International Conference on Haptic Interfaces for Virtual Environment and Teleoperator Systems (2004)
9. Liao, Y., Chen, Y., Lo, J., Liang, R., Chan, L., Chen, B.: EdgeVib: effective alphanumeric character output using a wrist-worn tactile display. In: Proceedings of the 29th Annual Symposium on User Interface Software and Technology, pp. 595–601 (2016)

Online Monitoring of Posture for Preventive Medicine Using Low-Cost Inertial Sensors

Karl-Heinz Kellner[✉], Hoang Le, Johannes Blatnik, Valentin Rosegger,
Robert Pilacek, and Albert Treytl

Center for Integrated Sensor Systems, Danube-University Krems, Viktor-Kaplan-Straße 2,
Wiener Neustadt, Austria
{karl-heinz.kellner,albert.treytl}@donau-uni.ac.at,
{hoang.le,johannes.blatnik,valentin.rosegger,
robert.pilacek}@vivaback.at

Abstract. People in many professions suffer from low back pain (LBP) due to wrong movements. Although this is anticipated by occupational medicine, the quality of evidence is low, since little objective measurements about the spine position in daily-use exist. The paper presents an ultra-flat posture monitoring system based on low-cost acceleration sensors, which can be very efficiently be used to measure the posture of the spine. First experiments (lab-based and in daily-use) showed a deviation of approximately 1° with a low standard deviation. Innovation is the suitability for daily-use by sensors having a height of 2,5 mm that allow a seamless usage even during positions applying pressure to the back such a leaned sitting on a chair.

Keywords: Spine posture · Low back pain · Inertial sensors
Online monitoring

1 Introduction

Extreme or awkward postures like bending or twisting of the back are presented as risk factors for developing low back pain (LBP) in several clinical guidelines (e.g. [1–3]). LBP patients have a reduced lumbar range of motion and move more slowly compared to people without low back pain [4]. Restriction in lateral flexion as well as reduced lumbar lordosis are also associated with increased risk of developing LBP [5].

Even though ergonomic interventions are key elements of physiotherapy and occupational medicine [6], the evidence for prevention of LBP is uncertain, because the quality of evidence is low [7, 8]. Recent systematic reviews cannot show (or disprove) a direct effect of extreme spine positions and a higher risk for LBP (e.g. [9–11]).

Application of sensors can help to increase evidence but at the same time it is necessary that such sensors are not only used during clinical studies but are also available in low-cost versions for wide-spread application in preventive and occupational medicine. This paper will introduce a low-cost, ultra-flat sensing platform that can measure spine posture during daily live without disturbing the movements of the patient wearing the sensor system.

© ICST Institute for Computer Sciences, Social Informatics and Telecommunications Engineering 2018
P. Perego et al. (Eds.): MobiHealth 2017, LNICST 247, pp. 67–74, 2018.
https://doi.org/10.1007/978-3-319-98551-0_8

2   State-of-the-Art

2.1   Measurement Principle and Medical Indication

Studies often assess the angle between thigh and trunk/pelvis (hip-flexion) as a measure for posture of the spine or simply quantify the angle between trunk and floor [10, 12–15]. This is also reflected by posture assessment tools of occupational medicine like OWAS (Ovako Working Posture Assessment System) REBA (Rapid Entire Body Assessment) or RULA (Rapid Upper Limb Assessment) that are widely used in scientific literature.

Nevertheless, this method has a serious flaw: The angle between the thigh and the trunk/pelvis is no measure for the position (curvature) of the back or even the position of the upper trunk in relation towards the floor, because bending forward can be done with a straight or flexed back (see Fig. 1). Forward bending should be evaluated assessing also the curvature of the back. Only few studies exist measuring the position (curvature) of the back with modern sensing methods during daily live [16].

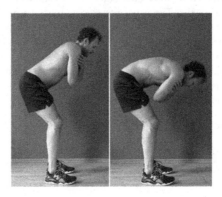

Fig. 1.   Curvature of spine: neutral spine (left) and flexed spine (right) position both showing the same amount of hip flexion. (Photos by Katharina Müller)

Even though there is no good evidence at the moment about correlation of extreme postures of the back and risk of back pain, some reviews show a dose-response relationship [12, 17, 18]. Hence, future occupational studies require to gather data under realistic daily-use circumstances for the full activity period instead of small time frames during a working day. A precise quantification of the position (curvature) of the back instead of using hip flexion or trunk position relative to the floor needs to be available to find medical evidence and derive therapeutically measures.

2.2   Measurement Methods

In order to determine the position (curvature) of the spine different approaches exist: Optical motion capture systems uses optical (infrared and visible light) markers attached to the person, which are scanned by external cameras [19]. These systems can be referred as the golden reference standard, yet are not further discussed, since they require dedicated test rooms and are therefore not suitable to monitor the spine movement in everyday situations.

Maier et al. [20] use strain gauges from Epionics applied over the full length of the spine and 3 axis accelerometers at the end of the gauges to determine the bending angel. The system connects the sensors via cables to a measurement device and requires dedicated band-aid that allow the movement of the strain gauges along the back of the patient. A disadvantage stems band-aid and from the fixed length gauges, since it cannot be adapted to different body sizes.

Dinu et al. [21] investigates the use of 17 inertial sensors (MVN Biomech system from Xsens) and compared it with a Vicon optical infrared marker system with eight camcorders to acquire the full body movement. Both systems only show a position difference of less than 6 mm. Problems are identified in the drift of acceleration sensors and the relative movement of the sensors on soft tissues of the subject. This relative movement might be due to relatively high weight of 16 g and size of $47 \times 30 \times 13$ mm^3. Additionally, the sensors have a battery lifetime of 6 h and require data recorded at 120 Hz to be continuously transferred to a base station. Similar systems are offered by Hocoma (valedotherapy.com) for bio-feedback of physical exercises using Bluetooth connected sensors. Yet, these sensors are designed for dedicated exercise and therefore short operation time of around 30 min before they need to be recharged.

Dorsavi [22] offer solutions based on 3D accelerometers, gyroscopes and a magnetometer designed for workplace application offering operation of 24 h and datastorage up to 72 h. Mjøsund et al. [23] compared the Dorsavi ViMove system to the Vicon system determine a RMS error of 0,71° up to 2,11° depending on the direction of flexion. To our analysis the Dorsavi system is very mature for an every-day use, yet it still uses relatively big sensors only slightly smaller than a match box.

Additionally, very simple sensors such as the acceleration sensor from Back-Track [24] or Lumolift [25] are available, yet these sensors only deliver the position compared to the earth magnetic or gravitation field (hip-flexion). Both sensors are either applied by a pouch or a magnetic clip on the side or front of the body.

3 Mobile Measurement System

Summarizing existing approaches there are two limitations identified: First, an important fact for all sensors applied to the skin is that the movement of soft tissue is influencing the measurement quality, since the measured position deviates from the position of the spine [26, 27]. In particular for overweight individuals this effect needs to be considered. Second, for everyday use in preventive and occupational medicine applications the thickness of the sensor is of high importance. Whereas many application in sports or therapeutic applications are in movement or without contact to hard surfaces, in preventive and occupational medicine positions like leaning or lying are more likely. If the sensor is too thick this will cause unnatural behavior. To overcome these limitations innovation is required to reduce the mass of the sensor as well as the thickness to suppress unnatural behavior and at the same time retaining a reasonable size to avoid artefacts of punctual tissue movement.

3.1 Inertial Sensor System

For the angular measurement of the spine, low cost inertial MEMS sensors where chosen. Aside the cost consideration the measurement of the earth magnetic field was excluded, since it is not reliable enough for accurate angular measurement. After evaluation of different sensor types (e.g. LSM9DS0, MPU9250) the LSM6DS3 was chosen in the version having a measuring ranges of ± 2 g (accelerometer) and $\pm 125°/s$ (gyroscope). The sensor is mounted on a 1,5 mm thick PCB giving the necessary stiffness and is encapsulated with epoxy resin resulting in an overall thickness of 2.5 mm. Experimental version with a chip embedded inside the PCB has been designed with reduce thickness but discarded due to complicated manufacturing. The sensor diameter was set to 25 mm as optimum between wearing comfort and suppression of soft tissue tilting and movement. The sensors are attached to the body using adhesive tape. Each sensor is connected to the device by a thin, flexible and robust I^2C cable providing distortion free transmission and the flexibility to use other sensor chipsets.

3.2 Recording Device

The recording device consists of a touchscreen, an AVR microcontroller, flash memory and a low cost WLAN module (see Fig. 2).

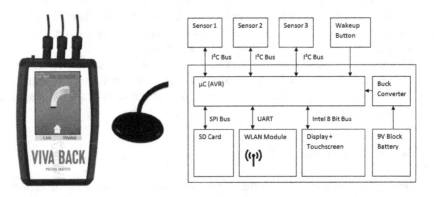

Fig. 2. Device in configuration mode with schematic spine (left), magnified sensor pad (middle) and block diagram (right)

There are three main modes: *setup, record* and *upload mode. Setup mode,* is dedicated to configuration and a guided calibration process determining maximum stretch and bend positions. For better positioning and verification of the three sensor pads a simple online spine model can be displayed (Fig. 2 left). In *record mode,* sensor data is processed and recorded on a flash memory. At any time the user can enter her current activity such as gardening, computer work or sport activity as well as a pain level to support posterior diagnoses. Finally, in the *upload mode* data can be transmitted to a designated FTP server over WLAN using an XML based encoding protected by a pre-shared WPA2 key. In the final device continuous upload is possible if a WLAN connection is available, but a doctor still can retrieve the data via *upload mode* if no connection during activity exists.

Special efforts in circuit design allowed to reduce the current consumption to approx. 5 mA in record mode easily allowing for a 24 h monitoring going beyond most of the state-of-the-art devices. Only during user interaction and WLAN upload, the current consumption raises to 100 mA primary due to the touch panel display, which is also activated during data upload. A Bluetooth Low-Energy chip will be integrated to reduce energy consumption further.

3.3   Data Processing and Algorithms

Data from the sensors is recorded at a speed of 20 Hz and the ground pointing vector of each sensor is calculated by fusion of gyroscope and accelerometer data. The gyroscope is slowly drifting and therefore only reliable at higher frequencies. The accelerometer is disturbed by quick movements, and more reliable at lower frequencies. So a first order complementary filter has been implemented with a cut-off frequency of 0,2 Hz. Two sensors, located at the skin over S2 of the sacrum and at the upper part of the sternum (sternum manubrium) are used to calculate the bending of the spine, whereas the third sensor is placed at the thigh and used for activity (sitting, standing, walking) tracking and as pedometer. Processed sensor data is stored on a flash memory for later diagnosis but also online alarms to give live feedback and help change erroneous posture patterns.

4   Device Characterization and Measurements

To measure the accuracy of the presented sensor system and algorithm following methods have been applied: (a) measurement of a reference dummy emulating the spine, (b) analysis in a 12 h practical daily-use example and (c) a comparison with an optical motion tracking system.

For the first test, the sensors were repeatedly positioned in a fixed angle to each other. The deviation from that constant value is the error that the device produces. Results of these measurements are shown in Fig. 3. On the left side. The mean error and the standard deviation were calculated for different cases. A particular resting position was recorded for 12 h to analyze if there are any long-term drift effects. No drift was observed during the measurements. Rotation of the sensor and linear movements as well as shocks were performed on the sensors in all rotational axis and directions.

Thereby the sensors were taken to their measure boundaries of ± 2 g and $\pm 125°/s$. Under extreme conditions exceeding the specification limits of the sensors, the precision deteriorated, especially, during rotation performed with 2 Hz and a range of $\pm 75°$ and shock performed in an interval of one second with more than 2 g acceleration.

For the second test, the sensor system was carried by a person in daily-use mostly consisting of office work, walking and relaxing. Two sensors have been applied on the

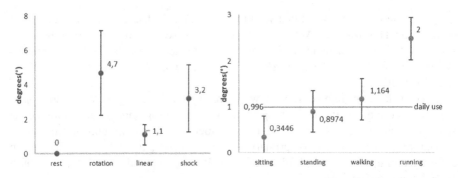

Fig. 3. Mean and standard deviation of measurement error for different disturbances (left) and mean and standard deviation for different activities (right)

lower back with a difference angle of zero degrees for a whole working day without removal. Thus, any value other than zero can be interpreted as a measurement error. In Fig. 3 (right side) the resulting error is plotted for different activities during the day. As expected the error is higher for dynamic movements yet significantly smaller than the static test values. Noteworthy is the very small overall deviation in the daily-use example of less than 1°. Only heavy shocks as occurring during running will result in higher values, yet are less frequent than during the rotation and shock tests.

As a last test the sensor values have been compared with the video motion tracking system Kinovea [28]. Two visual markers and one sensor has been attached to stiff plates and were attached to the lower back area and to the upper part of the chest.

Figure 4 shows first preliminary data obtained comparing the motion sensors and the optical references. It needs to be noted that the optical imaging software has a relatively high rate of false values, if the test person does not move exactly in the plane of the video and single optical marker are not (fully) visible. This is a principal problem caused by the diametric marker positions when using an optical system with a single camera. The preliminary deviation of 6.31° ± 4.76° degrees is therefore accounted mostly to the

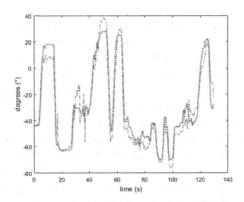

Fig. 4. Example measurement of optical system (blue) versus measurement of developed sensor based system (orange). (Color figure online)

bad optical situation and needs to be reinvestigated with multi-camera optical reference systems.

5   Outlook and Conclusions

The presented work shows that ultra-flat low-cost acceleration sensors can be very efficiently used to measure the posture. First experiments (lab-based and in daily-use) showed a deviation of less than 2° with a low standard deviation. Sensors having a height of 2,5 mm allow a seamless usage even during position applying pressure to the back such a leaned sitting. Yet, measurements also revealed that acceleration values especially during running are much higher than expected and cause outliers and higher deviations due to exceeding the sensor's measurement range.

Ongoing activities therefore focus on higher error reduction and clinical evaluation. First results backup the experimental results presented, but need to undergo a detailed evaluation not available when submitting this paper, since the clinical evaluation has not been finished. Next steps will be the evaluation of both sensors capable of switching to different measurement ranges and additional low-cost acceleration sensor to measure high accelerations. Research needs to be done to evaluate different sampling rates, energy consumption and algorithms to more precisely detect outliers and best to calculate interpolation values for continuous recording.

References

1. Goertz, M., et al.: Adult Acute and Subacute Low Back Pain, 15th edn. (2012)
2. Burton, A.K., et al.: European guidelines for prevention in low back pain. Eur. Spine J. **15**(Suppl 2), S136–S168 (2006). Chapter 2
3. Burton, A.K.: How to prevent low back pain. Best Pract. Res. Clin. Rheumatol. **19**(4), 541–555 (2005)
4. Laird, R.A., Gilbert, J., Kent, P., Keating, J.L.: Comparing lumbo-pelvic kinematics in people with and without back pain: a systematic review and meta-analysis. BMC Musculoskelet. Disord. **15**(1), 229 (2014)
5. Sadler, S.G., Spink, M.J., Ho, A., De Jonge, X.J., Chuter, V.H.: Restriction in lateral bending range of motion, lumbar lordosis, and hamstring flexibility predicts the development of low back pain: a systematic review of prospective cohort studies. BMC Musculoskelet. Disord. **18**(1), 179 (2017)
6. O'Sullivan, K., O'Sullivan, P., O'Sullivan, L., Dankaerts, W.: What do physiotherapists consider to be the best sitting spinal posture? Man. Ther. **17**(5), 432–437 (2012)
7. Steffens, D., et al.: Prevention of low back pain: a systematic review and meta-analysis. JAMA Intern. Med. **176**(2), 199–208 (2016)
8. Driessen, M.T., Proper, K.I., van Tulder, M.W., Anema, J.R., Bongers, P.M., van der Beek, A.J.: The effectiveness of physical and organisational ergonomic interventions on low back pain and neck pain: a systematic review. Occup. Environ. Med. **67**(4), 277–285 (2010)
9. Roffey, D.M., Wai, E.K., Bishop, P., Kwon, B.K., Dagenais, S.: Causal assessment of awkward occupational postures and low back pain: results of a systematic review. Spine J. **10**(1), 89–99 (2010)

10. Wai, E.K., Roffey, D.M., Bishop, P., Kwon, B.K., Dagenais, S.: Causal assessment of occupational bending or twisting and low back pain: results of a systematic review. Spine J. **10**(1), 76–88 (2010)
11. Kwon, B.K., Roffey, D.M., Bishop, P.B., Dagenais, S., Wai, E.K.: Systematic review: occupational physical activity and low back pain. Occup. Med. (Chic. Ill) **61**(8), 541–548 (2011)
12. Bernard, B., (ed.): Musculoskeletal disorders and workplace factors - a critical review of epidemiologic evidence for work-related musculoskeletal disorders of the neck, upper extremity, and low back. National Institute for Occupational Safety and Health. U.S. Department of Health and Human Services, Cincinnati (1997)
13. Jansen, J.P., Morgenstern, H., Burdorf, A.: Dose-response relations between occupational exposures to physical and psychosocial factors and the risk of low back pain. Occup. Environ. Med. **61**(12), 972–979 (2004)
14. Ng, Y.G., et al.: Risk factors of musculoskeletal disorders among oil palm fruit harvesters during early harvesting stage. Ann. Agric. Environ. Med. **22**(2), 286–292 (2015)
15. Lagersted-Olsen, J., Thomsen, B.L., Holtermann, A., Søgaard, K., Jørgensen, M.B.: Does objectively measured daily duration of forward bending predict development and aggravation of low-back pain? A prospective study. Scand. J. Work. Environ. Health **42**(6), 528–537 (2016)
16. Brandt, M., et al.: Participatory intervention with objectively measured physical risk factors for musculoskeletal disorders in the construction industry: study protocol for a cluster randomized controlled trial. BMC Musculoskelet. Disord. **16**(1), 302 (2015)
17. Ribeiro, D.C., Aldabe, D., Abbott, J.H., Sole, G., Milosavljevic, S.: Dose-response relationship between work-related cumulative postural exposure and low back pain: a systematic review. Ann. Occup. Hyg. **56**(6), 684–696 (2012)
18. Lis, A.M., Black, K.M., Korn, H., Nordin, M.: Association between sitting and occupational LBP. Eur. Spine J. **16**(2), 283–298 (2007)
19. Vicon (2017). https://www.vicon.com/. Accessed 18 June 2017
20. Maier, C., Altenscheidt, J., Kramer, M.: Non-invasive assessment of the lumbar spine motion and segmental velocities with Epionics SPINE. OUP **9**, 418–425 (2015)
21. Dinu, D., Fayolas, M., Jacquet, M., Leguy, E., Slavinski, J., Houel, N.: Accuracy of postural human-motion tracking using miniature inertial sensors. Procedia Eng. **147**, 655–658 (2016)
22. dorsaVi. http://eu.dorsavi.com/. Accessed 19 June 2017
23. Mjøsund, H.L., Boyle, E., Kjaer, P., Mieritz, R.M., Skallgård, T., Kent, P.: Clinically acceptable agreement between the ViMove wireless motion sensor system and the Vicon motion capture system when measuring lumbar region inclination motion in the sagittal and coronal planes. BMC Musculoskelet. Disord. **18**(1), 124 (2017)
24. Back-Track (2017). http://www.backtrack.co.uk/. Accessed 18 June 2017
25. Lumo-Lift (2017). http://www.lumobodytech.com. Accessed 18 June 2017
26. Consmüller, T., Rohlmann, A., Weinland, D., Druschel, C., Duda, G.N., Taylor, W.R.: Comparative evaluation of a novel measurement tool to assess lumbar spine posture and range of motion. Eur. Spine J. **21**(11), 2170–2180 (2012)
27. Consmüller, T., Rohlmann, A., Weinland, D., Druschel, C., Duda, G.N., Taylor, W.R.: Velocity of Lordosis angle during spinal flexion and extension. PLoS ONE **7**(11), 1–7 (2012)
28. Kinovea (2017). http://www.kinovea.org/. Accessed 17 June 2017

Energy Harvesting Based Glucose Sensor

Christoph Matoschitz[✉], Robert Lurf, and Manfred Bammer

Biomedical Systems, Austrian Institute of Technology GmbH,
Viktor-Kaplan-Str. 2, 2700 Wiener Neustadt, Austria
christoph.matoschitz@ait.ac.at

Abstract. Blood glucose self-monitoring plays an essential role in the life of diabetic people. A regular control helps diabetic persons to avoid acute complications, e.g. hypoglycaemic coma, and can reduce the risk of long-term consequences of diabetes. The implementation and usage of wireless technologies, e.g. NFC, in smartphones are a big step forward for diabetes home monitoring. Near Field Communication (NFC) is a wireless technology which allows the transmission of data and energy over short distances. The transmitted energy can be used for energy harvesting and in conjunction with low power electronic smart sensor solution reduced in size, weight and costs can be realized. We developed a smart glucose meter based on an amperometric measurement. The prototype is powered by the NFC interface of a smartphone. A user friendly mobile app completes the smart sensor system. The measured blood glucose is visualized on the smartphone and is stored in a diary automatically.

Keywords: Near Field Communication · NFC · Diabetes mellitus
Glucometer · Blood glucose self-monitoring · Mobile diagnostics

1 Introduction

Diabetes mellitus is a group of metabolic diseases whose main symptom is hyperglycemia, an increased blood glucose concentration. Diabetes is one of the most common metabolic disorders worldwide. According to the IDF Diabetes Atlas 2015 [1], around 415 million people worldwide suffer from diabetes mellitus. An unhealthy lifestyle, lack of exercise, hyper caloric nutrition and obesity favour diabetes. Over the last years the number of diabetics has grown rapidly.

There are four main types of diabetes in which type I and type II diabetes are the most common representatives. Type I diabetes is characterized by the impaired production of insulin of beta cells in the islets of Langerhans in the pancreas [2,4]. This leads to an absolute insulin deficiency. Type I diabetes affects about 5% to 10% of the diabetes patients worldwide and is most frequently diagnosed in children and in young adults [3,4].

Type II diabetes is the most prevalent form of diabetes mellitus [4]. Type II diabetes mellitus is characterized by insulin resistance of the tissue and by the

© ICST Institute for Computer Sciences, Social Informatics and Telecommunications Engineering 2018
P. Perego et al. (Eds.): MobiHealth 2017, LNICST 247, pp. 75–80, 2018.
https://doi.org/10.1007/978-3-319-98551-0_9

reduced insulin secretion (relatively insulin deficiency) [2]. Diabetes has acute and chronic effects on the patients' health. Acute complications can include hypoglycaemic and hyperglycaemic coma, ketoacidosis, fainting or death [4]. Chronic effects result from persistently high blood glucose concentrations; damage the retina, kidneys, nerves and circulatory system (micro- and macrovascular consequences) [2,4].

Blood glucose self-monitoring plays a crucial role in the life of diabetics. By controlling the blood glucose concentration help diabetic person to avoid acute hypoglycemic risks and can drastically reduce the likelihood of chronic effects [4]. A regular control of the blood glucose concentration helps patients to manage their disease successfully. In addition this increases the quality of life and the patient safety of diabetics. Furthermore, a good controlled blood glucose level will reduce the costs for the health care system. To maintain the health of type I diabetics they need to monitor their blood glucose concentration 5–6 times a day [4].

Nowadays smartphones are an integral part of our everyday life. The number of smartphone users is already quite high and is still increasing annually. The implementation and usage of the smartphones' wireless capabilities (e.g. Bluetooth, NFC) present a considerable progress for the blood glucose meters. In the case of NFC connectivity, the meter can be powered directly by the smartphone without an additional power source like a battery. Furthermore, size, weight and costs of the resulting device can be minimized.

2 Methods

2.1 Glucose Measurement

The most common glucose measurements are based on amperometric or photometric methods. Blood glucose meters based on amperometric measurement are currently state of the art [3]. The basic concept is that an immobilized enzyme, glucose oxidase (GOx) or glucose dehydrogenase (GDH), catalyzes the oxidation of glucose and uses one of three cofactors: PQQ, FAD, NAD. These two enzymes differ in redox potential, cofactors, turnover rate and selectivity for glucose [3,4]. Depending on the electron transfer mechanism; glucose biosensors were divided into different generations:

First generation glucose biosensors use the presence of oxygen to detect the concentration of hydrogen peroxide. Hydrogen peroxide is oxidized at a platinum electrode at an electrode potential of 0.7 V vs. Ag/AgCl electrode [5].

Second generation glucose biosensors use mediators to carry the electrons between the redox center and the electrode surface [6]. This biosensor does not require oxygen unlike the GOx method. Furthermore this biosensor results in faster electron transfer rates and the use of mediators reduce the required redox potential.

Third generation glucose biosensors do not require a regent [3]. The electron is transferred directly from glucose via the active side of the enzyme [3].

This type of biosensor is mainly used in continuous glucose measurement. Figure 1 shows the different glucose biosensor generations.

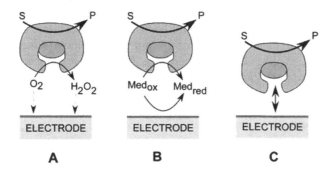

Fig. 1. Different glucose biosensors types: **A** first generation glucose biosensor, **B** second generation of glucose biosensor, **C** third generation of glucose biosensor [6]

2.2 Chronoamperometry

Chronoamperometry (CA) is an electrochemical technique to determine an analyte quantitatively in which a potential step is applied on the working electrode [7]. The resulting current from faradaic process occurring at the electrode is monitored as a function of time. The faradaic current is described in the Cottrell equation (1):

$$i = nFA\sqrt{\frac{D}{\pi t}}c_0 \tag{1}$$

where,

   i = current in A
   n = n the number of transferred electrons
   F = Faraday constant, 96.485 C mol^{-1}
   A = area of the electrode in cm^2
   c_0 = initial concentration of the analyte in mol cm^{-3}
   D = diffusion coefficient in cm^2 s^{-1}
   t = time in s

When an adequate amount of blood is applied on the test strip and the required redox potential is applied on the working electrode, a cascade of redox reaction takes place on the test strip [3]. The resulting current from the electrochemical reaction on the blood glucose test strip is direct proportional to the glucose concentration [3].

2.3 Near Field Communication

Near field communication (NFC) is wireless technology to transmit data and energy over short distances [8]. NFC is a future-oriented and upcoming technology well known in payment and access control. It also provides different application in the sensing and personal health monitoring area. NFC is based on RFID (Radio Frequency Identification) and uses inductive coupling between two devices (Fig. 2), like an air transformer. NFC operates at a frequency of 13.56 MHz and supports data rates of 106, 212 or 424 kbit/s [8].

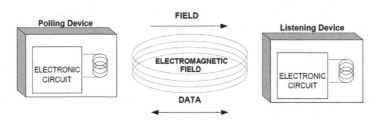

Fig. 2. NFC system [9]

A NFC system consists of an initiator (polling device or reader) and a target (listening device or transponder). Initiators actively generate an RF field that can power a passive target by using energy harvesting. NFC-enabled devices support three modes of operation: card emulation, peer-to-peer, and reader/writer. Peer-to-peer mode enables two active NFC-enabled devices to communicate with each other to exchange data [10]. In card emulation mode, the NFC-enabled device communicates with an external reader like a traditional contactless smart card [10]. Reader/writer mode enables NFC-enabled devices to read data stored on NFC tags [10]. The communication protocol is based on the ISO/IEC 18092 NFC IP-1, JIS X 6319-4 and ISO/IEC 14443 contactless smart card standards [8,10].

3 Results

3.1 NFC-Glucometer

The developed NFC-Glucometer is based on a multi-chip solution, containing NFC-frontend, low power microcontroller and measurement unit to measure blood glucose quantitatively (Fig. 3).

The NFC-frontend is an ISO/IEC 14443 (NFC-A) NFC forum tag type 2 with a dual access EEPROM. The NFC-frontend uses the transmitted energy for energy harvesting to power the electronics of the entire passive sensor tag.

The required redox potential of approximately 185 mV is supplied by a DAC of the low power microcontroller. A transimpedance amplifier (TIA) converts the resulting current to an equivalent voltage. This voltage is measured with an ADC of the low power microcontroller.

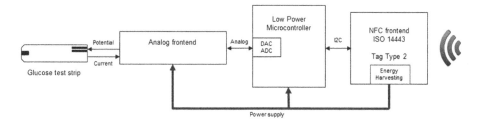

Fig. 3. NFC-Glucometer: Hardware architecture

The current NFC-Glucometer prototype is powered by the NFC interface of a smartphone. A user friendly and intuitive mobile app completes the smart glucose meter. The measured blood glucose concentration is visualized on the display and is stored in a diary automatically.

In contrast to a common glucose meter our NFC glucose sensor system take advantage of the versatile functionality of the smartphone. Therefore, only the blood glucose measurement is performed by the NFC-Glucometer. Data processing tasks, displaying the measured blood glucose concentration and data storage are performed by the NFC-enabled smartphone (Fig. 4).

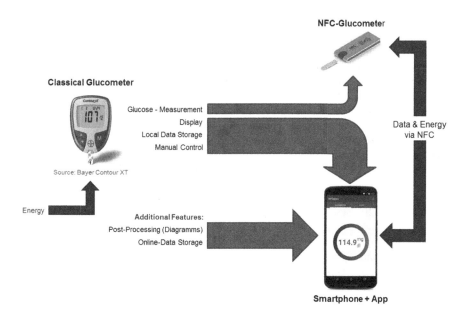

Fig. 4. Comparison of common blood glucose meter and NFC-Glucometer system

4   Discussion

According of the importance of blood glucose self-monitoring, the implementation of NFC in smartphones and the advantage of the versatile functionality of the smartphones present a considerable progress of diabetes home monitoring. The transmitted energy of the NFC field can be used for energy harvesting and allows to supply low power electronics. Therefore, size, weight and costs of the resulting device can be minimized. These smart sensor solutions enables the opportunity to measure diagnostic relevant parameters, e.g. blood glucose level, blood pressure, as well as therapeutic relevant parameters, e.g. medication compliance, time stamps of measurement, food intake, exercises and mood very easily and fast. The measured data can be stored local on the mobile device or on-line. Physician and patient itself have the opportunity to use the additional information to adjust the treatment, e.g. insulin treatment. An automatic diary function can reduce the risk of recording the measured blood glucose concentration incorrectly. Furthermore, a regular control of the blood glucose concentration can avoid acute complications, e.g. hypoglycaemic coma, and can reduce the risk of long-term consequences of diabetes. Finally this leads to an increased quality of life and patient safety of the diabetic persons.

References

1. International Diabetes Federation: IDF Diabetes Atlas, 7th edn. International Diabetes Federation, Brussels (2015)
2. Griebler, R., et al.: Zivilisationskrankheit Diabetes: Ausprägungen - Lösungsansätze - Herausforderungen. Österreichischer Diabetesbericht 2013. Bundesministerium für Gesundheit, Wien (2013)
3. Aggidis, A.: Investigating pipeline and state of the art blood glucose biosensors to formulate next steps. Biosens. Bioelectron. **74**, 243–262 (2015)
4. Heller, A., Feldman, B.: Electrochemical glucose sensors and their applications in diabetes management. In: Schlesinger, M. (ed.) Applications of Electrochemistry in Medicine, pp. 121–177. Springer, New York (2005). https://doi.org/10.1007/978-1-4614-6148-7_5
5. Newman, J.: Home blood glucose biosensors: a commercial perspective. Biosens. Bioelectron. **20**, 2435–2453 (2005)
6. Wang, J.: Electrochemical Glucose Biosensors. Chem. Rev. **108**, 814–825 (2008)
7. Princeton Applied Research, A Review of Techniques for Electrochemical Analysis. http://nanobioelectronics.weebly.com/uploads/3/8/8/6/38862535/review_of_techniques_for_electrochemical_analysis.pdf. Accessed 27 Jan 2017
8. Langer, J., Roland, M.: Anwendungen und Technik von Near Field Communication (NFC). Springer, New York (2011). https://doi.org/10.1007/978-3-642-05497-6
9. NFC Forum: Analog, Technical Specification Version 2.0. NFC Forum (2016)
10. NFC Forum: What It Does. http://nfc-forum.org/what-is-nfc/what-it-does/. Accessed 27 Jan 2017

Data Analysis

A Novel Algorithm to Reduce Machine Learning Efforts in Real-Time Sensor Data Analysis

Majid Janidarmian$^{(\boxtimes)}$, Atena Roshan Fekr, Katarzyna Radecka, and Zeljko Zilic

Electrical and Computer Engineering Department, McGill University, Montréal, QC, Canada
{majid.janidarmian,atena.roshanfekr}@mail.mcgill.ca,
{katarzyna.radecka,zeljko.zilic}@mcgill.ca

Abstract. In the fitness and health fields, wearable sensors generate massive amount of information in big data. The machine learning techniques use the data to assess individuals' health in real time and identify trends that may lead to better diagnoses and treatments. Applying efficient algorithms to learn from data can aid physicians to evaluate the state of human actions and diagnose the illnesses. The process of discerning valuable information from wearable sensors is a non-trivial task and is an on-going research area. Many research areas have focused on machine learning-based approaches to sensor data for better understanding and meeting people's needs. However, there are different challenges such as runtime complexity and the number of functions calls associated with these approaches limit us to reach an acceptable accuracy level. To reduce the computational costs of the feature extraction and classification, a novel algorithm is proposed to analyze the variations in the periodic signals. It reduces the learning efforts by detecting any significant changes in the signal. We used the idea of pheromone trail employed in the ant colony optimization algorithm to keep track of the signal updates. The findings of this paper enable the design of a highly effective real-time predictive model for wearable applications.

Keywords: Wearable sensors · Machine learning · Respiratory disorder
Ant colony optimization

1 Background

The wearable sensors, coupled with the advanced data processing and communication technologies have opened the window to a new era of cost-effective remote healthcare services. Recently, much of research has focused on machine learning approaches to sensor data for delivering more intelligence into different health and fitness applications. They enable the remote monitoring of physical activity, vital signals, the early diagnosis of serious conditions, and the remote control of medical treatments [1]. In real-time data analysis, the runtime complexity of the machine learning models and the number of functions calls are important challenges as the whole recognition procedure should quickly handle the online data processing requirements. Although the techniques presented in this paper can be used for different applications, we focus on building an efficient algorithm to analyze accelerometer sensor mounted on the rib cage while

© ICST Institute for Computer Sciences, Social Informatics and Telecommunications Engineering 2018
P. Perego et al. (Eds.): MobiHealth 2017, LNICST 247, pp. 83–90, 2018.
https://doi.org/10.1007/978-3-319-98551-0_10

capturing breathing patterns. The wearable motion sensor can be used to detect the small movements of the chest wall that occur during expansion and contraction of the lungs. It has been shown that with proper signal processing, this approach can produce results that closely match the measurements of nasal cannula pressure [2]. For example, the designed system in [3] used accelerometer sensors for diagnosis and treatment of patients with disordered breathing. This method shows a great potential to integrate the use of inertial sensors with machine learning techniques to model a broad range of human respiratory patterns including normal, Bradypnea [4], Tachypnea [5], Kussmaul [6], Cheyn–stokes [7], OSA [8], Biot's breathing [9], Sighing [10], and Apneustic [11] for the goal of cloud-based recognition of different respiratory problems. In addition, accelerometer-derived respiration signal has been proven itself particularly effective in providing an affordable platform for yogic breathing practices [12]. A disordered breathing pattern denotes inefficient oxygen inhalation and carbon dioxide expulsion from the body's tissues. The abnormal respiration is indicative of many diseases such as anemia, asthma, sleep apnea, sudden death syndrome, Chronic Heart Failure (CHF) and Chronic Obstructive Pulmonary Disease (COPD) [7]. For more details, the reader is referred to [1]. Figure 1 shows 30-s samples of eight respiration patterns derived from the accelerometer sensor. In this paper, we introduce an innovative technique that helps distinguish different patterns through analysis of dynamical characteristics of sensors data. It is an effective way to speed up the conventional recognition methods by reducing the number of calls of feature extraction and classification functions. It significantly reduces the usage of classification methods that require computationally expensive algorithms. The proposed algorithm is based on recurrence plot concept, which is the visualization of a square recurrence matrix of distance elements within a cut-off limit [13]. We use the higher-dimensional reconstruction by the method of time delays presented in [14]. From delayed coordinates of a signal $x(t)$, a pseudo-state space can be reconstructed as Eq. 1.

$$y(t_i) = \left[x(t_i), x(t_i + \tau), x(t_i + 2\tau), \ldots, x(t_i + (D-1)\tau) \right] \tag{1}$$

Where $y(t_i)$ is D-dimensional time-delayed vector of D points that are delayed or offset in time (τ). As shown in Fig. 2, the lag-reconstructed the acceleration vector will provide space-time information for nine breathing patterns performed by a subject. In this figure, each z-axis accelerometer signal is promoted into 3-dimensional space $(D = 3)$ and therefore plotted against itself twice delayed $(\tau$ and $2\tau)$ on a three-axis plot $(\tau = 0.6$ s). As seen, the shape of the trajectory shows the periodic nature and dynamic of breathing patterns. The embedding dimension (D) and delay (τ) between sequential time points in the 1-dimensional signal has to be chosen with a preceding analysis of the data. In this study, the Mutual Information (MI) method [15] and the False Nearest Neighbors (FNN) [16] are employed to estimate the time delay and the embedding dimension, correspondingly. The most common method for choosing a proper time delay is based on finding the first local minimum of the Mutual Information (MI), defined as Eq. 2.

$$M(\tau) = \int_t p(t, t + \tau) log \frac{p(t, t + \tau)}{p(t)p(t + \tau)} dt \tag{2}$$

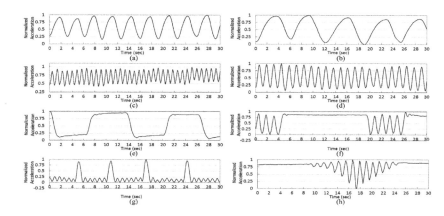

Fig. 1. (a) Normal, (b) Bradypnea, (c) Tachypnea, (d) Kussmaul, (e) Apneustic, (f) Biot's, (g) Sighing and (h) Cheyn-stokes breathing patterns from accelerometer sensor mounted on the subject's rib cage

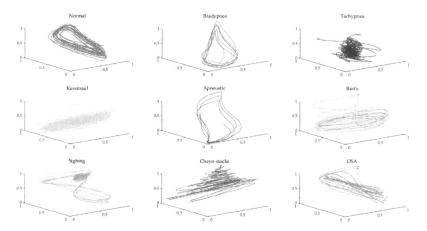

Fig. 2. Delay representation of normalized human breathing signals with embedding dimension 3 and tau 0.6 s.

Where $p(t, \tau)$ is the joint density function, and $p(t)$ and $p(t + \tau)$ are marginal density functions of $x(t)$ and $x(t + \tau)$, respectively [16]. The first minimum of the MI denotes the time delay, where the signal $x(t + \tau)$ adds maximal information to the knowledge obtained from $x(t)$ [15]. The time delay should be selected in a way that the reconstructed vector serves as independent coordinates while keeping the connection with each other. After finding a proper time delay, the embedding dimension can be calculated. In our algorithm, we used the nearest-neighbor methodology to find the embedding dimension. It steadily increases the embedding dimension and checks whether the neighborhood of all points in the phase space change. The algorithm stops where the amount of false nearest neighbors becomes almost unchanging. In another word, the information of the system has been completely maximized and no new information can be gained by trying higher dimension [16].

2 The Proposed Method

Algorithm 1 describes how we used embedding dimension (*dims*) and time delay (*taus*) parameters to optimize machine learning calls during real-time classification problems. According to the employed methods explained above, the time delay and embedding dimension for each label are determined in line 2. When a new sensor sample is ready at time $t > (D - 1)\tau$, a set of points, $\{points(t - (D - 1)\tau), \dots points(t - 2\tau), points(t - \tau), \dots, points(t)\}$ are defined in line 12. We use binary code to represent positive and negative directions for each point from time $t - 1$ to t. For example, if the changes in three points values lie in the $(-, +, +)$ directions, the binary coding for this will be (011) and the resulting decimal number is three (lines 11–17). The obtained decimal number denotes the state number and consequently there is a transition between states once a new sensor sample arrives. We expect to see very similar transitions over time while we are dealing with a periodic signal such as walking or normal breathing. To keep track of the previous recent changes, we use the idea of pheromone trail employed in ant colony optimization algorithm. For example, if the current state is three and the next changes lie in the $(+, -, +)$ directions, binary coding for the new state will be (101) which is five. Therefore, for the transition $3 \rightarrow 5$, a specific amount of pheromone, Δ, will be deposited in line 28. In our experiments, initially there is no pheromone associated to each transition and the pheromone trails in each iteration (every $\frac{1}{f}$ sec) are updated by applying the evaporation technique as follows (line 29):

$$pt_{i,j} \leftarrow (1 - \rho)pt_{i,j}, \forall(i, j) \tag{3}$$

Where $pt_{i,j}$ is the existing pheromone trail between state i and j. ρ is the pheromone evaporation coefficient which satisfies $0 < \rho \leq 1$ and is set to $\frac{1}{pt_{i,j}}$ in our study. The chosen value is high enough for a fair adaptation in the underlying problems. However, we believe that it should be experimentally determined under different scenarios. Thus, we read and write pheromones to track the signal behaviors, and more pheromones on each transition increase the probability of that transition being seen. Each new transition is counted, and accordingly, the number of unseen events (when there exists no pheromone associated with the new transition) is updated. However, we need to control the sensitivity of the system to avoid the transient noisy behavior. If the number of detected unseen events is more than the predetermined sensitivity, there exists a major change in the pattern, and the algorithm asks for running machine learning algorithms (*runClassifier*) in lines 22–27. The variable *freshWindow* (line 9 and line 23) is defined to control the number of calls as we have maximum one call for each new window of data according to the frequency and overlap value. If a new pattern keeps occurring, the algorithm will quickly adapt to new state transitions and stop calling the machine learning procedure until it detects a major change in the periodicity of the new pattern.

Algorithm 1: withSmartCalls

Input: *streamData, windowSize, overlap, freq, cModel,* $\Delta, \rho,$ *sensitivity, trainingData*
(labels, :), maxTau, minDim, maxDim; **output:** *improvement*

1. *newTransitions* ← 0; *smartCalls* ← 0; *preState* ← 1; *freshWindow* ← *false;*
   numberOfSamples ← 0;
2. [*taus, dims*] ← **Find_Taus_Dimensions** (*trainingData* (*labels,* :),
   maxTau, minDim, maxDim);
3. *samplesToWait* = **floor** (*windowSize* × *freq* × (1 − *overlap*));
4. **while** (~stop) { % It continues till sensor data is coming
5.   **while** (~ **ready** (*streamData.newInstance*));
       % Wait till there is a new sample of data (after resampling and filtering)
6.   *numberOfSamples* = *numberOfSamples* + 1;
7.   **if mod** (*numberOfSamples, samplesToWait*) == 0
       % If we have enough data to run the classifier again
8.   *endIndex* = *numberOfSamples;*
9.   *freshWindow* ← *true;*
10.   *conventionalCalls* ← *conventionalCalls* + 1;}
11.   **for** *i* = *1:dim* {
12.   *points* (*i*) ← (*end* − (*i* − 1) × *tau*);
        % The points values are increased by 1. "end" is the index of the last sensor
        instance.
13.   **if** *streamData* (*points* (*i*)) <= (*streamData* (*points* (*i*) - 1)
14.   *bin* (*i*) ← 0;
15.   **else**
16.   *bin* (*i*) ← 1; }}
17.   *nextState* ← **bin2Dec** (*bin*); % Convert binary to decimal
18.   **if** *transPheromones* (*nextState, preState*) == 0 {
19.   *newTransitions* ← **min** (*newTransitions* + 1, 10);
20.   **else**
21.   *newTransitions* ← **max** (*newTransitions* − 1, 0); }
22.   **if** *newTransitions* > 10 − *sensitivity*) && *freshWindow* {
23.   *freshWindow* ← *false;*
24.   *featuresVector* ← **featuresExtraction** (*streamData*
                (*endIndex* − *windowSize* × *freq* + 1: *endIndex*));
25.   *label* ← **runClassifier** (*cModel, featuresVector*);
26.   *tau* ← *taus* (*label*); *dim* ← *dims* (*label*);
27.   *smartCalls* ← *smartCalls* + 1; }
28.   *transPheromones* (*nextState, preState*) ← Δ;
        % Δ is the amount of pheromone deposited for the most recent state transition
29.   *transPheromones* (:, :) ← **max** ((1 − ρ) × *transPheromones* (:, :), 0) ;
30.   *preState* ← *nextState*; }
31. *improvement* ← ((*conventionalCalls* − *smartCalls*) / *conventionalCalls*) × 100
32. **return** *improvement;*

Algorithm 2: Find_Taus_Dimensions

> **Input:** *training Data (labels, :), maxTau, minDim, maxDim*; **output:** *taus, dims*
> 1. **for** *i = labels* {
> 2.   *MI* ← **mutualInformation** (*trainingData (i, :), maxTau*);
> 3.   *valleysLocations* ← **valleysFinder** (*MI*);
> 4.   *taus (i)* ← *valleysLocations* (1) ; % First local minimum of the mutual information
>   (MI)
> 5.   *dims (i)* ← **falseNearestNeighbors** (*trainingData (i, :), minDim, maxDim*); }
> 6. **return** *taus, dims*;

3   Experimental Results

The evaluation was performed on data from 10 healthy volunteers, five males and five females aged 27 to 48 with (Mean $\pm$ SD) 34.80 $\pm$ 6.89. The tests lasted for about 35 min per subject. The ethical approval was received from McGill University Ethics Committee. All participants were informed about the experimental procedures before starting the trial sessions. The subjects were asked to perform nine introduced breathing patterns, each for 1 min in sitting position (torso at about 90° angle to the floor). For simulating apnea in Cheyn-stokes, Biot's and OSA breathing exercises, the subjects paused their breathing for at least 10 s. We asked the participants to prolong their inspiration and expiration during Apneustic maneuver for at least 5 s. Finally, for the Sighing pattern, they performed normal breathing, which is followed by deep periodic of inspiration every 3–7 s. OSA breathing pattern is similar to Biot's breathing pattern; however, it has a different phase shift between chest and abdomen compared to Biot's breathing. The SPR-BTA spirometer [17] is also used in all tests to make sure that the subjects were not over emphasizing the breathing movements. The LIS3DH 3-axis accelerometer with 12-bit resolution is used and secured by a soft and elastic strap which is easy to attach and comfortable to wear. The sensor is mounted on the subject's chest in the middle of sternum region. In our tests, the sensor is sampling with 50 Hz. The proposed algorithm is validated on breathing disorder classification in which we deal with 1D motion signal (z-axis). Figure 3 plots a raw breathing signal for three different patterns. In this example, the time delay $\tau = 2$ s is selected for the phase space reconstruction. Given the time delay, we take the embedding dimension as 4 for the windowed breathing signal. Therefore, we have $2^4 \times 2^4$ states. This figure also shows the amounts of pheromones ($\Delta = 12$) in each transition at nine different moments. The proposed technique can detect any major changes or motion artifacts in the signal. Figure 4 shows the improvement in number of machine learning functions calls in each breathing pattern performed by different subjects. In average, the number of functions calls reduced by in average 52.75%, 47.37%, 42.71%, 48.35%, 19.28%, 10.69%, 20.21%, 9.51%, 20.43% for Normal, Bradypnea, Tachypnea, Kussmaul, Apneustic, Biot's, Sighing, Cheyn-stokes and OSA breathing patterns, respectively. The results indicated an average improvement of more than 31% on all different breathing maneuvers with no reduction in classification accuracy.

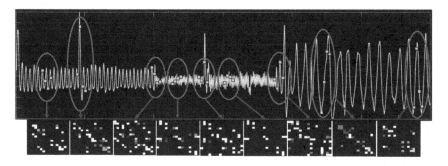

Fig. 3. Raw breathing signal for three different patterns and the pheromone trail updates during the procedure. We show the *transPhermone* updates at nine different moments. As the embedding dimension is four in this test, the size of *transPhermone* is 16×16.

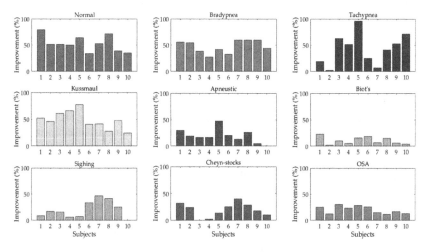

Fig. 4. The improvement in number of machine learning functions calls in each breathing pattern performed by each subject

4 Conclusion

We proposed an innovative approach to speed up the conventional recognition methods by reducing the number of calls of feature extraction and classification functions. It is a very fast algorithm to analyze the dynamical characteristics of sensor data at each sample to detect any significant change in the signal. When working with breathing data derived from the accelerometer sensor, an average improvement of more than 31% was obtained. This finding enables the design of a highly effective real-time predictive model for wearable applications.

References

1. Janidarmian, M., Roshan Fekr, A., Radecka, K., Zilic, Z.: Multi-objective hierarchical classification using wearable sensors in a health application. IEEE Sens. J. **17**(5), 1421–1433 (2017)
2. Bates, A., Ling, M.J., Mann, J., Arvind, D.K.: Respiratory rate and flow waveform estimation from tri-axial accelerometer data. In: International Conference on Body Sensor Networks (BSN), pp. 144–150 (2010)
3. Roshan Fekr, A., Janidarmian, M., Radecka, K., Zilic, Z.: A medical cloud-based platform for respiration rate measurement and hierarchical classification of breath disorders. Sensors **14**, 11204–11224 (2014)
4. Kou, Y.R., Shuei Lin, Y.: Bradypnea. In: Lang, F. (ed.) Encyclopedia of Molecular Mechanisms of Disease, pp. 241–243. Springer, New York (2009). https://doi.org/10.1007/978-3-540-29676-8
5. William, H., Myron, L., Robin, D., Mark, A.: Current Diagnosis and Treatment in Pediatrics, 21st edn, p. 989. McGraw-Hill Professional, New York (2002)
6. Kaufmann, P., Smolle, K.H., Fleck, S., Lueger, A.: Ketoacidotic diabetic metabolic dysregulation: pathophysiology, clinical aspects, diagnosis and therapy. Wien. Klin. Wochenschr. **106**, 119–127 (1994)
7. Brack, T., Thüer, I., Clarenbach, C.F., et al.: Daytime cheyne-stokes respiration in ambulatory patients with severe congestive heart failure is associated with increased mortality. Chest J. **132**(5), 1463–1471 (2007)
8. Hofsoy, D.A., Clauss, J.F., Wolf, B.: Monitoring and therapy of sleep related breathing disorders. In: Proceedings of the 6th International Workshop Wearable Micro and Nano Technologies for Presonalized Health, pp. 41–44, June 2009
9. Farney, R.J., Walker, J.M., Boyle, K.M., Cloward, T.V., Shilling, K.C.: Adaptive servoventilation (ASV) in patients with sleep disordered breathing associated with chronic opioid medications for non-malignant pain. J. Clin. Sleep Med. **4**, 311–319 (2008)
10. Aljadeff, G., Molho, M., Katz, I., Benzaray, S., Yemini, Z., Shiner, R.J.: Pattern of lung volumes in patients with sighing breathing. Thorax J. **48**, 809–811 (1993)
11. Respiratory center, The American Heritage R_Medical Dictionary (2007)
12. Janidarmian, M., Fekr, A.R., Radecka, K., Zilic, Z.: Haptic feedback and human performance in a wearable sensor system. In: 2016 IEEE-EMBS International Conference on Biomedical and Health Informatics (BHI), Las Vegas, NV, pp. 620–624 (2016)
13. Webber, C.L., Zbilut, J.P.: Recurrence quantification analysis of nonlinear dynamical systems. In: Riley, M.A., Van Orden, G.C. (eds.) Tutorials in Contemporary Nonlinear Methods for the Behavioural Sciences, National Science Foundation, Arlington, VA, pp. 26–95 (2005)
14. Takens, F.: Detecting strange attractors in turbulence. In: Rand, D., Young, L.-S. (eds.) Dynamical Systems and Turbulence, Warwick 1980. LNM, vol. 898, pp. 366–381. Springer, Heidelberg (1981). https://doi.org/10.1007/BFb0091924
15. Fraser, A.M., Swinney, H.L.: Independent coordinates for strange attractors from mutual information. Phys. Rev. A **33**, 1134 (1986)
16. Kennel, M.B., Brown, B., Abarbanel, H.D.I.: Determining embedding dimension for phase-space reconstruction using a geometrical construction. Phys. Rev. A **45**, 3403–3411 (1992)
17. Spirometer. http://www.vernier.com/products/sensors/spr-bta/

A Method for Simplified HRQOL Measurement by Smart Devices

Chishu Amenomori, Teruhiro Mizumoto$^{(\boxtimes)}$, Hirohiko Suwa,
Yutaka Arakawa, and Keiichi Yasumoto

Nara Institute of Science and Technology, Ikoma, Nara 630-0192, Japan
teruhiro.mizumoto@ieee.org
http://ubi-lab.naist.jp/

Abstract. Health-related quality of life (HRQOL) is a useful indicator that rates a person's activities in various physical, mental and social domains. Continuously measuring HRQOL can help detect the early signs of declines in these activities and lead to steps to prevent such declines. However, it is difficult to continuously measure HRQOL by conventional methods, since its measurement requires each user to answer burdensome questionnaires. In this paper, we propose a simplified HRQOL measurement method for a continuous HRQOL measurement which can reduce the burden of questionnaires. In our method, sensor data from smart devices and the questionnaire scores of HRQOL are collected and used to construct a machine-learning model that estimates the score for each HRQOL questionnaire item. Our experiment result showed our method's potential and found effective features for some questions.

Keywords: Health related quality of life (HRQOL)
WHOQOL · Biological information · Location information

1 Introduction

Worldwide concern is growing over the issue that increases in hard work and stress are reducing people's abilities to perform various physical, mental, and social activities. People experience declines in their physical and mental functions when they continue to perform stressful activities for a long time, and they might even experience the following: melancholy [1], cognitive decline [2], and lifestyle-related diseases [3]. To prevent a performance decline in physical and mental activities, we must identify its early signs to prevent it. In particular, many Japanese people tend to rank their own personal satisfaction lower than other countries [4]. This attitude could cause a decline of activities.

Quality of Life (QOL) is an indicator that assesses the satisfaction and quality of our daily lives. Health-related quality of life (HRQOL), which is one element of QOL, is a useful indicator that evaluates the quality of life in such domains as physical and psychological health, social relationships, and economic and vocational status. We believe that HRQOL is an appropriate indicator to find the

© ICST Institute for Computer Sciences, Social Informatics and Telecommunications Engineering 2018
P. Perego et al. (Eds.): MobiHealth 2017, LNICST 247, pp. 91–98, 2018.
https://doi.org/10.1007/978-3-319-98551-0_11

signs of decline in physical, mental, and social activities. If we can automatically and continuously measure HRQOL, we may be able to detect the signs of its decline early and prevent that decline. However, since HRQOL measurements require users to answer many questions every day, its daily measurements impose a heavy burden. In existing research, even though many studies are estimating HRQOL using smart devices, they remain unimplemented [5,6].

In this paper, for the continuous measurement of HRQOL, we propose a simplified HRQOL measurement method which reduces the burden for answering a questionnaire and makes estimates from actually measured data. In our proposed method, we collect sensor data from a wrist-type sensor and a smartphone as well as the scores of the questionnaire items of WHOQOL-BREF, which is one HRQOL measurement method. We construct a machine-learning model from the collected data to estimate the score of each HRQOL questionnaire item with the Random Forest algorithm and use the collected sensor data and the questionnaire scores as features and correct answers, respectively.

To evaluate the accuracy of the models, we conducted a leave-one-out cross-validation and collected data from one participant for 15 weeks. In the evaluation, we also analyzed the effect of the features on each questionnaire item. We achieved an F-score of up to 87.9% and found that each questionnaire item has specific effective features. We also found that accuracy can be improved by feature selection. This paper makes two contributions. First, it proposes the first method that easily measures HRQOL by smart devices. Second, we analyzed the effects of the features extracted from the data measured by smart devices for each questionnaire item.

2   HRQOL Overview

2.1   Definition

The World Health Organization (WHO) defines QOL as "an individual's perception of their position in life in the context of the culture and value systems in which they live, and in relation to their goals, expectations, standards and concerns" [7]. Spilker classified QOL under five domains: (1) physical status and functional abilities; (2) psychological status and well-being; (3) social interactions; (4) economic and/or vocational status; and (5) religious and/or spiritual status [8]. Each domain contains associated components: daily behavior and medical institutions for (1), body appearance and self-evaluation for (2), human relationships and social supports for (3), economic resources and transportation for (4), and such activities as faith, worship, and memberships in organizations for (5). QOL can be classified into health-related quality of life (HRQOL) and non-health related quality of life (NHRQOL).

HRQOL represents a QOL that is directly influenced by health, disease, and medical intervention. Existing methods ask questions that correspond to each domain of QOL to measure HRQOL. NHRQOL represents a QOL that is not directly influenced by medical intervention, such as the environment, the economy, and politics [9].

Since our final goal in this study is the early detection of the signs of stress and its prevention, we focus on measuring HRQOL, which is strongly related to physical and mental health states.

2.2 HRQOL Evaluation Method

The answering scale differs depending on the individual, because HRQOL is an indicator of the personal satisfaction felt by individuals. Even for the same person, the scale changes depending on her context, such as her mental state. Various methods for quantitatively evaluating HRQOL have been proposed, including the Sickness Impact Profile (SIP), Short Form-36 (SF-36), WHOQOL [10], WHOQOL-BREF [11], etc. Even though WHOQOL is recognized worldwide, its questionnaires have too many items. So WHOQOL-BREF was developed by a simplified WHOQOL. Since WHOQOL-BREF's policy resembles our method that aims to continuously and simply measure HRQOL, we propose a simpler measurement method based on WHOQOL-BREF.

3 Related Work

Many surveys have addressed the relationship between HRQOL and such individual attributes as activity and ability. Brown et al. [12] revealed the relationship between HRQOL and physical activity and collected physical activity data and answers to four questions related to HRQOL developed by the U.S. Centers for Disease Control and Prevention from 175,850 adults. However, the questionnaire survey was only given once to the participants, unlike our method that measured for long time. Sörensen et al. [13] identified the relationship between HRQOL and the working capacity of middle-aged men in blue-collar occupations. They measured the working capacity index (WAI) and HRQOL scores by Rand-36 from 196, 40–60 year old men. They found a relationship between HRQOL and working capacity and suggested that improving the latter might benefit QOL. However, this study just focused on physical health.

Some studies have used smart devices to measure stress levels. Garcia-Ceja et al. [14] used the accelerometer data of smartphones to detect stress in a working environment and achieved a maximum overall accuracy of 71% for user-specific models. Sano et al. [15] used wrist sensors and smartphones to recognize stress. They collected Three-axis accelerometer data and skin temperatures and conductance from wrist sensors and the usage of smartphones of 18 subjects over five days. They achieved over 75% accuracy of low and high perceived stress recognition using a combination of mobile phone usage and sensor data. However, these indicators for evaluating stress were not constructed based on any standard method for stress measurement.

As shown above, since almost all HRQOL surveys have been carried out using questionnaires, they have not done to continuously conduct long-term QOL measurements. Some studies used smart devices to make their own evaluation standards and focused on a specific activity or mental state. In this study, we achieved a simple and continuous method for HRQOL estimation with high accuracy under globally established evaluation standards.

4   Simplified HRQOL Measurement Method

4.1   Overview

We propose a simplified HRQOL measurement method to estimate HRQOL scores from life log data that are measured and collected by a wristband and a smartphone (Fig. 1). The HRQOL estimation model is constructed by the Random Forest algorithm, which is one machine-learning algorithm. This method reduces the burden of questionnaire responses and enables real-time measurements.

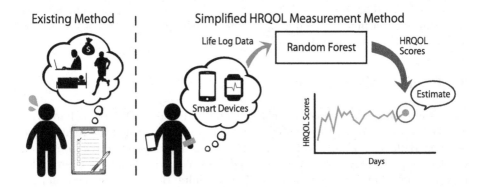

Fig. 1. Method's overview

4.2   Devices and Features

We used an E4 wristband [16] and a smartphone to measure the life log data. An E4 wristband is a smart device that can measure acceleration (ACC), electro-dermal activity (EDA), blood volume pulse (BVP), heart rate (HR), inter-beat interval (IBI), and skin temperature (TEMP). The following are the sampling frequencies of each sensor: BVP, 64 Hz; ACC, 32 Hz; EDA, 4 Hz; HR and TEMP, 1 Hz. IBI irregularly gets data.

First, we identified the sleeping time and the activity (rising) time as status. Next we calculated the following seven features for each of six kinds of sensor data measured by the E4 wristbands: total, average, median, standard deviation, variance, maximum, and minimum. Moreover, we calculated the BVP-LF/HF ratio [17] and the HR-LF/HF ratio every five minutes and used four features: total, maximum, minimum, and the number of times the average was exceeded.

The smartphone collects location data at ten minute intervals and generates six features: total moving distance, moving distance around the home, time staying at home/workplace, sleeping place, and farthest distance from the wake-up position based on location data.

4.3 HRQOL Estimation Model

We constructed an HRQOL estimation model using machine learning with the Random Forest algorithm. The model was implemented using scikit-learn, which is one type of Python library.

In the basic model, the 109 input features are explained in Sect. 4.2. As the training data, we used the WHOQOL-BREF questionnaire results answered by the participant. We applied the leave-one-out cross-validation method and evaluated the estimation accuracy.

5 Preliminary Results

In this section, we evaluate the accuracy of our proposed estimation model through preliminary experiments.

5.1 Purpose

The purpose of our experiment is to evaluate the accuracy of the proposed model and show the feasibility of the simplified measurement method that reduces the burden of questionnaire responses. We investigated the accuracy of HRQOL estimation based on the log data obtained from the smart devices as well as important features that affect the estimation accuracy.

5.2 Overview

Life log data were collected for 15 weeks from a 23-year-old male participant with a wearable device and a smartphone. He answered a WHOQOL-BREF questionnaire every day based on the actual activities of his day. The WHOQOL-BREF question items are shown in Table 1. WHOQOL-BREF has four domains: physical health (PHY), psychological (PSY), social relationships (SOC), and environment (ENV).

During the experiments, we placed no limitations on any aspect of his behavior; just instructed him to answer the questions every day. The dataset was created by removing the daily data if participant forgot to answer the questions or there was data lost from the smart devices. As a result, the dataset contains 100 days of data.

The HRQOL estimation model, which was constructed by Random Forest based on the dataset, was validated by the leave-one-out cross-validation method.

5.3 Results

The 3rd to 5th columns of Table 1 respectively show the Precision, Recall, and F-scores when estimating the scores of each questionnaire item. The 6th column shows the variance of the scores for each item. Each item was answered from among five values: 1: not at all, 2: slightly, 3: moderately, 4: very, 5: extremely.

Table 1. WHOQOL-BREF

Item	Domain	Precision	Recall	F score	Variance	Question item [11]
Q1	-	0.423	0.490	0.440	0.927	How would you rate your quality of life?
Q2	-	0.552	0.571	0.550	0.797	How satisfied are you with your health?
Q3	PHY	0.348	0.357	0.351	0.783	To what extent do you feel that physical pain prevents you from doing what you need to do?
Q4	PHY	0.417	0.520	0.425	0.742	How much do you need any medical treatment to function in your daily life?
Q5	PSY	0.401	0.429	0.412	0.780	How much do you need any medical treatment to function in your daily life?
Q6	PSY	0.419	0.429	0.423	0.750	To what extent do you feel your life to be meaningful?
Q7	PSY	0.290	0.327	0.299	0.671	How well are you able to concentrate?
Q8	ENV	0.437	0.541	0.470	0.603	How safe do you feel in your daily life?
Q9	ENV	0.413	0.480	0.409	0.753	How healthy is your physical environment?
Q10	PHY	0.451	0.480	0.457	0.810	Do you have enough energy for everyday life?
Q11	PSY	0.519	0.602	0.522	0.475	Are you able to accept your bodily appearance?
Q12	ENV	0.787	0.878	0.830	0.129	Have you enough money to meet your needs?
Q13	ENV	0.735	0.857	0.791	0.241	How available to you is the information that you need in your day-to-day life?
Q14	ENV	0.364	0.367	0.363	0.969	To what extent do you have the opportunity for leisure activities?
Q15	PHY	0.417	0.469	0.436	1.070	How well are you able to get around?
Q16	PHY	0.270	0.327	0.283	0.851	How satisfied are you with your sleep?
Q17	PHY	0.450	0.520	0.479	0.632	How satisfied are you with your ability to perform your daily living activities?
Q18	PHY	0.331	0.449	0.315	0.789	How satisfied are you with your capacity for work?
Q19	PSY	0.417	0.510	0.412	0.644	How satisfied are you with yourself?
Q20	SOC	0.464	0.469	0.419	0.606	How satisfied are you with your personal relationships?
Q21	SOC	0.843	0.918	0.879	0.081	How satisfied are you with your sex life?
Q22	SOC	0.609	0.724	0.629	0.267	How satisfied are you with the support you get from your friends?
Q23	ENV	0.735	0.857	0.791	0.173	How satisfied are you with the conditions of your living place?
Q24	ENV	0.806	0.898	0.850	0.093	How satisfied are you with your access to health services?
Q25	ENV	0.752	0.867	0.806	0.131	How satisfied are you with your transport?
Q26	PSY	0.560	0.561	0.487	0.844	How often do you have negative feelings such as blue mood, despair, anxiety, depression?

The estimation accuracy of such question items in the SOC and ENV domains as Q12, Q13, Q21, Q22, Q23, Q24, and Q25 exceeds the question items of the PHY and PSY domains. One possible reason is that the answers for the SOC and ENV items do not change very frequently. In fact, their variance is smaller than the other items. In our data, changes in those items appeared when the participant went on a business trip. Therefore, for SOC/ENV, it will be effective to sent questionnaire prompts only when triggers for the changes appeared, e.g., business trips.

On the other hand, since the estimation accuracy is low in the PHY and PSY domains, perhaps some unrelated features should have been used to train the model. So we focused on two items (Q3 and Q5) and re-estimated them using some selected features. For feature selection, we added features one by one in the order of their importance with the Gini coefficient method and repeated it until the estimation accuracy became maximum.

Q3 is in the PHY domain. Q3's accuracy improved from 0.351 to 0.502 as a result of selecting seven features. We selected these five features in the activity time: EDA and HR medians, EDA and HR averages, HR minimum, and two sleep time features: average and maximum TEMP.

Q5 is in the PSY domain. Q5's accuracy improved from 0.412 to 0.547 as a result of selecting ten features. Four of the selected features were based on location data: farthest distance from his wake-up position, total moving distance and staying time at home/workplace; three activity time features: total of composite acceleration, HR median, and BVP variance; three features in the sleep time: maximum of BVP-LF/HF ratio, standard deviation of TEMP, and BVP total.

We found that the features that improved the estimation accuracy were different among the question items. Thus, we must select suitable features for each question item. Extracting suitable features for all 26 items and estimating their accuracy is future work.

6   Conclusion

In this paper, we proposed a simplified HRQOL measurement method that reduces the burden of answering questionnaires to achieve continuous HRQOL measurements. The proposed method utilizes sensor data from smart devices and the questionnaire scores of HRQOL and constructs a machine-learning model to estimate the score for each questionnaire item by the Random Forest algorithm.

In the experiment, we estimated the questionnaire response values from life log data, obtained estimation accuracy that was higher in the social relations and the environmental domain, and achieved an F-score of up to 87.9%. We also improved the estimation accuracy by feature selection for each question item.

Future work will improve the accuracy by feature selection for each questionnaire item. Moreover, based on the user's situation, we will investigate how much the user burden can be reduced by changing the frequency of the questionnaires. We will also apply the proposed method to larger datasets obtained from many diverse participants.

Acknowledgment. This work is partly supported by JSPS KAKENHI Grant Number 16H06980, Grants-in-Aid for Humanophilic Innovation Project, and Health and Labor Sciences Research Grants (201621010A).

References

1. Larun, L., Nordheim, L.V., Ekeland, E., Hagen, K.B., Heian, F.: Exercise in prevention and treatment of anxiety and depression among children and young people. The Cochrane Library (2006)
2. Biddle, S.: Physical activity and mental health: evidence is growing. World Psychiatry **15**(2), 176–177 (2016)

3. Babazono, A., Kame, C., Ishihara, R., Yamamoto, E., Hillman, A.L.: Patient-motivated prevention of lifestyle-related disease in Japan: a randomized, controlled clinical trial. Dis. Manage. Health Outcomes **15**(2), 119–126 (2007)
4. Cabinet Office, Government of Japan: International Survey of Youth Attitude (2013). http://www8.cao.go.jp/youth/english/survey/2013/pdf_index.html
5. van Uem, J.M.T.: A viewpoint on wearable technology-enabled measurement of wellbeing and health-related quality of life in parkinson's disease. J. Parkinson's Dis. **6**(2), 279–287 (2016)
6. Gonçalves, J., Faria, B.M., Reis, L.P., Carvalho, V., Rocha, Á.: Data mining and electronic devices applied to quality of life related to health data. In: 10th Iberian Conference on Information Systems and Technologies (CISTI) 2015, pp. 1–4. IEEE (2015)
7. The WHOQOL Group. The development of the world health organization quality of life assessment instrument (the WHOQOL). In: Orley, J., Kuyken, W. (eds.) Quality of Life Assessment: International Perspectives. Springer, Heidelberg (1994). https://doi.org/10.1007/978-3-642-79123-9_4
8. Spilker, B.: Quality of Life and Pharmacoeconomics in Clinical Trials, pp. 1–10. Lippincott Williams & Wilkins, New York (1996). Chapter Introduction
9. Kirita, T., Omura, K. (eds.): Oral Cancer. Diagnosis and Therapy, vol. 3. Springer, Tokyo (2015). https://doi.org/10.1007/978-4-431-54938-3
10. THE Whoqol GROUP: The world health organization quality of life assessment (WHOQOL): development and general psychometric properties. Soc. Sci. Med. **46**(12), 1569–1585 (1998)
11. World Health Organization et al. WHOQOL-BREF: Introduction, Administration, Scoring and Generic Version of the Assessment: Field Trial Version, December 1996 (1996)
12. Brown, D.W., et al.: Associations between recommended levels of physical activity and health-related quality of life findings from the 2001 behavioral risk factor surveillance system (BRFSS) survey. Prev. Med. **37**(5), 520–528 (2003)
13. Sörensen, L.E., Pekkonen, M.M., Männikkö, K.H., Louhevaara, V.A., Smolander, J., Alén, M.J.: Associations between work ability, health-related quality of life, physical activity and fitness among middle-aged men. Appl. Ergon. **39**(6), 786–791 (2008)
14. Garcia-Ceja, E., Osmani, V., Mayora, O.: Automatic stress detection in working environments from smartphones' accelerometer data: a first step. IEEE J. Biomed. Health Inf. **20**(4), 1053–1060 (2016)
15. Sano, A., Picard, R.W.: Stress recognition using wearable sensors and mobile phones. In: 2013 Humaine Association Conference on Affective Computing and Intelligent Interaction (ACII), pp. 671–676. IEEE (2013)
16. Real-time physiological signals - e4 eda/gsr sensor. https://www.empatica.com/e4-wristband
17. Malik, M.: Heart rate variability. Ann. Noninvasive Electrocardiol. **1**(2), 151–181 (1996)

An Open, Labeled Dataset for Analysis and Assessment of Human Motion

Andre Ebert$^{(\boxtimes)}$, Chadly Marouane, Christian Ungnadner, and Adrian Klein

Mobile and Distributed Systems Group, Institute for Computer Science,
Ludwig-Maximilians-University, Oettingenstrasse 67, 80538 Munich, Germany
andre.ebert@ifi.lmu.de

Abstract. Analysis of human activity, e.g., by tracking and analyzing motion information or vital signs became lots of attention in medical as well as athletic appliances during the last years. Nonetheless, comprehensive and labeled datasets containing human motion information are only sparsely accessible to the public. Especially qualitatively labeled datasets are rare, although they are of great value for the development of concepts concerning qualitative motion assessment, e.g., to avoid injuries during athletic workouts or to optimize a training's success.

Therefore, we provide an open and qualitative as well as quantitative labeled dataset containing acceleration and rotation data of 8 different body weight exercises, conducted by 26 study participants. It encompasses more than 11,000 exercise repetitions of which we extracted 8,576 into individual segments. We believe, that due to its structure and labeling our work is suitable to serve for development, benchmarking, and validation of new concepts for human activity recognition and qualitative motion assessment (Publication notes: The dataset will be published at http://github.com/andrebert/body-weight-exercises together with this paper's presentation on the MobiHealth conference 2017, taking place in Vienna, 14–16 November.).

Keywords: Machine learning · Activity recognition
Motion assessment

1   Introduction

Automated monitoring and analysis of human motion by using motion sensors gained great attention during the last years. Reasons for that are the ubiquitous availability of powerful, portable, and small computing devices, e.g., smartphones, as well as the distribution of robust and cheap sensor platforms capable of motion tracking. This enables the analysis of complex and also spatially distributed human motion without being bound to a fixed area or tracking system, e.g., in contrast to the usage of cameras for visual analysis approaches. An important field for automated monitoring and motion assessment are medical appliances as well as the athletic context and physical exercises. Apps like Freeletics[1] provide detailed instructions for challenging workouts and exercises

---

[1] http://www.freeletics.com.

© ICST Institute for Computer Sciences, Social Informatics and Telecommunications Engineering 2018
P. Perego et al. (Eds.): MobiHealth 2017, LNICST 247, pp. 99–106, 2018.
https://doi.org/10.1007/978-3-319-98551-0_12

as well as features for exercise tracking, such as counting of repetitions or distances. But these challenging exercises are often conducted by amateur athletes without being monitored or advised by professional instructors. Unfortunatly, incorrect execution of physical exercises may not only lead to less successful training results, it can also lead to serious harm and injuries [1, 4, 6]. We believe, that automated monitoring, analysis and assessment of human motion will enable the development of proactive feedback systems, which are capable of reducing such injuries and optimize training results. Moreover, the assessment of human motion is also of use within other areas, e.g., in a medical context to monitor ambulant patients, for gait analysis, for workflow optimization, and others.

To address this challenge, we developed a distributed sensor system called SensX [3]. Subsequently, we designed a study for our concept's evaluation and recorded more than 11,000 individual repetitions of 8 different body weight exercises. In our context, body weight exercises are defined as physical exercises which are conducted only with an athlete's own body weight and without the use of artificial training equipment, e.g., Sit-ups or Squats [5]. Moreover, we developed different approaches for activity recognition and generic qualitative assessment of human motion in [2].

Besides our own concepts concerning human motion analysis, there may be lots of new approaches and ideas of other researchers which can be tested and evaluated by using our dataset as a basis. Therefore, we publish all data recorded during our study, which is publicly available at GitHub[2]. Besides the raw data of all sensors, we also extracted single exercises into individual segments of adaptive length and labeled them regarding their class of quality as well as regarding their type of exercise. This paper provides an overview concerning the used sensor system, the data structure, and the describing meta data and is meant to function as a manual for the provided dataset.

2   Dataset

All in all, we recorded 11,087 individual repetitions of 8 different body weight exercises, of which we were able to extract 8,576 repetitions into individual segments of adaptive length. Subsequently, all details concerning the study design, the sensor system, the recording process itself, and the data structure are presented.

2.1   Study Design

In context of our study we recorded data of 26 athletes by using the SensX sensor system, which is presented in [3]. In prior to the collection of data we designed a workout plan encompassing 8 body weight exercises, scheduled to stress an athlete's body consistently. An overview across these exercises is depicted in Fig. 1. Namely these were (1) Crunches (cr), (2) Lunges (lu), (3) Jumping Jack

---

[2] https://github.com/andrebert/body-weight-exercises

(ha), (4) Bicycle Crunch (bi), (5) Squat (kn), (6) Mountain Climber (mo), (7) Russian Twist (ru), and (8) Push-ups (li). The exercises are numbered in order of their execution during the study – their abbreviations are used for storing them in our file system and are originating from the German exercise terms. All athletes had to complete 3 sets containing 20 repetitions for each exercise. In between all sets, a mandatory break of 30 seconds was scheduled. All exercises were introduced in prior to their first execution with a professional instruction video. All exercises were taped on video during their execution. Additionally, the participants were urged to fill out a questionnaire containing several questions concerning their age, their profession and their habits regarding the conduction of physical exercises. Moreover, we captured the amount of repetitions which each individual athlete was able to execute and encouraged all participants to make a subjective rating concerning the overall quality of their exercise sets within a range of 1 to 5. Thereby, 1 symbolized *very good*, 2 *good*, 3 *medium*, 4 *bad*, and 5 *very bad* in terms of quality.

2.2   Study Participants

Within the scope of this study we recorded the acceleration and rotation data of 6 female and 18 male participants. Their average age was 27.15 years while the average weight of all participants was 67.04 kg. The oldest participant was 53 years old, while the youngest was 20. All participants were coerced to provide information concerning the individual frequency with which they are doing sports as well as a self-assessment regarding their level of fitness. The rating scale for both, frequency and level of fitness, ranged from 1 to 5. Corresponding to the rating's range in Sect. 2.1, 1 symbolizes *never* or *very low* while 5 symbolizes *every day* or *very high*.

2.3   Sensor System

The sensor system used for tracking the athletes consists of 4 external sensor platforms which are attached to the athlete's wrists and ankles and an additional central computation unit (CCU), e.g., a smartphone, which is attached to the participant's chest. For fastening the CCU, a common GoPro harness (see Fig. 1) was used. All devices are tracking acceleration as well as rotation information in X-, Y-, and Z-dimension, respectively. This makes an overall count of 30 individual signals which are available to describe an athlete's movements. The CCU is used to (1) gather the signals of all connected external sensor units and (2) to store them with a synchronized timestamp on its internal storage together with its own sensor data. Within the studies conduction, we used two different CCU setups: the first two athletes were tracked within a preliminary test cycle by using a LG Nexus 5x running Android 5.0 Lollipop, while the main study was conducted with a HTC One (M7) running Android 6.0.1 Marshmallow. Reason for that was, that the second setup was capable to record significantly more balanced sampling rates for the external sensors. Thereby, the LG setup operated with an average sampling rate of 200 Hz for the CCU and an inconsistent rate

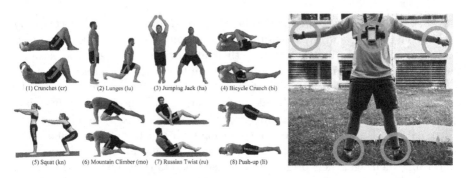

Fig. 1. All exercises which were included in our study plus their abbreviations (left) and the SensX sensor system carried by a study participant (right).

of 20 Hz–40 Hz for external devices, while the HTC setup achieved 100 Hz for the CCU and a relatively consistent rate of 40 Hz for external sensors. The main reason for that may be the manufacturer dependent implementation of Bluetooth Low Energy (BLE), which is used to connect the external sensors with the CCU. Our experiments showed, that different implementations offer different sampling rates when connecting multiple BLE devices at the same time.

2.4   Labeling

In general, the data set is labeled for two different purposes: (1) activity recognition and (2) qualitative motion assessment. All segmented repetitions are labeled implicitly by the folder structure used for storing their data files (see Sect. 2.6), which indicates the underlying type of activity (e.g., Sit-up, Push-up, Squat, etc.). A second, active labeling provides information concerning the actual quality of a conducted exercise and can be found within the INFO file, which is placed in the root folder of each participant's exercise sets. The qualitative labeling was implemented for the exercises 1–6 (see Fig. 1) and in the frame of the qualitative assessment described in [2], while the exercises 7 and 8 are not labeled qualitatively. The second last row tagged with the Index key maps the quality ratings which are stored within the last row to specific exercise repetitions; the key used to identify the last row containing the ratings is named Rating. E.g., the rating related to the first Push-up within a set of Push-ups is the first value of the last row, while the rating of the second Push-up corresponds to the last row's second value (see also Sect. 2.6).

The qualitative labeling was undertaken by analyzing each single exercise repetition on basis of the recorded video material. To maximize the qualitative rating's accuracy, this step was done together with sports professionals especially skilled for body weight workouts and endurance training. At the beginning of the rating process, each individual exercise repetition is labeled with an initial start value of $p_s = 1$, which represents the highest quality (*very good*). Subsequently, a penalty value p_a is added to p_s for each anomaly a (mistakes, malpositions, etc.)

made by the participant during an exercise's execution. If the characteristics of a specific anomaly are significant, p_a has a value of 1, for an anomaly of medium significance we add 0.5, and in case of a minor mistake it is 0.25. The amount of detected p_a was within a range of 7–13 incidents i, depending on the specific exercise. As soon as the score is reaching a value of 5, we stop adding any more penalty points, which means the rating scale's spectrum ranges from 1 till 5 (very good, good, medium, bad, very bad). In case that the final score is not an integer value, it became rounded commercially. Thus, the process of creating a qualitative label L for an individual exercise repetition r without rounding it may be defined as

$$L_r = p_s + \sum_{n=0}^{i} p_a, \text{ if } L_r > 5 : L_r = 5$$

Due to the sheer addition of penalty points without respecting specific causes we achieve a generic quality notation: L_r tells us about the quality of a specific exercise repetition r in terms of good or bad, though it does not contain any information concerning the cause for a specific rating.

2.5 Descriptive Statistics

All in all we provide 8,576 adaptively segmented and qualitatively labeled exercise repetitions. Table 1 gives a descriptive overview across these quantities. Additionally, all raw data without qualitative labeling and segmentation can be found within each exercise set's root folder. It is significant, that a great number of the individually segmented repetitions were rated at least medium or even better. Reasons for that may be the relatively low average age of our participants as well as the fact that most of them do sports regularly and thus were not completely unskilled. Concerning Bicycle Crunches and Russian Twists, the dataset contains roughly half of the amount of repetitions (in contrast to all other exercises) – the reason for that is, that we decided to count a left-sided and the following right-sided execution together as one instance.

Table 1. Qualitative rating and quantitative amounts of all segmented exercise repetitions.

	cr	lu	ha	bi	kn	mo	ru	li
Overall quantity	1,315	1,345	1,394	692	1,379	1,227	660	564
Label *very good* (1)	554	592	235	150	458	439	-	-
Label *good* (2)	367	421	749	204	660	409	-	-
Label *medium* (3)	293	180	347	257	137	244	-	-
Label *bad* (4)	101	131	58	81	112	123	-	-
Label *very bad* (5)	-	21	5	-	12	12	-	-

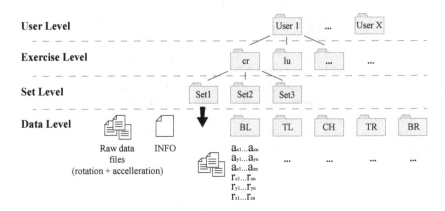

Fig. 2. The dataset's folder structure and the 4 different organization levels.

2.6   Folder and Data Structure

In the following we provide insights into the file and data storage system. The sensor data itself was stored by using the metrics which were returned by the specific sensor platforms. This means that data is stored in m/s^2 (minus earth gravitation) and rad/s for the CCU (Android API standard), while the external Metawear sensors return their measurements in gravitational force (g) and deg/s (for acceleration and rotation). All in all, our dataset is organized in four levels namely the (1) user level, (2) the exercise level, (3) the set level and (4) the data level (see Fig. 2). The first level encompasses the folders of all 26 athletes which participated on our study. These are named by an individual code consisting of two abbreviating characters. Within the second level the exercise folders named by their German abbreviation can be found: (1) Crunches (cr), (2) Lunges (lu), (3) Jumping Jack (ha), (4) Bicycle Crunch (bi), (5) Squat (kn), (6) Mountain Climber (mo), (7) Russian Twist (ru), and (8) Push-up (li). Within the following third level the data is structured by the three individual workout sets, which each study participant had to conduct for each exercise (e.g., *Set1, Set2*, etc.). Each of these set folders encompass an instance of the fourth level, namely the raw data files of each exercise set, the segmented repetitions, and an INFO file with some meta information. The raw data files are named by the first two chars of the recording sensor platform's MAC address plus an indicator for acceleration (*acc*) or rotation (*rot*). The raw data files of the CCU are labeled with *CH* (chest) plus the rotation or acceleration tag. Furthermore, each raw data file is mapped to a specific body extremity:

- C6_acc, C6_rot: raw motion data of the left arm (*top-left*, abbr. TL)
- EE_acc, EE_rot: raw motion data of the left leg (*bottom-left*, abbr. BL)
- D1_acc, D1_rot: raw motion data of the right arm (*top-right*, abbr. TR)
- CF_acc, CF_rot: raw motion data of the right leg (*top-right*, abbr. BR)
- CH_acc, CH_rot: raw motion data of the chest (abbr. CH)

Next to the INFO file and the raw data files the data level contains 5 containers which are inhabiting the segmented repetitions of each set. They are named by the abbreviations introduced above and indicate from which sensor position the encompassed data originates (TL, BL, etc.). The files inside a specific sensor folder are named by the *acc*-tag or *rot*-tag plus the dimension of its content (x, y, or z) and an index number of the specific repetition, e.g., acc-x-1. This means that one single repetition of an exercise consists of 30 different data sources, e.g., the 10th repetition of a set is described by the following files, mapped to the five individually tracked parts of a participants bodies:

- right arm: TR/acc-x-10, TR/acc-y-10, TR/acc-z-10, TR/rot-x-10, TR/rot-y-10, TR/rot-z-10
- right leg: BR/acc-x-10, BR/acc-y-10, BR/acc-z-10, BR/rot-x-10, BR/rot-y-10, BR/rot-z-10
- chest: CH/acc-x-10, CH/acc-y-10, CH/acc-z-10, CH/rot-x-10, CH/rot-y-10, CH/rot-z-10
- left arm: TL/acc-x-10, TL/acc-y-10, TL/acc-z-10, TL/rot-x-10, TL/rot-y-10, TL/rot-z-10
- left leg: BL/acc-x-10, BL/acc-y-10, BL/acc-z-10, BL/rot-x-10, BL/rot-y-10, BL/rot-z-10

Data Structure of Segmented Exercise Repetitions. The data within the files of segmented repetitions, e.g., acc-x-10, is organized as follows: the first row contains a vector of acceleration or rotation information; the second row contains a corresponding timestamp for each value counting the milliseconds of a repetition from start to end (for metrics see Sect. 2.6).

Raw Data Structure. As stated in Sect. 2.6, each exercise set is described by ten files of raw data. Within these files an individual number of data rows with 4 columns can be found. The first column contains its timestamp in UNIX epoch milliseconds, the following three columns contain acceleration or rotation information in X-, Y-, and Z-direction.

Data Format Within the INFO File. The INFO file contains additional meta information concerning individual exercise sets. Besides the average sampling rate of each single sensor platform it contains the following information:

- the amount of *Raw* data repetitions
- the number of segmented *Repetitions*
- the *Length* of a set in seconds
- the *Index* for the *Rating* for each single segmented exercise.

All keys are separated with an ":" from their content. Ratings and their indices are separated with an "-" in between the individual values.

2.7   Metadata

In order to enable an easy distribution and findability of our dataset, we defined meta information corresponding to a recommendation for dataset markups published by Google[3].

2.8   Adaptive Segmentation

All adaptively segmented exercise repetitions were created by using the segmentation approach described in [2].

3   Conclusion

Within this paper, we present an open dataset encompassing 11,087 repetitions of 8 different body weight exercises in raw data format. Moreover, 8,576 of these exercises were extracted into segments of adaptive length and labeled qualitatively as well as quantitatively. Subsequently they were stored in a suitable data structure for further analysis. Some promising results concerning human activity recognition and qualitative assessment of human motion on basis of this dataset were published in [2] and encourage further analysis. Multiple new analysis methods, e.g., neural networks, were not used for dataset examination, yet. Moreover, a detailed anomaly detection and description of specific error classes as well as advances for decision certainty concerning activity recognition and qualitative assessment are still missing. By publishing this dataset, we hope to promote further advances within human motion analysis, e.g., to optimize motion sequences and to detect malpositions or injuries within medical as well as athletic appliances.

References

1. Brady, T.A., Cahill, B.R., Bodnar, L.M.: Weight training-related injuries in the high school athlete. Am. J. Sports Med. **10**(1), 1–5 (1982)
2. Ebert, A., Beck, M.T., Mattausch, A., Belzner, L., Popien, C.L.: Qualitative assessment of recurrent human motion. In: European Signal Processing Conference (EUSIPCO), 2017 25th. IEEE (2017)
3. Ebert, A., Kiermeier, M., Marouane, C., Linnhoff-Popien, C.: Sensx: About sensing and assessment of complex human motion. In: 14th IEEE International Conference on Networking, Sensing and Control (ICNSC) 2017. IEEE (2017)
4. Jones, B.H., Bovee, M.W., Harris, J.M., Cowan, D.N.: Intrinsic risk factors for exercise-related injuries among male and female army trainees. Am. J. Sports Med. **21**(5), 705–710 (1993)
5. Lauren, M., Joshua, C.: Fit ohne Geräte: Trainieren mit dem eigenen Körpergewicht. Riva (2011)
6. Leaf, J.R., Keating, J.L., Kolt, G.S.: Injury in the australian sport of calisthenics: a prospective study. Aust. J. Physiotherapy **49**(2), 123–130 (2003)

---

[3] https://developers.google.com/search/docs/data-types/datasets.

Watchful-Eye: A 3D Skeleton-Based System for Fall Detection of Physically-Disabled Cane Users

Mona Saleh Alzahrani[1,2(✉)], Salma Kammoun Jarraya[2],
Manar Salamah Ali[2], and Hanêne Ben-Abdallah[2]

[1] College of Information and Computer Science,
Al Jouf University, Sakaka, Saudi Arabia
mszahrani@ju.edu.sa
[2] Faculty of Computing and Information Technology,
King Abdulaziz University, Jeddah, Saudi Arabia
{smohamadl,mali,hbenabdallah}@kau.edu.sa

Abstract. In this paper, we present *Watchful-Eye*, a 3D skeleton-based system to monitor a physically disabled person using a cane as a mobility aid. Watchful-Eye detects fall occurrences using skeleton tracking with a Microsoft Kinect camera. Compared to existing systems, it has the merit of detecting various types of fall under multiple scenarios and postures, while using a small set of features extracted from Kinect captured video streams. To achieve this merit, we followed the typical machine learning process: First, we collected a rich fall detection dataset. Second, we experimentally determined the most relevant features that best-distinguish fall from non-fall frames, and the best performing classifier. As we report in this paper, the offline evaluation results show that Watchful-Eye reached an accuracy between 87.2% and 94.5% with 5.5% to 12.8% error rate depending on the used classifier. Furthermore, the online evaluation shows that it can detect falls with an accuracy between 89.47% and 100%.

Keywords: Physically disabled · Computer vision · Machine learning
Fall detection · Skeleton tracking · Features selection · Kinect

1 Introduction

Computer vision research is actively contributing in building smart applications by providing for image/video content "understanding". Among the various application domains, this paper is interested in the contribution of computer vision to the development of applications to provide care for physically disabled people. More specifically, this paper proposes a computer vision based system to detect falls of physically disable people using canes as a means of assistance. Such a system is vital given the fall consequences on these people and the fall occurrence rates.

© ICST Institute for Computer Sciences, Social Informatics and Telecommunications Engineering 2018
P. Perego et al. (Eds.): MobiHealth 2017, LNICST 247, pp. 107–116, 2018.
https://doi.org/10.1007/978-3-319-98551-0_13

Indeed, according to statistics from the World Health Organization (WHO)[1] in 2016, one out of three 65-year-old people falls each year and, as age increases to 80, the fall occurs each year. Furthermore, falls constitute the second leading cause of accidental or injury deaths after injuries of road traffic. These statistics call for efficient and practical/comfortable means to monitor physically disabled people in order to detect falls and react urgently.

In fact, several researches have proposed systems and/or methods for fall detection using computer vision techniques [1–4]. Our investigation of the recent systems showed that the most of them use the Microsoft Kinect camera, and some of them [1, 5, 6] also use smart sensors mounted on the person in an effort to increase the fall detection rate. In addition, these systems do not cover all types nor scenarios of fall, and they may depend on the distance of the person from the camera. Furthermore, our investigation highlighted the need for a benchmark dataset to assist in the development of new fall detection methods and the comparison of existing ones. As such, this paper has a two-fold objective. First, it proposes a dataset that contains data covering a large spectrum of fall types and scenarios. Secondly, it proposes a new system called Watchful-Eye for fall detection of physically disable people using canes. Compared to existing systems, it has the merit of detecting various types of fall under multiple scenarios and postures, while using a small set of features extracted from Kinect captured video streams. To achieve this merit, we followed the typical machine learning process: First, we collected a rich fall detection dataset. Second, we experimentally determined seven most relevant features that best-distinguish fall from non-fall frames, and RandomForest as the best performing classifier. As we report in this paper, the offline evaluation results show that Watchful-Eye reached an accuracy between 87.2% and 94.5% with 5.5% to 12.8% error rate, depending on the used classifier. Furthermore, the online evaluation shows that it can detect falls with an accuracy between 89.47% and 100%.

The remainder of this paper is organized as follows: Sect. 2 overviews the Kinect-based literature studies. Section 3 presents the proposed Watchful-Eye system and details its building steps—dataset collection, features' extraction and selection, and system setting and development. Section 4 discusses the experimental evaluation results, and Sect. 5 summarizes the presented work and outlines its extensions.

2   Kinect-Based Fall Detection

Several recent studies [1–3], classified under vision-based approaches, use Kinect for developing Fall Detection (FD) systems. In 2013, Lee and Lee [2] present a system to detect falls and notify health care services. They use the Kinect depth camera as the input sensor and Microsoft Kinect SDK to collect skeleton data. Among the collected skeleton data, they chose to track only the hip joins which they process with two functions that check the position and velocity of the center of mass. They achieve a 90% accuracy FD rate. Nonetheless, they have a list of false positive postures such as

---

[1] http://www.who.int/mediacentre/factsheets/fs344/en/.

sitting on the floor with both legs folded behind, kneeling on the floor, squatting, bending down to wear shoes or tie shoelaces. In addition, they cannot detect when the user falls off a chair, which is relatively a very common scenario.

In 2014, in an effort to reduce the number of false alarms by collecting more information, Kwolek and Kepski [1] add to the Kinect a wearable smart device containing accelerometer and gyroscope sensors; this smart device is worn near the pelvis region of the monitored person. They use a triaxial accelerometer to indicate both a potential fall and whether the person is in motion. Their proposed system operates as follows: If the measured acceleration is higher than an assumed threshold value, the system extracts the person on the basis of the depth reference maps, calculates some depth features, and executes the SVM-based classifier to authenticate the fall alarm. This system acquires depth images using the OpenNI (Open Natural Interaction) library. It achieves 98.33% accuracy when using accelerometer and depth data, and 90% accuracy and 80% specificity when using depth only which is the worst result compared to other techniques in their research.

In 2015, Stone and Skubic [3] develop a two-stage FD system for detecting falls in the homes of older adults using the Microsoft Kinect. The first stage characterizes the vertical state of a 3D object for an individual frame, it then segments on ground events from the vertical state time series. The second stage utilizes a set of decision trees and a set of features extracted from an on-ground event to generate a confidence that a fall preceded it. As a preprocessing step, this system segments 3D foreground objects from each depth frame using dynamic background subtraction. When the falls are near the sensor and not significantly occluded, this system can achieve 98%, 70%, and 71% accurate detection of standing, sitting, and lying falls, respectively; however, when the falls are far to the sensor and significantly occluded, the system can achieve 79%, 58%, and 5% accurate detection of standing, sitting, and lying falls, respectively.

Overall, existing fall detection systems using Kinect [1–3] differ in their performance: Some do not cover many fall types and/or scenarios; others have high false alarm rates when operating on particular postures; yet others have low accuracy when the faller is far from the Kinect. In addition, those trying to improve the fall detection rate use wearable sensors, which may hinder daily activities and/or make the person uncomfortable. Furthermore, the proposed systems' performance evidently depends on the features used. However, the feature differences (in nature and number) and the lack of a benchmark dataset hinders a systematic evaluation of the performance of existing systems.

As such, the aim of this paper is to propose a fall detection method that: suits physically disabled people using canes, relies solely on Kinect, and can determine various types of falls in different postures with a high accuracy and a low false alarm. Such a method highly depends on the selection of the appropriate features. Towards this end, this paper's second contribution is the elaboration of a dataset that can be used as a benchmark to both identify the features and compare existing/future methods.

3 Overview of the Skeleton-Based Fall Detection

The development of Watchful-Eye proposes three main contributions to the domain of fall detection of physically disabled people:

1. Proposition of a new fall dataset that covers all fall types and scenarios. The dataset is available in all the image-based streams provided by the Kinect camera.
2. Identification of the features best describing fall scenarios of cane users; besides accounting for all fall types and scenarios, the identified features overcome the challenges incurred by the distance between the Kinect and the faller.
3. Proposition of new skeleton-based method that: detects the different fall types and scenarios, imposes minimum restrictions on the people with physical disabilities (i.e. pose or calibration), overcomes the natural scene conditions (e.g., lighting), requires no prior knowledge about the rooms, is suitable for physical disabled people using canes, and minimizes the false alarm rate.

The above contributions are detailed in the next subsections, and the experimentally evaluated performance of the developed system is discussed in Sect. 4.

3.1 The Fall Detection Dataset

The current FD datasets [1–3] are not suitable for this study for the following reasons: either they targeted healthy people only, they did not provide skeleton data streams, did not cover most of the scenarios, or they are not made accessible. These reasons prompted us to record a new dataset that: is made especially for the physically disabled people using canes as mobility aid; provides all the Kinect image-based streams (RGB color, depth, skeleton, infrared and body index); covers almost all the fall scenarios suggested by Noury et al. [7]; is accessible by contacting the authors and will be available soon at web.

To include all fall types and scenarios in [1–3, 7], we prepared a large dataset that contains 392 videos. These videos include 208 fall videos that cover backward, forward, lateral fall to the right and to the left. In addition, they include 184 non-fall videos composed of 115 videos of pseudo fall situations and 69 videos of ADL (Activities of Daily Living). This dataset was recorded using Kinect v2 for two male subjects in a frame rate of 30 fps. In each testing room, Kinect was set at 1 m high from the floor.

A dataset with real fall cases would be much more valuable but it is actually impracticable to test the fall situations with physically disabled people. So, the subjects simulated the cane user's walking pattern introduced by Melis et al. in [8]. Sample images of the dataset are shown in Fig. 1.

3.2 Features Extraction and Selection

In order to prepare the learning data for the detection system, we first extracted, from all videos' frames, the 3D positions of the 25 joints obtained from Kinect v2, which represent the skeleton. Second, for each frame, we preprocessed the joints' positions in three different ways: (i) *Original* positions (W) without any preprocessing;

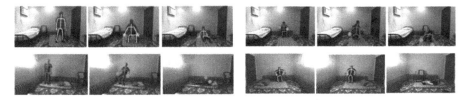

Fig. 1. Dataset samples.

(ii) *Translated* positions (T) by translating the mid spine joint to Kinect origin along with the other joints depending on it; and (iii) *Normalized* positions (N) using the torso-centered method [9]. These preprocessing ways overcome the difference of the faller size, distance and position. After each preprocessing method, we calculated three feature sets as follow:

1. Distances (D) of the joints from the Kinect [10]: 75 features (25 from the original skeleton, 25 from the translated skeleton, and 25 from the normalized skeleton).
2. Velocities (V) of the joints in the direction normal to the floor plane [4]: 75 features (25 from the original skeleton, 25 from the translated skeleton, and 25 from the normalized skeleton).
3. Angles (A) [11]: 45 features (15 from the original skeleton, 15 from the translated skeleton, and 15 from the normalized skeleton).

Because of the large number of features (195 features), we conducted three selection trials to eliminate irrelevant features, using two filter methods (Relief-F and Information Gain) and wrapper methods using two classifiers (C4.5 and IBk). From the union of all the features resulting from these methods, we took the most relevant features that gave us the best results.

In each of the three trials, we changed the way of classifying the fall frames. In Trial 1, the fall frame was *any* frame belonging to a fall video. In Trial 2, the fall frames were divided into two classes as indicated in [1]: (i) *Temporary-pose* frames when the faller starts falling until s/he reaches the floor; and (ii) *Fall* frames when the faller hits the floor, and stays on it. Finally, in Trial 3, the fall frame was the temporary pose and the fall frames from Trial 2. Tables 1, 2 and 3 summarize these three trials. Figures 2, 3 and 4, respectively, show the most relevant features obtained from the three trials.

Furthermore, to identify the most appropriate/performing features, we evaluated the results of each trial using a C4.5 classifier to measure its performance. As seen in Table 4, the best results were obtained from the seven relevant features in Trial 3 with a 91.53% accuracy. These features belong to the upper body part, which makes sense because this part is the main part used to support the cane before a fall happens.

3.3   Proposed Skeleton-Based Fall Detection Method and Its Setting

The conceptual architecture of the Watchful-Eye system receives the skeleton stream captured through the Kinect and transferred through USB to a laptop running the FD method. This latter first extracts the skeleton and normalizes a copy of it. Afterward, from the original data, it extracts features: right shoulder distance, right hand and right

Table 1. The conducted Trial 1 of the feature selection experiment.

Training data	4960 frames; 2480 for each class	
Classes	• 1 (Fall): if the frame from fall video classifies as fall • 0 (Non-fall): if the frame from non-fall video classifies as non-fall	See Fig. 2
Best features	**5 features calculated from 7 joints:** 1. Original angle of (left hip, base spine, right hip) 2. Original head velocity 3. Translated left ankle distance 4. Translated angle of (shoulder spine, mid spine, base spine) 5. Normalized mid spine distance	
Accuracy	77.29%	

Table 2. The conducted Trial 2 of the feature selection experiment.

Training data	4959 frames; 1653 for each class	
Classes	• 2 (Temporary pose): from fall video, the frame when the person starts fallen classify as a temporary pose • 1 (Fall): from fall video, the frame after the person are fallen and laying in the floor classify as fall • 0 (Non-fall): if the frame from non-fall video classifies as non-fall	See Fig. 3
Best features	**4 features calculated from 3 joints:** 1. Original left shoulder distance 2. Original head velocity 3. Normalized left shoulder distance 4. Normalized left thumb distance	
Accuracy	74.8%	

Table 3. The conducted Trial 3 of the feature selection experiment.

Training data	4960 frames; 2480 for each class	
Classes	• 1 (Fall): from fall video, the frame when the person starts fallen until he fallen and laying in the floor classify as fall • 0 (Non-fall): if the frame from non-fall video classifies as non-fall	See Fig. 4
Best features	**7 features calculated from 6 joints:** 1. Original right shoulder distance 2. Original right hand velocity 3. Original right thumb velocity 4. Normalized left hand distance 5. Normalized left shoulder distance 6. Normalized left thumb distance 7. Normalized right thumb distance	
Accuracy	91.53%	

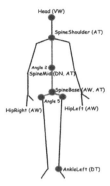

Fig. 2. Mapping of the best features representing the fall from Trial 1.

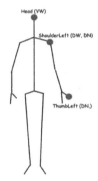

Fig. 3. Mapping of the best features representing the fall from Trial 2.

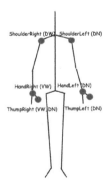

Fig. 4. Mapping of the best features representing the fall from Trial 3.

thumb velocities. From the normalized data, it extracts the rest features: left hand, left shoulder, left thumb and right thumb distances (features retained from Trial 3) and it feeds them to the appropriate classifier. Finally, based on the frames' classification results, it decides whether there is a fall, in which case it triggers an alarm. To

Table 4. The online evaluation results.

Fall type	Video number	Weaker side	F	TP	FN	SE
Backward fall	1	Left	79	75	4	94.9%
	2	Any	63	57	6	90.5%
Forward fall	3	Right	49	49	0	100%
	4	Any	31	31	0	100%
Lateral fall to the right	5	Left	76	68	8	89.47%
	6	Any	49	49	0	100%
Lateral fall to the left	7	Right	77	72	5	93.5%
	8	Any	52	49	3	94.23%

determine the appropriate classifier, we conducted a set of experiments whose results we discuss in the next section.

During the development of Watchful-Eye, we supposed that the system is to operate under the following settings/hypotheses:

1. It is set to monitor a room containing the disabled person in real-time;
2. It uses Kinect v2 for Windows with the free tool of Kinect SDK to detect and track the body/skeleton of the disabled person;
3. The Kinect sensor is placed 1 m high from the floor, as we did in the dataset. Its field of view should be able to cover both the room and the monitored person. In addition, the depth range of Kinect, which could reach 4.5 m [4] is also considered in the detection process;
4. The tracked joints are the six extracted from Trial 3 of the feature selection experiment.

4   Experimental Results

In this section, we analyze the detection performance of Watchful-Eye through an offline and online experimental evaluations. The two subjects from the recorded dataset were engaged in both experiments.

Experiment 1: Offline Evaluation. This first experiment aims to identify the appropriate classifier. Towards this end, we prepared a sample of 4960 frames from the recorded data with 2480 fall frames and 2480 non-fall frames. The frames used during the offline experiment correspond to the whole range of the captured 392 videos. We used 70% of this data (3472 frames) for training and 30% (1488 frames) for testing.

To determine the best classifier to build the classification model, we tested the data using different classification algorithms: C4.5, Logistic Model Trees (LMT), RandomForest, RandomTree, REPTree, and Instance-Based k (IBk) used with their default parameters as suggested by [12]. Based on the obtained results, we concluded that RandomForest is the best classifier (**Accuracy = 94.5%**, **Sensitivity = 92.8%**, **Specificity = 96%** and **AUC** (Area Under the ROC Curve) = **0.9858**) to use in Watchful-Eye and the online experimental evaluation.

Experiment 2: Online Evaluation. For the online evaluation, we developed the Watchful-Eye program that we operated with real-time videos of the two subjects as captured directly from Kinect. In this experiment, we used eight different fall videos (V) representing the following types of falls:

1. Backward fall from standing ending lying.
2. Backward fall from sitting on chair with no back ending lying.
3. Forward fall from standing ending on the knees.
4. Forward fall from sitting with forwarding arm protection.
5. Lateral fall to the right from standing ending lying flat.
6. Lateral fall to the right from lying on bed.
7. Lateral fall to the left from standing ending lying flat.
8. Lateral fall to the left from lying on bed.

Table 4 shows the experimental results where F and SE are the Total Video Frames, and the Sensitivity, respectively. In addition, "Weaker side" represents the weaker side of the physically disabled person. If s/he has left weaker side, then s/he was holding the cane by his other stronger side (right) as explained by Melis et al. in [8]. The videos with (*Any*) weaker side, that means the subject did not need to hold a cane because her/his postures (sitting or lying), and this situation could happen to the physically disabled person with *any* (left or right) weaker side.

From these experimental results, we notice that the offline evaluation results show that Watchful-Eye reached an accuracy between 87.2% and 94.5% with 5.5% to 12.8% error rate depending on the used classifier. Furthermore, the online evaluation shows that it can detect falls with an accuracy between 89.47% and 100%.

5 Conclusion

In this work, we presented Watchful-Eye, a skeleton-based monitoring system to monitor a physically disabled person using a cane and to detect fall occurrences. To develop such system, we constructed a dataset that can serve as a benchmark for evaluating and/or developing fall detection methods. This dataset has the merit of using the latest Kinect version, containing rich collected data, and covering a large spectrum of fall types and scenarios. In addition, we experimentally identified seven relevant features and appropriate classifier (RandomForest) classify frames into fall or non-fall. Finally, we experimentally showed that thus-developed system offers accuracy between 87.2% and 94.5% with 5.5% to 12.8% in offline evaluation, while in online evaluation shows that it can detect falls with an accuracy between 89.47% and 100%. In our future works, we will focus on improving Watchful-Eye by training it to detect falls from frame sequences in order to increase its accuracy and reduce its false alarm rates.

References

1. Kwolek, B., Kepski, M.: Human fall detection on embedded platform using depth maps and wireless accelerometer. Comput. Methods Programs Biomed. **117**, 489–501 (2014)

2. Lee, C.K., Lee, V.Y.: Fall detection system based on Kinect sensor using novel detection and posture recognition algorithm. In: Biswas, J., Kobayashi, H., Wong, L., Abdulrazak, B., Mokhtari, M. (eds.) ICOST 2013. LNCS, vol. 7910, pp. 238–244. Springer, Heidelberg (2013). https://doi.org/10.1007/978-3-642-39470-6_30

3. Stone, E.E., Skubic, M.: Fall detection in homes of older adults using the Microsoft Kinect. IEEE J. Biomed. Health Inf. **19**, 290–301 (2015)

4. Kawatsu, C., Li, J., Chung, C.: Development of a fall detection system with Microsoft Kinect. In: Kim, J.H., Matson, E., Myung, H., Xu, P. (eds.) Robot Intelligence Technology and Applications 2012. AISC, vol. 208, pp. 623–630. Springer, Berlin, Heidelberg (2013). https://doi.org/10.1007/978-3-642-37374-9_59

5. Kozina, S., Gjoreski, H., Gams, M., Luštrek, M.: Efficient activity recognition and fall detection using accelerometers. In: B, Juan A., Álvarez-García, J.A., Fujinami, K., Barsocchi, P., Riedel, T. (eds.) EvAAL 2013. CCIS, vol. 386, pp. 13–23. Springer, Heidelberg (2013). https://doi.org/10.1007/978-3-642-41043-7_2

6. Abdali-Mohammadi, F., Rashidpour, M., Fathi, A.: Fall detection using adaptive neuro-fuzzy inference system. Int. J. Multimed. Ubiquit. Eng. **11**, 91–106 (2016)

7. Noury, N., Fleury, A., Rumeau, P., Bourke, A., Laighin, G., Rialle, V., et al.: Fall detection-principles and methods. In: 2007 29th Annual International Conference of the IEEE Engineering in Medicine and Biology Society, pp. 1663–1666 (2007)

8. Melis, E., Torres-Moreno, R., Barbeau, H., Lemaire, E.: Analysis of assisted-gait characteristics in persons with incomplete spinal cord injury. Spinal Cord **37**, 430–439 (1999)

9. Rhemyst and Rymix. Kinect SDK Dynamic Time Warping (DTW) Gesture Recognition, 30 July 2011–2 January 2017. http://kinectdtw.codeplex.com/

10. Pterneas, V.: Measuring Distances using Kinect – The Right Way, 29 October 2016. http://pterneas.com/2016/08/11/measuring-distances-kinect/

11. Le, T.-L., Nguyen, M.-Q.: Human posture recognition using human skeleton provided by Kinect. In: 2013 International Conference on Computing, Management and Telecommunications (ComManTel), pp. 340–345 (2013)

12. Hall, M., Frank, E., Holmes, G., Pfahringer, B., Reutemann, P., Witten, I.H.: The WEKA data mining software: an update. ACM SIGKDD Explor. Newsl. **11**, 10–18 (2009)

A Virtual Reality-Based Physical and Cognitive Training System Aimed at Preventing Symptoms of Dementia

Sara Arlati[1,2(✉)], Luca Greci[2], Marta Mondellini[2],
Andrea Zangiacomi[2], Simona G. Di Santo[3], Flaminia Franchini[3],
Mauro Marzorati[4], Simona Mrakic-Sposta[4], and Alessandra Vezzoli[4]

[1] Dipartimento di Elettronica, Informazione e Bioingegneria,
Politecnico di Milano, Milan, Italy
sara.arlati@polimi.it
[2] Institute of Industrial Technologies and Automation,
National Research Council, Milan, Italy
{luca.greci,marta.mondellini,
andrea.zangiacomi}@itia.cnr.it
[3] IRCCS Fondazione Santa Lucia, Rome, Italy
{s.disanto,f.franchini}@hsantalucia.it
[4] Institute of Molecular Bioimaging and Physiology,
National Research Council, Segrate, MI, Italy
{mauro.marzorati,simona.mrakic,
alessandra.vezzoli}@ibfm.cnr.it

Abstract. This work presents a physical and cognitive training program, based on virtual reality technologies, designed with the aim of preventing the occurrence of symptoms of dementia in elderly with Mild Cognitive Impairment (MCI). The system foresees a physical task to be performed on a cycle-ergometer and two virtual environments for cognitive stimulation. In this paper, results of different validation phases conducted on both healthy and MCI subjects are described. The presented validation path allowed to implement, in parallel, the two current versions of the setup: the former, optimized to assess the efficacy of the intervention in a randomized clinical trial, which will take place in the next future, and the latter, more experimental, which foresees the employment of immersive environments to increase subjects' engagement and motivation.

Keywords: Mild cognitive impairment · Physical training
Cognitive stimulation · Virtual reality · Oxidative stress

1 Introduction

Patients with Alzheimer's Disease (AD) may initially be affected by the so-called Mild Cognitive Impairment (MCI), that is the presence of an impairment in at least one cognitive domain, without a significant deterioration of autonomy in activities of daily living [1]. MCI population has an increased risk to develop dementia, even if a

© ICST Institute for Computer Sciences, Social Informatics and Telecommunications Engineering 2018
P. Perego et al. (Eds.): MobiHealth 2017, LNICST 247, pp. 117–125, 2018.
https://doi.org/10.1007/978-3-319-98551-0_14

consistent percentage remain stable or reverse to normality during the years [2]. Therefore, subjects with MCI represent a reasonable target population for interventions aimed at halting and reducing AD progression, in particular for strategies centered on modifiable risk factors for dementia [3].

Several clinical trials have been conducted in recent years to identify non-pharmacological interventions capable of reducing the risk or, at least, slowing down the occurrence of the symptoms of dementia. Though there is still uncertainty on the efficacy of such interventions, promising results seem to be provided by either the separate or concurrent provision of cognitive stimulation (CS) and physical activity (PA) [4]. Starting from these evidences, the presented system was developed with the aim of providing elderly with minor cognitive disorders with an effective and easy accessible technological tool for physical, cognitive and functional stimulation, in order to prevent the occurrence of new symptoms of dementia. Virtual Reality (VR) has been used as the enabling technology due to its capabilities of reproducing controlled training environments with high ecological validity and of engaging and motivating the patients [5, 6]. In the following paragraphs, the system and the validation path followed to test and improve the first-designed setup are presented.

2 The Training System

The system was designed to allow MCI patients to both perform physical exercise and train their cognitive abilities with a single experimental setup. To facilitate the transfer of the capabilities acquired during the training into real life, three VR-based scenarios representing activities of daily living were implemented. In details, they simulate the following activities: (1) riding a bike in a park, (2) crossing roads - avoiding cars – and (3) making the grocery shopping in a supermarket. The first scenario is dedicated to the accomplishment of the PA, whereas scenarios (2) and (3) are designed to provide the CS and, in particular, to train visuospatial abilities, which correspond to one of the domains commonly impaired in AD and thus require proper stimulation.

The hardware devices composing the training system are: a cycle-ergometer (Ergosana Eurobike 320), a smart garment (Wearable Wellness System, Smartex) – aimed at measuring the hearth rate in real time, a finger touch projector (EB-1430WI, Epson) and a PlayStation controller anchored on the cycle-ergometer handlebars. The choice of the cycle-ergometer was motivated by safety reasons, since, with respect to a treadmill (the only other equipment allowing an easy modification of the workload), is associated with a lower risk of injury, especially in case of an elderly user.

2.1 Physical Activity

While performing the physical task (scenario 1), the patient rides the cycle-ergometer, facing the projected screen and wearing the smart garment, as shown in Fig. 1. Exercise intensity is chosen as to correspond to about 65–70% of individual maximal heart rate (HR), previously determined on the basis of the age-predicted value.

During the training session, the work rate is adjusted in real-time, through a digital controller, which tunes the workload to make the subject maintain the target HR. The

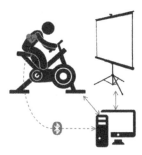

Fig. 1. The system setup. The dashed line represents Bluetooth connection; continuous line represents connections through cables.

Virtual Environment (VE) represents a trail in a park (Fig. 2, top-left) that flows according to the pedals velocity. The VE has the aim of increasing the user's engagement and of providing him/her with the information needed to control the exercise, such as speed, covered distance, round-per-minute, time elapsed and heart rate.

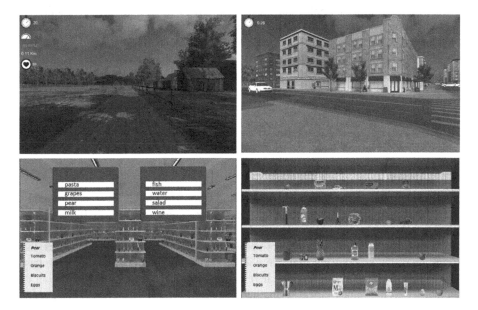

Fig. 2. Screenshots of the developed VEs: above, the park (left) and the crossing-road (right) scenarios; below, the two tasks of the supermarket scenario: aisle (left) and shelf (right).

2.2   Cognitive Stimulation

The CS starts after a predefined time lapse (15 or 20 min), when the park displayed on the projected screen turns into an urban route. In this second scenario, the user has still to ride the cycle-ergometer, but the task is not more physical (the workload is set to 0), but cognitive: he/she, in fact, has to face the crossing of five traffic-congested and non-regulated crosswalks.

The trial participant has thus to perform different visuospatial and attentional tasks: (1) pedaling to reach the border of the sidewalk, (2) brake when being near it, (3) check on both sides if there are cars moving closer and, if not, (4) restart pedaling to reach the following cross. Braking and turning the point of view can be accomplished using, respectively, the X button and the joystick of the PlayStation controller. This choice was motivated by the impossibility of implementing a real brake by accessing the wheel compartment without affecting the CE certification of the ergometer.

After the completion of this first cognitive task, the user reaches the entrance of a supermarket (scenario 3) and has to get down from the cycle-ergometer and do the shopping of some grocery items indicated on the shopping list that the system generates randomly. To buy a product, the user has first to find and tap on the projected screen the aisle whose sign is containing the name of product (*aisle task*) and then tap on the right product, placed on the shelves in a random position, among other distractors (*shelf task*, see Fig. 2).

Different levels of difficulty were implemented for both tasks. The increase in difficulty is obtained mainly by the increase of *distractors* and of their similarity. For the aisle task, a further complication to promote language and attentional training is obtained by the introduction of a word that is orthographically or semantically similar to the target object name. For the shelf task, higher levels are characterized by the presence of different formats and discounted versions of the same product, so that the attentional and visuospatial demands are increased.

For both the described tasks, if the user commits an error or does not interact with the VE for more than 45 s, the system intervenes providing a hint to help him/her proceed to the next task.

3 Validation Path

For the validation of the designed intervention, different phases have been already accomplished and others will be completed in the next future (see Fig. 3). In particular, with respect to the previously presented achievements this work adds the results from the preliminary tests on the immersive version of the system and includes the description of the randomized trial that will be held using the third version. Each past phase – described in the subparagraph hereinafter – allowed collecting different kind of data that led to the improvement of the hardware devices and of the VEs' design and functionalities.

3.1 Phase 1: Preliminary Tests

First experiments on the developed system were performed enrolling healthy subjects. For the PA, a cardiologist tested the algorithm that regulates the cycle-ergometer workload according to the user current and his/her maximal heart rate [7]. Thanks to his suggestions, modifications were made to the controller to adjust the slope with which

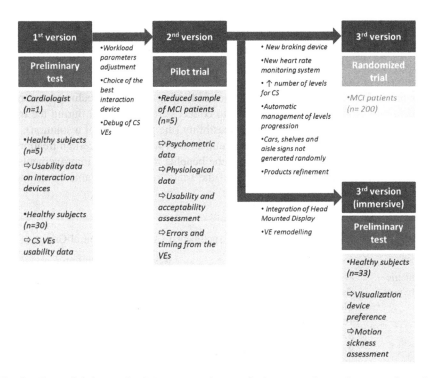

Fig. 3. The validation path: the setup version used, the type of experiment performed, its outcomes (indicated by arrows) and the subsequent modification to software and hardware devices. Grayed-out blocks indicate that the trial is currently ongoing.

the increase or decrease of the workload is made, to avoid too sharp variations in the users' HR.

Dealing with the CS environment, two different experiments were performed. The former, described in [8], allowed to define the best interaction device for selecting the aisle and the grocery items from the shelves. The touch-projected screen resulted the best in terms of intuitiveness and fatigue, with respect to Kinect-based solutions, Leap Motion and 3D mouse in tests conducted on 5 healthy subjects. The latter experiment involved 30 healthy participants with the aim of identifying potential criticalities in the supermarket scenario. Each subject was asked to perform the shopping tasks and then to fill in a questionnaire assessing the usability of the system and to provide suggestions for improvement. The collected feedback led to the replacement of certain products, which resulted confounding due to the screen resolution or to potential ambiguity (i.e. Grana Padano vs. Parmigiano Reggiano) and to the modification of the clickable area in the aisle scenario: the entire aisle was turned into a button, after it was observed that many users clicked the lane area instead of the aisle sign.

3.2   Phase 2: The Pilot Trial

After the validation on healthy subjects, the developed system was tested in a first randomized pilot trial conducted on elderly with MCI. Ten subjects responding to inclusion criteria (age $\geq$ 65 years, one or more test scores indicating compromised visuospatial abilities, one or more test scores indicating cognitive decline) were randomized in two groups. A set of variables to collect before, after and during the trial, was defined with the aim of assessing the feasibility (the practicality of a solution), the acceptability (the social, psychological and ethical acceptability of a certain treatment) and providing first insights of the efficacy (the benefits measured by improvements in health) of the designed program. Results of the trials, reported in Table 1, are more extensively described in [9, 10].

Table 1. Results of the pilot trial. EG: Experimental Group, CG: Control Group.

Outcomes	Assessment methodology	Results and conclusion
Psychometric tests (pre/post)	Mini-Mental State Test, Rey-Osterrieth Complex Figure Test, Clock Drawing Test, Trail Making Test-A/B, Frontal Assessment Battery, Word and Non-Word Repetition Task, Verbal fluency tests, Functional Assessment Questionnaire.	EG showed improvements in the MMSE, in visual-constructive and visuospatial tests, while the CG worsened. The EG had a greater improvement in the executive, memory and verbal functions. No difference was statistically significant, reasonably due to the small sample and its heterogeneity. However, the highlighted tendency can be considered encouraging.
Oxidative stress measurement (pre/post)	Detection of Reactive Oxygen Species (ROS) concentration by Electron Paramagnetic Resonance, antioxidant status and oxidative damage [11, 12].	The EG after training intervention showed statistically ($p < 0.05$) lower ROS production rate. The training may help to delay neurodegenerative damage caused by oxidative stress.
Software data (acquired during the training)	Durations of the PA and CS. Accident, errors and hints occurred during the CS.	Good adherence to both PA and CS. Levels of CS training were indeed of increasing difficulty, but too easy to complete for patients with only mild cognitive impairments. Few products were confounding.
Subjective evaluation (post intervention)	Questionnaire on satisfaction, desire to continue, enjoy and comfort. Suggestions for improvements through open questions.	EG reported high levels of engagement and motivation, enabled mainly by VR technologies. Feedbacks on the VEs revealed appreciation: participants would continue with the program also at home.

Despite positive feedback from the experimental subjects, the observations of the sessions and the collection of the psychologists and the patients' comments highlighted a few critical aspects to be improved in a third version of the system (Fig. 3). A 3D-printed braking device, equipped with a potentiometer, was anchored on the cycle-ergometer handles to allow a more natural interaction; the smart garment was replaced with more practical heart rate monitor (a finger pulse oximeter), which allows more participants to use the same equipment. The software was made able to handle automatically the level selection, excluding potential errors committed by operators. Moreover, all the road crossing, the aisle and the shelf tasks proposed are now previously computed and just loaded during the sessions, so that more precise and comparable data will be available for further analyses.

The resulting third version, improved according to the feedback collected during the pilot study and thanks to the promising results obtained on MCI patients, will be tested in the next months in a multicenter randomized controlled trial (§4).

3.3 Phase 3: Preliminary Test on the Immersive Version

Another aspect that would have been interesting to address in order to improve the second version is the possibility to provide the users with a more immersive experience. Solving this issue requires the replacement of the projected screen with a Head Mounted Display (HMD), whose use often causes physical drawbacks [13]. Therefore, there is the need of testing the immersive solution on healthy subjects before integrating it into an elderly/frail people-dedicated system. Due to this reason, an alternative version of the system was developed in parallel to the non-immersive third setup. The park and road crossing VEs were adapted to be visualized using the Samsung GearVR headset; an *ad-hoc* client/server application, which allowed the data exchange between the cycle-ergometer and the VEs running on the Android smartphone placed in the GearVR, was implemented.

A within-subject experiment comparing the projected screen and the HMD was then conducted on a sample of 33 healthy young adults, who were asked to answer the Simulator Sickness Questionnaire (SSQ) [14] and to select the device they prefer after 10 min of cycling in the two VEs. Preliminary results revealed that SSQ total scores were significantly higher using the HMD ($p < 0.001$, $z = -4.79$). However, most of the subjects ($n = 24$, $\chi^2 = 9.64$, $p < 0.05$) reported to prefer the experience with the HMD, indicating that subjects are capable of tolerating small malaises in exchange of a more involving and engaging experience. Only subjects who reported a high number of symptoms (≥ 4), in fact, preferred the projected screen; moreover, they often reported discomfort in this less-immersive condition too.

4   Conclusion and Future Works

This paper presents a system developed to provide MCI patients with physical and cognitive training and describes three different validation phases and the technical and methodological improvements implemented after each phase. In the next future, the last non-immersive version (#3) will be part of a multicenter randomized clinical trial, involving about 200 MCI patients. Further studies will be performed also on the immersive environments, which are more engaging and more intuitive, trying to improve the VEs design with the aim of reducing as much as possible the physical drawbacks. When the navigation and the interaction while wearing an HMD will be comfortably tolerated by a population of young adults, first tests on elderly will be conducted taking into account the proper safety equipment (e.g. harness).

Acknowledgments. This work has been partly funded by MIUR under the "Progetto di interesse Invecchiamento CNR: Goji". The authors wish to acknowledge their gratitude and appreciation to the project partners for their contribution during the development of this research.

References

1. Petersen, R.C., Smith, G.E., Waring, S.C., Ivnik, R.J., Tangalos, E.G., Kokmen, E.: Mild cognitive impairment: clinical characterization and outcome. Arch. Neurol. **56**(3), 303–308 (1999)
2. Mariani, E., Monastero, R., Mecocci, P.: Mild cognitive impairment: a systematic review. J. Alzheimer's Dis. **12**(1), 23–35 (2007)
3. Beydoun, M.A., Beydoun, H.A., Gamaldo, A.A., Teel, A., Zonderman, A.B., Wang, Y.: Epidemiologic studies of modifiable factors associated with cognition and dementia: systematic review and meta-analysis. BMC Public Health **14**(1), 643 (2014)
4. Andrieu, S., Coley, N., Lovestone, S., Aisen, P.S., Vellas, B.: Prevention of sporadic Alzheimer's disease: lessons learned from clinical trials and future directions. Lancet Neurol. **14**(9), 926–944 (2015)
5. García-Betances, R.I., Jiménez-Mixco, V., Arredondo, M.T., Cabrera-Umpiérrez, M.F.: Using virtual reality for cognitive training of the elderly. Am. J. Alzheimer's Dis. Other Dement. **30**(1), 49–54 (2015)
6. Coyle, H., Traynor, V., Solowij, N.: Computerized and virtual reality cognitive training for individuals at high risk of cognitive decline: systematic review of the literature. Am. J. Geriatr. Psychiatr. **23**(4), 335–359 (2015)
7. Kawada, T., Ikeda, Y., Takaki, H., Sugimachi, M., Kawaguchi, O., Shishido, T., Sato, T., Matsuura, W., Miyano, H., Sunagawa, K.: Development of a servo-controller of heart rate using a cycle ergometer. Heart Vessel. **14**(4), 177–184 (1999)
8. Greci, L.: GOJI an advanced virtual environment for supporting training of physical and cognitive activities for preventing the occurrence of dementia in normally living elderly with minor cognitive disorders. In: 12th EuroVR Conference (2015)
9. Arlati, S., Zangiacomi, A., Greci, L., di Santo, S.G., Franchini, F., Sacco, M.: Virtual environments for cognitive and physical training in elderly with mild cognitive impairment: a pilot study. In: De Paolis, L.T., Bourdot, P., Mongelli, A. (eds.) AVR 2017. LNCS, vol. 10325, pp. 86–106. Springer, Cham (2017). https://doi.org/10.1007/978-3-319-60928-7_8
10. Marzorati, M., et al.: Supporting physical and cognitive training for preventing the occurrence of dementia using an integrated system: a pilot study. In: Perego, P., Andreoni, G., Rizzo, G. (eds.) MobiHealth 2016. LNICST, vol. 192, pp. 367–374. Springer, Cham (2017). https://doi.org/10.1007/978-3-319-58877-3_46
11. Mrakic-Sposta, S., Gussoni, M., Montorsi, M., Porcelli, S., Vezzoli, A.: A quantitative method to monitor reactive oxygen species production by electron paramagnetic resonance in physiological and pathological conditions. Oxidative Med. Cell. Longev. **2014**, 10 (2014). Article ID 306179, https://doi.org/10.1155/2014/306179

12. Mrakic-Sposta, S., et al.: Effects of mountain ultra-marathon running on ROS production and oxidative damage by micro-invasive analytic techniques. PLoS One **10**(11), e0141780 (2015)
13. Nichols, S., Patel, H.: Health and safety implications of virtual reality: a review of empirical evidence. Appl. Ergon. **33**(3), 251–271 (2002)
14. Kennedy, R.S., Lane, N.E., Berbaum, K.S., Lilienthal, M.G.: Simulator sickness questionnaire: an enhanced method for quantifying simulator sickness. Int. J. Aviat. Psychol. **3**(3), 203–220 (1993)

Design for Healthcare

Improved Patient Engagement in Self-management of Health, a Key to Sustainable Preventative Healthcare Systems

Adriana Alexandru[✉], Marilena Ianculescu, and Dora Çoardos

National Institute for Research and Development in Informatics, 8-10 Averescu Avenue,
011455 Bucharest, Romania
adriana_alexandru@yahoo.com

Abstract. The use of mobile health together with the Internet of Things (IoT) technology and wireless networks have the potential of reshaping the healthcare systems towards the patient-centred and preventative ones. Better empowered patients which are familiar with smart technology represent a viable way for raising the quality of the self-management of health. Usability is a key factor for a successful acceptance of mHealth solutions. This paper presents the results of the heuristic evaluation of two mHealth apps that support self-healthcare revealed several important usability problems which have to be fixed in the further versions.

Keywords: mHealth · IoT · Patient engagement · Personalized healthcare
Usability inspection · Heuristic evaluation

1 Introduction

Mobile technology in medical care (mHealth) has grown throughout the world over the last few years. This technology changes the way healthcare is provided shifting it towards a patient-centred approach which means that the "care that is respectful of and responsive to individual patient preferences, needs, and values and [ensures] that patient values guide all clinical decisions" [1]. mHealth supports a better engagement of the patients and health professionals aiming to ensure preventive actions and healthier life styles, and to improve health outcomes and health system efficiency.

The concept of self-management of patients is associated with a better empowerment of them and an improved responsibility in taking the most appropriate choices regarding a personal management of the disease.

In a digitalized healthcare system, wearable and in-home sensors collect health data, facilitate analysing and finding insights in the huge amount of stored data and provide real-time actions of healthcare providers.

For a broader acceptance of mHealth usability evaluation has to be performed even from the development process for meeting the patients' demands and necessities.

This paper presents two case studies, TactioHealth app and iMHere app. These are mHealth apps that provide useful information for supporting people in self-care

© ICST Institute for Computer Sciences, Social Informatics and Telecommunications Engineering 2018
P. Perego et al. (Eds.): MobiHealth 2017, LNICST 247, pp. 129–137, 2018.
https://doi.org/10.1007/978-3-319-98551-0_15

activities. The results of the usability inspection of both of them using heuristic evaluation are described.

2   The Potential of mHealth to Remodel the Self-management of Health Processes

The worldwide current healthcare systems aim to provide complex, high quality, cost efficient, accessible and patient-centred care. New healthcare delivery models based on the latest medical research have emphasized the intensive link between the early identification of a disease and the successful treatment results. Thus, a preventative approach of the healthcare services have lately become an increasing demand, imposing a shift in care from treating a disease to prevent or slow down it.

Preventative healthcare can be classified in primary (avoiding the occurrence of a disease), secondary (controlling a disease from the early stages by minimizing its impacts) and tertiary (identifying the most appropriate management of a chronic disease for raising the quality of life of the patient).

Preventative healthcare systems imply both a proactive and a predictive tackling as specified in [2]: "Proactive care solutions stratify at-risk individuals based on known algorithms and ensure that preventive action is taken to intervene well before the onset of symptoms. Predictive care solutions leverage cutting-edge technologies and sophisticated machine learning data algorithms to predict risk and intervene even further upstream".

Continuous changes at the societal level and the huge technological advances enforce a shift towards a more comprehensive patient empowerment. The tremendous role of information communication technology in the healthcare systems and the broader access to knowledge have sustained the emergence of a new category of patients, digitally active and having quite well established demands and expectations regarding integrated patient-centred healthcare services.

Digitalisation has also facilitated an increased role of the patient in his/her self-health management, with many benefits like: better engagement with healthcare providers, greater confidence, enhanced safety, improved health outcomes, cost and time efficiency. mHealth has proved to be a successful tool for better engaged patients looking for smarter healthcare.

The most appropriate domains for mHealth applications comprise: self-monitoring of health parameters (in conjunction with wearable devices and IoT), remote consultations, emergency management, health data acquisition, storing and processing, comprehensive and limitless access to health knowledge.

According to [3], 36% of respondents believe the use of app-enabled patient portals is the most effective tool in patient engagement.

To get the most out of the mHealth targeting the self-management of health, the most appropriate, familiar and personalised user interface design has a key role in a broader acceptance of these health services, together with a more consistent use of interoperability standards, more pervasive ways to collect, analyse health data in order to transform it into improved knowledge, and also with better issues of privacy and security in order to increase the confidence of the patient-users.

The continuous emerging of newer mHealth based solutions and technology, the integration of smart devices into everyday life and the increased degree of the patients' acceptance accelerates the reshaping of the healthcare systems.

3   The Internet of Things - Facilitators of for Improving Patient Engagement and Personalized Healthcare

The IoT can provide early detection of abnormal health data and rapid response to medical emergencies, support patients' adherence to often-complex medication regimens, and offer a greater confidence. The emergence of wireless networks in healthcare applications gains momentum by increasing the number of vital signalling sensors and localization tags that can track both medical staff and patient status/location continuously in real time [4].

"IoT is the network of physical objects or "things" embedded with electronic devices, software technologies, sensors and networked connections, which facilitates the collection and exchange of data to benefit from various services" [5]. IoT is a concept reflecting a connected set of anyone, anything, anytime, anyplace, any service, and any network. IoT is a technology for interconnection of uniquely identifiable smart objects and devices within today's internet infrastructure with extended benefits.

With IoT, many medical applications can be generated, such as remote health monitoring, health programs, chronic illness [6].

Wireless health care systems can be used together with IoT systems. These systems include health sensors, smart phone devices and server system for information control and management [5]. The sensors contain input values that they transmit to the server using the smartphone. The server processes the data and informs the patients. These health systems help patients make decisions based on what their application transmits.

The monitoring system is mainly based on two types of sensors: *wearable sensors* that are attached to the patient to measure vital parameters and *in-home sensors* embedded in and around the different parts of the patient's room [7].

IoT allows a variety of health care services where each *service* offers a set of health care solutions. Of the types of IoT-based healthcare services we mention: Ambient Assisted Living (AAL), The Internet of m-Health Things (m-IoT), Adverse Drug Reaction (ADR), Community Healthcare (CH), Children Health Information (CHI), Wearable Device Access (WDA), Semantic Medical Access (SMA), Indirect Emergency Healthcare (IEH), Embedded Gateway Configuration (EGC), Embedded Context Prediction (ECP).

Figure 1 shows the operation of wireless networks used to help patients. It consists of sensors attached to the human body, wireless devices, server system and doctors and hospitals that provide patient services [5].

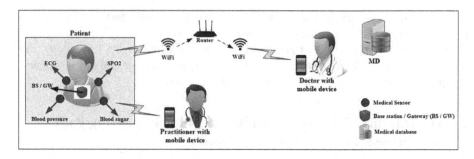

Fig. 1. Wireless sensor networks for healthcare

4   Usability Evaluation of mHealth Apps Supporting Self-care

The ISO 9241-11 standard defines usability as "the extent to which a product can be used by specified users to achieve specified goals with effectiveness, efficiency and satisfaction in a specified context of use" [8]. Poor usability is a major obstacle to health information adoption and a clear cause of medical error [9]. Usability is a key determinant to the adoption and success of mHealth into disease self-management [10].

Usability evaluation aims at finding, documenting, and reporting usability problems for refining the design of the system to address the problems found. Usability evaluation methods are classified in: inspection methods and user testing [11]. *Usability inspection* is done by experts that are testing the user interface with the goal to anticipate usability problems. The most widely used inspection method is the *heuristic evaluation* [12], where an expert reviewer assesses the tested user interface with a set of universally accepted usability principles (heuristics). Table 1 illustrates the 11 principles of the heuristic evaluation for mHealth apps that are in accordance with the 10 principles proposed by Nielsen [13], and the last is from Karat et al. [14].

Table 1. Principles of good interface design (heuristics).

No.	Heuristics
1	Visibility of system status
2	Match between system and the real world
3	User control and freedom
4	Consistency and standards
5	Error prevention
6	Recognition rather than recall
7	Flexibility and efficiency of use
8	Aesthetic and minimalist design
9	Help users recognize, diagnose, and recover from errors
10	Help and documentation
11	Intuitive visual layout

4.1   mHealth Apps: Case Studies

The objective of the presented case studies was to evaluate the usability of two mHealth apps that enhance the quality of life by empowering the patient with self-care possibilities:

1. *TactioHealth app* consists in mobile proactive applications suited for helping people to manage a healthy lifestyle. Tactio software apps provides a better health management without requiring medical expertise. There are apps dealing with Diabetes (see Fig. 2), Obesity, Hypertension, Atherosclerosis, COPD, CHF, and Pregnancy. Patients are empowered to manage a wide range of health data from simple manual logging to self-tracking apps connected to medical devices. Reference ranges are provided by incorporated science-based rules and can be used on every data: weight, steps, nutrition, activity, sleep, mood, blood pressure, pulse, glucose, cholesterol, temperature and oximetry [15].

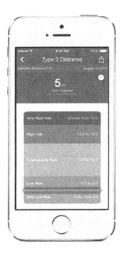

Fig. 2. Tactio Type 2diabetes mHealth Apps

2. *iMHere (Internet Mobile Health and Rehabilitation)* is a mHealth system developed to support self-care and adherence to self-care regimens for individuals with spina bifida and other complex conditions who are vulnerable to secondary complications [16]. The system allows clinicians to monitor a patient's condition and send a treatment plan for each patient to a smartphone designed to empower patients to do preventive self-care and adapted to user's disabilities. The five apps that constitute the iMHere support preventive self-care for managing medications (MyMeds), neurogenic bladder (TeleCath) and bowel (BMQs), skin breakdown (SkinCare), and mood (Mood) as presented in Fig. 3. It is possible to generate self-created reminders with customized alarm tones and messages prompted individuals to perform tasks related to self-care at home.

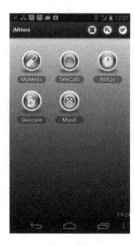

Fig. 3. iMHere mHealth App - Home screen for suite of apps

4.2   Results of Heuristic Evaluation of mHealth Apps

In order to address any issues concerning the use of mHealth apps inspected in the two case studies, a group of users (acting as patients) was introduced to the usability study. Previous studies from HCI literature found that 80% of usability problems can be detected with only 5 subjects [17, 18], and almost all of high-severity usability problems with only 3 subjects [17]. In this study, 5 evaluators (3 women and 2 men) specialised in: web design, medical care, healthy lifestyle, psychologist, caregiver tested the selected mHealth apps independently and reported the usability problems found for each of the six main themes emerged from usability literature [19]: Presentation of health information; Aesthetic and minimalist design; Flexibility and efficiency of data input; Task feedback; Intuitive design; and App stability. None of the evaluators has severe intellectual disability and any problem in vision, hearing, speech, or hand moving which would affect operation of a smartphone device. All subjects were smartphone users prior to be included in the study. Two evaluators are usability experts and three are patients.

Before starting the evaluation, each evaluator received the evaluation themes, the set of usability heuristics, and two papers with examples of usability inspection. The usability inspection has been done independently by each expert using his/her own smartphone during 90 min.

According to the potential effect on the theme, the severity of the detected usability problems has been assessed as severe, moderate and minor.

Each evaluator detected between 5 and 9 usability problems and specified each of them on an Excel table. After removing the false ones and analysing each problem in order to agree on the severity, 13 usability problems in TactioHealth app and 12 in iMHere app resulted as important. The usability evaluation results are presented in Table 2.

Table 2. Usability problems per task and severity

Theme	TactioHealth app				iMHere app			
	Total	Severe	Moderate	Minor	Total	Severe	Moderate	Minor
1	2	0	1	1	6	1	3	2
2	2	0	2	0	1	0	1	0
3	3	1	2	0	1	0	1	0
4	2	0	2	0	1	0	1	0
5	3	0	1	2	2	0	1	1
6	1	0	1	0	1	0	1	0
Total	13	1	9	3	12	1	8	3

The two severe problems are related to the big quantity of input data in TactioHealth app and to the small dimension of some activity buttons at the top of the screen diminishing users' access capabilities in iMHere app.

Most of the moderate problems are related to the findings presented in Table 3.

Table 3. Usability results for the two case studies (moderate severity)

No.	Theme	Key usability problems in TactioHealth app	Key usability problems in iMHere app
1	Presentation of health information	– Too small dimension of graphs for seeing trends over time	– Light text colour such as white or yellow on a light background (e.g., grey) causing reading difficulties; – Narrow width of the scrollbar leading to under-completion of the data – Difficulties in understanding the meanings of certain words (e.g. alias)
2	Aesthetic and minimalist design	– Overcrowded screens – Obstructive decorative elements competing with relevant content	– Overcrowded screens
3	Flexibility and efficiency	– Lack of flexibility in entering data	– Not patient centred design leading to not appropriated remainders, and scheduling – Errors in tasks procedures by not using of in-app directional notes
4	Task feedback	– Too much input data requested by apps and no feedback provided – Lack of feedback to state the completion of an action	– Non appropriate use of words in dialog with the users
5	Intuitive design	– Difficulties in understanding how to use an app	– Lack of different colours for different apps
6	App stability	– Occasional apps breakdowns	– Certain problems for sending data if 4G signal is unstable

5   Conclusion

Inside the healthcare systems, mHealth has proved to bring value and an increased quality both from the point of view of healthcare services and of a more comprehensive and involved self-health management performed by the patients. A preventative approach of lifestyle and health supported by smart technology and patient-centred solutions have transformed the passive patients into active engaged actors. Despite the tremendous development of smart health technology, a greater importance has to be put on designing more familiar and personalised mHealth solutions for increasing their degree of integration in patients' everyday life. Usability evaluation of mHealth solutions can reveal the issues that might restrain their acceptance, use and the positive impact on self-management of patients' health as it has demonstrated inside this paper.

Acknowledgement. This work has been developed under the framework of *"Using Big Data Technologies in Government Computer Systems"* and *"ICT in healthcare: A comparative analysis of the eHealth solutions in Member States and successful models in the world"* projects funded by the Romanian Ministry of Communication and Information Society (2015-2017).

References

1. Institute of Medicine: Crossing the Quality Chasm. National Academies Press, Washington (2001)
2. Wise, A.: Transforming Health: Shifting from Reactive to Proactive and Predictive Care (2016). https://www.marsdd.com/news-and-insights/transforming-health-shifting-from-reactive-to-proactive-and-predictive-care/
3. HIMSS Mobile Technology Survey (2015). http://www.himss.org/2015-mobile-survey
4. Omogbadegun, Z.O., Ayo, C.K.: Impact of mobile and wireless technology on healthcare delivery services. In: 3GSM & Mobile Computing: An Emerging Growth Engine for National Development (2007)
5. Sreekanth, K.U., Nitha, K.P.: A study on health care in Internet of Things. IJRITCC **4**(2), 044–047 (2016). ISSN: 2321-8169
6. Pang, Z.: Technologies and architectures of the Internet-of-Things (IoT) for health and well-being, Doctoral Thesis in Electronic and Computer Systems KTH. Royal Institute of Technology (2013)
7. Srijani, M., Koustabh, D., Soumya, K.D.: Patient health management system using e-Health monitoring architecture. In: IEEE International Advance Computing Conference (IACC) (2014)
8. International Organization for Standardization. ISO 9241-11 Ergonomic requirements for office work with visual display terminals (VDTs) — Part 11: Guidance on usability (1998). https://www.iso.Org/obp/ui/#iso:std:iso:9241:-11:ed-l:vl:en
9. Coutu-Nadeau, C.: Evaluating the Usability of Diabetes Management iPad Applications. Weill Medical College of Cornell University (2014)
10. Arsand, E., Froisland, D.H., Skrovseth, S.O., Chomutare, T., Tatara, N., Hartvigsen, G., Tufano, J.T.: Mobile health applications to assist patients with diabetes: lessons learned and design implications. J. Diabetes Sci. Technol. **6**(5), 1197–1206 (2012)
11. Cockton, G., Lavery, D., Woolrych, A.: Inspection-based evaluation. In: Jacko, J.A., Sears, A. (eds.) The Human-Computer Interaction Handbook, LEA, pp. 273–292 (2003)

12. Nielsen, J., Molich, R.: Heuristic evaluation of user interfaces. In: Proceedings of ACM CHI 1990, pp. 249–256 (1990)
13. Nielsen, J., Blatt, L.A., Bradford, J., Brooks, P.: Usability Inspection, pp. 413–414 (1994)
14. Karat, C.-M., Campbell, R., Fiegel, T.: Comparison of empirical testing and walkthrough methods in user interface evaluation. In: Proceedings of the SIGCHI Conference on Human Factors in Computing Systems, pp. 397–404. ACM, Monterey (1992)
15. TactioHealth Group https://www.tactiohealth.com/health-tracking-apps/
16. Parmanto, B., Pramana, G., Yu, D.X., Fairman, A.D., Dicianno, B.E., McCue, M.P.: iMHere: a novel mHealth system for supporting self-care in management of complex and chronic conditions. JMIR mHealth uHealth 1(2), e10 (2013)
17. Virzi, R.A.: Refining the test phase of usability evaluation: how many subjects is enough? Hum. Factors 34(4), 457–468 (1992)
18. Nielsen, J.: Why You Only Need to Test with 5 Users? (2000). http://www.useit.com/alertbox/20000319.html
19. Lewis, J.R.: Sample sizes for usability tests: mostly math, not magic. Interactions 13(6), 29–33 (2006)

NESTORE: A Multidomain Virtual Coach for Active and Healthy Ageing

Maria Renata Guarneri[1]([✉]), Alfonso Mastropietro[2], and Giovanna Rizzo[2]

[1] Politecnico di Milano, Milan, Italy
Mariarenata.guarneri@polimi.it
[2] Istituto di Bioimmagini e Fisiologia Molecolare, CNR, Segrate, MI, Italy

Abstract. Technology can play a key role in support of the needs of the ageing population. In this direction, the rapid development of the ICT, and in particular mobile technologies, offers an important opportunity to address the development of an integrated solution to support active and healthy ageing. Whilst technology can potentially have a significant impact on health and wellbeing, to date uptake of digital health technologies has been problematic in a number of wide-scale studies. Literature has cited confidence, the stigmatizing aesthetics of products, meaningfulness of technology in the broader context of the persons' life, ease of use and integration into everyday routines as important factors of non-acceptance. With the aim of overcoming the above limitation, we have gathered a multi-disciplinary consortium to develop an integrated solution that, strongly leveraging user participation and co-design as well as state-of-the-art technologies, offers a virtual coach service to elderly people so that they can maintain wellbeing and independence. The solution, in addition to being multi-technology, has the ambition of addressing wellbeing in a holistic manner taking into consideration several dimensions. NESTORE has started in September 2017 and will last three years. NESTORE involves 16 partners from 7 European countries. The paper presents the approach to the research and the envisaged results.

Keywords: Healthy ageing · Wellbeing · Smart objects · Interaction design
User empowerment · Self-management

1 Introduction

The NESTORE (Non-intrusive Empowering Solutions and Technologies for Older people to Retain Everyday life activity) project has been recently funded by the H2020 Programme under Strategic Challenge 1 "Health, demographic change and wellbeing" in response to the call on healthy ageing.

The aim of the project is to develop a companion - NESTORE - that, as the mythological Nestor, can give advice to older people so that they can maintain their wellbeing and their independence at home, based on **experience** and on **understanding the current situation**. The experience of our modern NESTORE is based on well-grounded psychological and behavioural theories jointly with relevant know-how on the ageing process, while the current situation is understood on the basis of a comprehensive

© ICST Institute for Computer Sciences, Social Informatics and Telecommunications Engineering 2018
P. Perego et al. (Eds.): MobiHealth 2017, LNICST 247, pp. 138–146, 2018.
https://doi.org/10.1007/978-3-319-98551-0_16

sensors' system able to monitor the different key parameters. An intelligent system, based on a cloud and leveraging Decision Support logics, will deliver "advice and coaching", which will be offered via the companion, embodied in a smartphone or an intelligent tangible object, according to the user's preferences and interests.

The core idea of NESTORE is linked to the design of pathways that, according to user preferences and inclinations, leverage existing personal capabilities to support healthy lifestyles and overall wellbeing.

The paper presents first an overview of the wellbeing dimensions covered by NESTORE; the core of the paper focuses on the key concept and on the approach to be followed in the development of the solution. An overview of the validation approach will then be presented.

2   The Five Key Dimensions of Wellbeing

Ageing is a multi-dimensional and multi-directional process. It involves the social, economic, physical, psychological and cognitive spheres and all these characteristics of a person and its context is strongly interconnected. Crucial factors that affect the well-being and along which the solution proposed by NESTORE will be developed are: (i) physiological status and physical activity behaviour, (ii) nutrition, (iii) cognitive capabilities, (iv) mental and psychological wellbeing, and (v) social interaction.

Physiological Status and Physical Activity Behaviour. Ageing is characterized by motor function impairment such as coordination difficulty, slowing of movements, and difficulties with balance and gait [1]. These deficits may have a negative impact on the ability to perform daily activities and may result in a reduced independence and self-confidence, thus increasing the risks of traumatic events (i.e., falls) and social exclusion. Progressive and generalized **loss of skeletal muscle mass and strength** (i.e., sarco-penia) is physiologically associated with ageing and has an important impact on well-being [2]. **Physical activity** is a most effective intervention to counteract skeletal muscle impairment [3]. The aerobic and anaerobic physical activities should be tailored to the older people in order to retain or improve their cardiovascular fitness, muscle strength and overall balance.

Nutrition. The process of ageing involves a steady decay of the metabolic flexibility [4]. The whole metabolism is more sensitive to unbalanced diets and to **suboptimal nutrition**. Ageing also involves the senescence of tissues and metabolic processes, which results in altered absorption of nutrients together with decreased capacity in detoxifying by-products. Therefore, during this period of life, a **balanced diet together with optimal dietary patterns** is key in order to maintain the whole body homeostasis and to overcome the naturally occurring physiological limitations of the subject.

Cognitive Capabilities. Ageing is also related to **cognitive decline**, one of the most worrying age-related changes in later adulthood [5]. Whereas more knowledge-driven domains tend to be maintained relatively well, the more biologically-driven fluid abilities show average decline throughout adulthood, with accelerated decline late in life and prior to death. Cognitive training interventions are known to be successful in improving the trained abilities, with little evidence for transfer to unrelated areas or real life [6] The trainings, to be successful, need to engage older adults in novel tasks that are ecologically valid and easily integrated into the daily life routines.

Mental and Psychological Wellbeing. Other important aspects are the preservation of **mental wellbeing** of older people [7]. In order to ensure a mental wellbeing, interventions should focus on **psychological factors** (participation in activities that are relevant to an individual's personal goals, emotionally close personal relations, protection of a positive sense of self through prevention of discrimination), socioeconomic factors (i.e., financial security to meet one's personal goals), and physical health (i.e., successful management of physical conditions to ensure high subjective health).

Social Wellbeing. Strictly related to the previous dimension, another important aspect is the preservation of the **social capital** provided by older people. The socio-economic status, social integration and high personal competencies are related to higher subjective wellbeing [8]. The quality of the social contacts and the availability of emotionally meaningful social relations is, as well, an important factor to consider for a better wellbeing. There is evidence that voluntary work, as well as the educational and **social activity group interventions,** can improve the mental health and prevent social isolation and loneliness among older people.

3   The NESTORE Concept

With the objective of addressing the five dimensions described above with an integrated holistic approach, the solution will be developed in co-design with the users and will the potential of ICT to meet their needs. Co-design will ensure that users can be emotionally involved, thus achieving a significant step ahead in the empowerment of citizens and in promoting and actively sustaining active ageing.

3.1   The NESTORE Vision

The vision proposed is that of NESTORE as a friend and a companion. As a trusted friend, NESTORE can also be accepted as a coach.

NESTORE knows me and understands my emotions. We have only recently met, but it is as if we have known each other for our entire life. It is really an empathic and emotional relation that has been developed. I know you can count on him for the right support, for that one hint of encouragement when my will is not strong. Now it is really much more fun to take a walk, to perform those boring exercises needed to keep in good shape; thanks to NESTORE my social life is still active and I have even met new friends. Occasionally we play together and that also exercises my brain. He is there when I need him, but he also understands when I want to be left on my own. NESTORE really is the "answer" to my needs.

NESTORE is capable of valorising the capabilities of the person and helps him/her to select the vocational path along the five dimensions of the well-being profile, i.e.

nutrition, physical activity, cognitive, social and mental. NESTORE is also aware of the family ties and leverages them to add a human touch to the technology based service offering.

3.2 The NESTORE Services

This section provides an overview of the potential services NESTORE can provide to the target audience, and what is meant by "pathways of wellbeing". NESTORE is designed to address the needs of the older people of tomorrow, therefore the solution must be flexible to include technologies yet to come, and it must offer open and standardised interfaces so that new services – meeting new needs and preferences - can be offered by third parties. Computer literacy and capabilities to use technologies will also increase in the future. To better understand the users, the consortium will conduct focus groups, not only with people that today are in target (i.e. over 65) but also with people that today are in their 50ies, to understand how they see their future and what would be on target in 15 years and more from the present time.

Typical users of NESTORE are people that are familiar with modern technologies, are in a reasonably good health, have recently retired or about to retire and have a social life they want to keep. They remain users of NESTORE throughout the process of ageing. With age, NESTORE knows the person, becomes aware of possible degradation of functional capabilities and provides suggestions and services to compensate such shortcomings.

To start the initial definition of services, NESTORE works on the assumption that older people recently retired want or need to find new interests: new life, new challenges! They also have finally time to cultivate better existing interests. The theoretical base for the design of the solution starts from the Selection, Optimization and Compensation (SOC) model [9] that outlines general-purpose processes of specialization by selection of developmental pathways, preferences or goals. According to SOC, the goal of NESTORE is to empower the latent reserve capacity of older people to limit the age-related loss of skills, in relation to the 5 dimensions addressed by NESTORE. To foster motivation, NESTORE helps the user to select and identify a final purpose "*the wellbeing pathway*" (based on the risk perception, self-efficacy and outcome expectancies); it then facilitates the action planning and the maintenance of self-efficacy through the provision of a set of actions aimed at the achievement of the goal. Finally, NESTORE monitors the user's progresses in order to propose recovery actions in case of impediments or actual loss of motivation.

Adopting SOC, NESTORE will define specific pathways that meet user preferences and whose aim is to allow reaching, by the older people, the maximum capacity of their latent reserve, that guarantees an active and healthy ageing. Such definition is related to the **Selection** component of the SOC model. It will then identify the building blocks that specify each pathway; this is related to the acquisition, application and integration of resources involved in attaining a higher level of functionality (internal or external) in all the dimensions (**Optimization**). Such building blocks can be represented as possible actions that the user shall perform to pursue its pathway and that are suggested, monitored and provided by the Virtual Coach. Finally, NESTORE monitors the user's level of motivation and engagement and intervenes to restore and manage impediment or loss of motivation (**Compensation**).

Following the approach described above, the following example of service provision scenario can be devised:

John is 65 and has recently retired. He loves gardening and now that he is free, he would like to spend more time in his garden. Mary, his wife, has in mind some renovations that have been postponed due to lack of time, bad weather, etc. In addition, doing some exercise in the garden will help to keep fit.

Gardening is the topic of the coaching activity selected by John. NESTORE has learned about the interest in gardening on the basis of John's profile and John has confirmed this. By means of the profile data and other data coming from observing the user, NESTORE sets quantitative goals that optimize John's health and wellbeing status according to the NESTORE Integrated Wellbeing Model and proposes a set of activities that foster the achievement of the defined goals. NESTORE then monitors John's progresses in order to outline and manage the possible loss of motivation. The services proposed by NESTORE come from a combination of required activities according to the Integrated Wellbeing Model, i.e. the need to perform certain physical exercises to keep muscle strength or to maintain the cardio-respiratory function, to ensure a certain level of social activities, etc.; these services will support the user in performing them within the topic of gardening, making them more pleasurable for the user. As John performs the activities proposed by NESTORE, he can gain points on the NESTORE system that will reward him with new services, such as e.g. discounts. Indeed, offering open interfaces to third parties, service providers may join the NESTORE network, so that they can advertise their services directly on the platform, and join the stakeholders' network. Within NESTORE we will develop a limited number of potential pathways, based on the results of the focus groups. Such pathways will be demonstrated and tested in the pilots.

3.3 The NESTORE Technologies

In order to achieve such an ambitious vision, the research brings together different technologies and resources from several European partners and leverages the most advanced state of the art technologies. With a bottom-up approach, the following areas of research are addressed:

- **Information gathering technologies, to learn things about the user.** Here we include Sensing Technologies with a wide approach, including passive and active monitoring, based on a pervasive IoT. We aim at knowing the user "intimately" therefore we want to understand habits, feelings and emotions, the environment, the social life and other key information about the user, including – of course – the health status. According to a human model that covers the five dimensions of the NESTORE interventions, we will investigate several conventional and unconventional sensing technologies that can generate data about the user achieving advanced personalisation of the solutions and related service offerings. Such technologies include wearable sensors, cameras, environmental sensors, social networks, games, etc. The actual selection will be guided by the results of focus groups with users.

- **Technologies for information analysis to understand the user and to generate the appropriate feedback.** NESTORE will support the development of pathways of wellbeing, proposing different actions and services and then coaching the user so that motivation can be sustained in time. The data collected are analysed by a decision support system (DDS) that determines the type of intervention. The NESTORE DSS will be based on a three-layer structure: (1) a short-term analysis that analyses data on a daily basis; (2) a long-term analysis that looks at trends and is able to detect change and adapts the coach in the long term, following the changing needs of people as they age; (3) a combined short and long-term analysis to provide personalized plans as part of the Coaching function.

- **Technologies to convey the feedback to the users, i.e. the Coaching System, the embodiment of NESTORE.** From the point of view of the user interaction NESTORE combines different modalities (tangible voice and touch) and different devices (smartphones, tablets, PCs, smart TV, etc.). Within the project we will investigate the use of tangible objects that may favour an affective interaction, supporting the user in a continued use of the system. Gamification mechanics will be used to support motivation, rewarding the users for positive behaviours.

- **Technologies to deploy and control sensing environments: Pilot Sites.** All the technologies used and developed will be integrated to offer an intelligent system easy to configure, deploy and replicate in various pilot sites. Existing IoT platforms and cloud infrastructures represent today a viable solution to implement features envisioned by Smart Environments concept. Cloud services will be beneficial for two reasons: (1) there are fewer components deployed at home/site. (2) A unified view is offered for geographically distant sites. The management and configuration of the pilot site are simplified because less local interventions are required. The intelligence of the system is deployed in the cloud and the Control Centre interacts with the cloud to transparently tune or upgrade the system.

4   The NESTORE Methodology

4.1   Co-design and Participatory Approach

The methodological approach followed in NESTORE provides for users to be involved in the design of the solution throughout the project duration. The methodology adopted draws on the value of 'thinking with things' as a means to build an understanding of the factors end-users identify as being important in the design of digital health services and devices.

Literature highlights that the reason for non-acceptance of health technologies is complex. The role of the design is to better understand the broader physical and social environments in which services and technologies will operate and how they relate to the contexts of the end users' lives. NESTORE will adopt co-design tools and methods that will seek to engage and elicit information related to perception, acceptance and usability of technology to support healthcare. Such methods have been shown to be beneficial in the evaluation and design of health-care interventions [10].

4.2 Development of the Solution

Development of a multi-domain unobtrusive monitoring system, to monitor physiological and behavioural data related the five domains of wellbeing. Technical solutions based on advanced non-invasive monitoring systems, such as wearable and environmental sensors (indoor/outdoor), multifunction tangible objects, serious games, will be optimized and integrated. The *Wearable monitoring system* includes sensors suitable for end-user self-operating and allowing for an accurate assessment of meaningful physiological parameters. The *Environmental monitoring* system includes sensors for indirect monitoring of behavioural information, related for instance to nutrition, daily living activities patterns, physical activity, etc. *Multifunction tangible objects* include sensors suitable for indirect recognition of emotional and mental status. The *Serious games* integrate sensors suitable for monitoring cognitive abilities, such as memory performance or verbal fluency.

Development of an intelligent and innovative ICT Decision Support System (DSS), able to analyse the seniors' behaviour, tracking changes and compliance to active ageing guidelines, providing personalized target behaviours towards the adoption and maintenance of healthy lifestyle. For such a system to work effectively as a DSS, person's goals, overall cognitive/physical/mental and social status need to be assessed together with a profile of a person's daily life activities monitored using technology-based tracking systems in order to provide a reference frame and basis for the DSS that includes an individualized real-life approach rather than a mere population-based approach based on maximum performance laboratory-based assessments.

Development of an active coaching system, which, based on the user profile and needs, stimulates and engages older people with personalized coaching activities in a single or multiple wellbeing domains, following the Selection, Optimization and Compensation (SOC) model [9]. The coach will provide the necessary information to appropriately support the different phases of the behaviour change intervention, following the health action process approach (HAPA) [11]. The coach will be developed as a conversational agent able to assume different forms. In particular, it can be embodied in a physical companion that aims at establishing a trustful and affective communication with the user through multimodal communication channels. The emotionality of the communication can be supported by affective interactions with the coach, both through physical interactions with the tangible embodiment of the coach and through the semantic analysis of the conversations between the user and the coach.

System Validation. The solution will be investigated with the target user communities in three EU locations (Spain, Italy and The Netherlands) in order to take into account differences concerning nutrition habits and lifestyles as well as the cultural and social environment. The system will be tested in terms of usability and ease of user interaction, acceptability and effectiveness.

4.3 Validation of Solution Through Pilots in Real-Life Settings

Because of their different social organisation, end-user's recruitment will be based on participation of different entities and networks of each piloting sites, such as: older people associations, senior networks and volunteers' associations, primary care centres, and general practitioners, neighbourhood nurses, third age universities, social care providers, seniors' centres.

Different tools will be used in the piloting phase to collect the user's needs and preferences that the resulting ICT platform should take into account. The results of these tools execution will be considered including different functionalities and/or components of the platform. The first user testing will be focused on showing to the user the implemented functionality considering the requirements collected from the questionnaires and focus groups, on finding out if the User interface design (UI) concept was understandable and on verifying if they see the resulting service as something necessary and usable. This testing validated the functionality included in the prototype and allowed a refinement of the requirements collected in the focus groups and questionnaires, involving new functionalities and changes/additions of architecture components.

To evaluate the correctness of the measurements provided by the NESTORE's monitoring system, a measurement validation process will be carried out comparing measures obtained by sensors and devices with standardized measures including the same type of information obtained by standardized and validated tools.

The effectiveness of the coaching activity proposed by NESTORE will be evaluated in a sub-study. We will add some other assessment variables to analyse the impact in each one of the 5 domains included in NESTORE. Some complementary measurements will help to provide information on possible positive effects on the body produced by using the NESTORE platform.

5 Conclusions

NESTORE has the ambition to offer a solution that addresses healthy ageing with a wide-reaching and integrated approach, and by testing such solution in real-life settings in order to accelerate the process for digital innovation and to achieve wide acceptance by the target audience. The proposal has also the ambition to contribute to some aspects of the strategy of Triple Win for Europe, with specific attention to the older population.

- **Improve the health and quality of life of citizens**; by providing a solution along the concept of "wellbeing pathways" supporting senior citizens not only to keep their health but also to improve their quality of life with personalized and meaningful suggestions that encounter their preferences and fulfill self-achievement.
- **Support the long-term sustainability and efficiency of health and social care systems**; by providing a solution that allows people to live longer in their homes and a system that eases communication with the surrounding social.
- **Enhance the competitiveness of EU industry creating economic growth opportunities and jobs in the Silver Economy**; NESTORE aims at providing an open solution that allows the provision of services by third parties by means of open API.

In this manner novel services can be designed by innovative companies to reach a market that through NESTORE can offer loyalty programs. NESTORE therefore offers growth opportunities to innovative SMEs in the health and social care field.

Acknowledgments. NESTORE is co-funded by the European Commission under the H2020 program, GA769643. The authors wish to thank all the project partners for their contribution to the project.

References

1. Nelson, M.E., Rejeski, W.J., Blair, S.N., et al.: Physical activity and public health in older adults: recommendation from the American College of Sports Medicine and the American Heart Association. Med. Sci. Sports Exerc. **39**(8), 1435–1445 (2007)
2. Di Tano, G., Fulle, S., Pietrangelo, T., Bellomo, R., Fanò, G.: Sarcopenia: characteristics, genesis, remedies. Sport Sci. Health **1**(2), 69–74 (2005)
3. Freiberger, E., Sieber, C., Pfeifer, K.: Physical activity, exercise, and sarcopenia – future challenges. Wien Med. Wochenschr. **161**(17–18), 416–425 (2011)
4. Calçada, D., Vianello, D., Giampieri, E., Sala, C., Castellani, G., de Graaf, A., Kremer, B., van Ommen, B., Feskens, E., Santoro, A., Franceschi, C., Bouwman, J.: The role of low-grade inflammation and metabolic flexibility in aging and nutritional modulation thereof: a systems biology approach. Mech. Ageing Dev. **136–137**, 138–147 (2014)
5. Harada, C.N., Natelson Love, M.C., Triebel, K.: Normal cognitive aging. Clin. Geriatr. Med. **29**(4), 737–752 (2013)
6. Klimova, B., Valis, M., Kuca, K.: Cognitive decline in normal aging and its prevention: a review on non-pharmacological lifestyle strategies. Clin. Interv. Aging **25**(12), 903–910 (2017)
7. Steptoe, A., Deaton, A., Stone, A.A.: Psychological wellbeing, health and ageing. Lancet **385**(9968), 640–648 (2015)
8. Charles, S., Carstensen, L.L.: Social and emotional aging. Ann. Rev. Psychol. **61**, 383–409 (2010)
9. Freund, A.M., Baltes, P.B.: The orchestration of selection, optimization and compensation: an action-theoretical conceptualization of a theory of developmental regulation. In: Perrig, W.J., Grob, A. (eds.) Control of Human Behavior, Mental Processes, and Consciousness: Essays in Honor of the 60th Birthday of August Flammer, pp. 35–58. Lawrence Erlbaum, Mahwah (2000)
10. Schmittdiel, J.A., Grumbach, K., Selby, J.V.: System-based participatory research in health care: an approach for sustainable translational research and quality improvement. Ann. Fam. Med. **8**(3), 256–259 (2010)
11. Schwarzer, R.: Self-efficacy in the adoption and maintenance of health behaviors: theoretical approaches and a new model. In: Schwarzer, R. (ed.) Self-efficacy Thought Control of Action, Washington, DC, pp. 217–242. Hemisphere (1992)

GeriatricHelper: Iterative Development of a Mobile Application to Support Geriatric Assessment

Rafael Pinto[(✉)], Ilídio C. Oliveira, and Samuel Silva

IEETA/DETI, University of Aveiro, Aveiro, Portugal
rafaelfelgueiras@ua.pt

Abstract. Clinical assessment scales for specific medical subareas include domain knowledge that may not be of general awareness among practitioners, hindering the adoption of best practices. In this context, we propose a pocket guide for comprehensive geriatric assessment as a mobile application. The GeriatricHelper is an Android mHealth application developed under an iterative, User-Centered Design approach. Feedback from a broad set of users including domain experts has been obtained throughout and a functional prototype is currently being tested in a Portuguese hospital, allowing for any clinician to apply the otherwise experts-limited geriatric assessment.

Keywords: mHealth · Geriatrics · Comprehensive geriatric assessment
Android · Patient follow-up · Pocket guide · User Centered Design

1 Introduction

The Comprehensive Geriatric Assessment (CGA) [1, 2] is a multidimensional and interdisciplinary evaluation of the elderly. It is composed of mental, functional, nutritional and social areas of assessment, each one containing several related scales. Its main objectives are to reach a precise and full diagnose and facilitate prevention and follow up. CGA is applied to people over 75 years old, or over 65 if in risk situations, such as lack of social support, multiple pathologies, chronic disease or institutionalization. Being a multidisciplinary evaluation, it would ideally be applied by physicians, nurses, social services technicians, gerontology doctors and physiotherapists. It should be performed on a regular basis to better adjust to the decaying health conditions of some patients.

The inexistence of a formal medical specialty in Geriatrics, in Portugal, makes it difficult to widely apply CGA in routine, due to the lack of awareness and training to this kind of evaluation. There are only three medical centers in Portugal in which CGA is performed by a multidisciplinary team (nutritionist, doctor and pharmaceutical). For the remaining locations, CGA is applied by a single person, mainly an internal medicine doctors or general practitioner, filing a paper form. In the current practice, doctors need to calculate the result for each scale by hand.

After performing the scales relevant to the appointment, a health professional may need to prescribe medicine. The Start/Stopp [3] and Beers [4] criteria make up a

© ICST Institute for Computer Sciences, Social Informatics and Telecommunications Engineering 2018
P. Perego et al. (Eds.): MobiHealth 2017, LNICST 247, pp. 147–154, 2018.
https://doi.org/10.1007/978-3-319-98551-0_17

valuable tool, since they advise on drugs that should or should not be prescribed to the elderly. However, these encompass large lists that would profit from easier access.

In this paper, we describe the development of a mobile application to act as a pocket guide to assist any practitioner to apply the CGA scales, applying a User-Centered Design approach.

2 Related Work

Currently, there are some mobile solutions focused on assessing the elderly. PT-Measures [5] includes one scale from the mental area and five from the functional area, which are grouped by their respective area; each scale includes some associated textual info; scales can't be performed for a patient, instead, after performing each scale individually, the doctor inserts the patient's personal information; this application doesn't include any clinical criteria.

Indicators of dependence [6] contains eleven scales, from mental, functional and social areas, but scales aren't grouped into areas; there is detailed information on how to perform each scale, their scoring outcomes and associated bibliography; scales can't be associated to a patient, only saved with a keyword.

iGeriatrics [7] was developed by the American Geriatrics Society, doesn't include information on how to perform CGA, but instead covers a wide range of topics related to older adults, such as vaccinations and prevention of falls. It doesn't allow to perform scales, but contains the Beers criteria.

OncoScale [8] includes mental, functional and nutritive scales, grouped into areas; there is info about a scale's bibliography and how to perform it. As a side-note, none of these apps allows tracking patient's medication.

As we can see, some of them implement only part of the required functionalities. It is important to stress out that CGA is performed i.e., it can assess multiple areas and contain multiple scales or tests, while these apps only allow to perform one test at a time.

3 GeriatricHelper

Motivated by the abundance of smartphone devices, mainly Android, and the convenience for a technology-oriented CGA, we propose GeriatricHelper, an Android mobile application that implements a mobile-oriented CGA, act as a guide on how to perform CGA, and includes the clinical criteria that may aid health professional prescribing drugs for the elderly.

3.1 Methods

To implement this solution, we opted for User Centred Design (UCD) [9], based on the end-user characterization, example workflows and requirements, so the objective was to obtain a final product with high usability standards.

For requirements elicitation, in a first instance, Personas were built and scenarios defined for the context of interest. Personas provide examples of representative users, for better capturing not only the roles, but also the motivations of users in using the technology in their daily activities. Personas include a description of tasks, expectations, and user profiling information, to "humanize" actors.

Being an iterative process, we opted for short cycles of prototyping followed by evaluation adjusted to the current stage of development.

3.2   Users and Scenarios

The first stage of the development process consisted of a brainstorming session with a doctor from the Geriatric Studies Center (*Núcleo de Estudos de Geriatria* -GERMI) [10], of the Portuguese Society of Internal Medicine (*Sociedade Portuguesa de Medicina Interna*). During this session, some use cases were established, for the application, who would use it and in which context, as well as which high-level features should be implemented.

Then, we created four Personas, corresponding to two doctors and two patients (not provided here in full for compactness). One of the Personas is a doctor profile, Albert, a 55 years old Family Doctor. He performs the CGA daily. To view a patient's progress, he must consult the previous paper records and that can be quite cumbersome. Sometimes he uses his tablet to store notes about his patients.

One of the "patient" Personas is 82 years old Laura. She had a brain vascular accident which led to problems in locomotion and right side dexterity. Very often she experiences some level of depression. She has already taken some drugs to help her, but very frequently she finds herself questioning her daily life and feeling alone. She would like to feel more well fit into society.

Based on the Personas and on the information collected during the initial brainstorming session, scenarios were proposed. As an example, we have "Laura's monthly appointment". To reevaluate her, Albert decides it is better to redo every CGA test. He opens her patient profile in the app and creates a new evaluation for her. The doctor thinks that Laura has been sadder recently, so conducts a test for tracking depression. He checks her temporal evolution for that test and sees that the results got worse, so he should prescribe some medicine for that.

Albert consults the app and inserts the name of the medicine he has in mind. The app informs him that this medicine should be avoided for a health issue Laura already has. He searches another drug by using the Start criteria that inform which drugs are best for certain conditions.

3.3   User Requirements

The system requirements dictated the features included on each prototype. As expected, these changed along with the development of the application, since, after each evaluation, the overall performance results and participant feedback were discussed leading to ideas for new and refined requirements. Table 1 contains a list of the requirements considered for each of the prototypes (P1, P2 and P3).

Table 1. Requirements for each of the prototypes. New requirements that were added to each list appear in bold, strikethrough requirements weren't implemented on the prototype.

Prototype version	Subset of the original requirements list implemented
P1	1. Possibility to create new patients
	2. View a patient's profile
	3. Must allow to track the patient's progress
	4. Create new evaluations
	5. Act as a guide for choosing the best medicine for a given patient
	6. ~~Patients data must remain confidential always~~
	7. Store information relative to patients and evaluations
P2	**8. Act as a guide on how to conduct a CGA evaluation**
P3	**9. Export a session's result into a PDF file**
	10. Save drugs prescribed to a patient

3.4 Evolving Prototypes

Three prototypes were developed, beginning with a requirements elicitation and the outcomes of each iteration were subject of user assessment (Fig. 1).

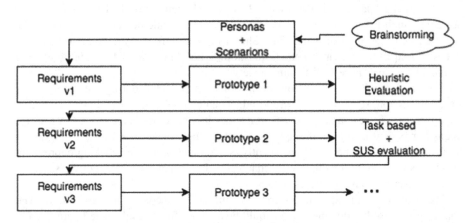

Fig. 1. Iterative design and development approach, integrating User-Centered Design, and multiple cycles of requirement elicitation, prototype development and evaluation.

3.4.1 First Iteration

The first prototype was based on the initial system requirements (Table 1). This prototype (P1) allowed to conduct public and private CGA sessions (Fig. 2a), consult medical criteria (Fig. 2d), and manage patient's profiles (Fig. 2c), along with their respective sessions.

The iterative method followed considers that the evaluation type should be adapted to the current stage of development. The objective for P1 evaluation was mainly to

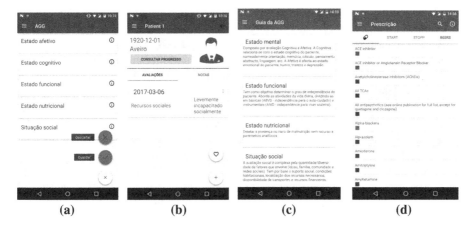

Fig. 2. Screenshots of the first (a), (b) and second (c), (d) prototype running on a smartphone. (a) displays an ongoing CGA session, (b) is a patient's profile, (c) the CGA guide and (d) a list of drugs.

expose issues concerning general usability guidelines, focusing on platform and context specific methods in later stages of the usability evaluation process. Being a broader evaluation, Nielsen's heuristics [11] were chosen as the evaluation method. Considering the general purpose of this first stage of evaluation, the users who participated in the evaluation were not yet domain experts, but five students from a Computer Science degree (at University of Aveiro) who had previous knowledge about Nielsen's heuristics. Besides those heuristics, we also considered as important the *Competency* concept from Health-ITUEM [12] and *Pleasurable and respectful interaction* and *Privacy* heuristics from the heuristics proposed for mobile interfaces [13].

Most of the usability problems found were not severe to the point to make it impossible for a user to use the application. The heuristic that had more flaws was Aesthetic and minimalist design, in both versions of the app (smartphone and tablet), with comments such as "There is too much text" or "Text is too small".

3.4.2 Second Iteration

The second prototype (P2) added the possibility to register in the app, contained improvements to patients and sessions management, allowed adding textual notes to a patient, the application could run on more devices, sessions appeared in a dedicated menu entry, made it easier to quickly check which type of requirements were associated to a drug, and allowed to consult tests information as a pocket guide (Fig. 2c).

P2's evaluation aimed to detect additional usability issues that become apparent when trying to reach concrete goals. Think aloud was the chosen evaluation method, since it is based in tasks and goals. Goals consisted of 15 tasks which the user will perform based on the workflows identified for the app from the devised scenarios such as "Check patient's progress relative to Clock Drawing scale" or "Consult Start criteria associated with Metformin". The participants in this evaluation were eleven individuals with knowledges of Human Computer Interaction (HCI) and/or mobile applications development.

Besides measuring the time taken to complete a task and the success rate, we deemed as necessary to have concrete values about usability and easiness while handling the application. Popular questionnaires include Software Usability Measurement Inventory (SUMI), Post-Study System Usability Questionnaire (PSSUQ), and the System Usability Scale (SUS) [14]. The first one requires purchasing a license so it was dismissed from the start. PSSUQ should be used carefully as it is susceptible to the "acquiesce bias" (people are more likely to agree with a statement than to disagree with it). Since all questions in the PSSUQ are positively worded this may occur.

SUS avoids this acquiesce bias, so it was chosen. The original version is in English, but, when applying it to Portuguese users, some of them may not be as capable of understanding the language as others. Therefore, since there is already a validated translation of this scale to Portuguese, we chose to use it [14].

Overall, the participants were able to complete the tasks (average success rate of 89%) although a few required more time to get acquainted with the application and exceeded the initial time given (see Fig. 3). Regarding SUS results (Fig. 4), the average was 78.4, the lowest 57.5 and the highest 97.5. SUS scores present an average of 68 [15], so, with an average score of 78.4, GeriatricHelper can already be considered as providing a good usability.

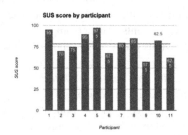

Fig. 3. SUS scores for P2's evaluation

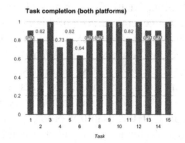

Fig. 4. Task completion for P2's evaluation

After the evaluation, and after solving some of the usability problems reported during the think aloud, a brainstorming session was conducted with a clinician, presenting the current state of the application and collecting suggestions that further informed the creation of the third prototype.

3.4.3   Third Iteration

The third prototype (P3) is currently in development. The main corrections and improvements to be included were: displaying a summary of each CGA area when conducting a CGA session; an increase in font size for some screens; the user was warned when trying to leave a scale without having answered every question; added feedback to actions that were lacking it and increased feedback time for key actions; added more contextualization for the user; and made more use of the bigger screen on the tablet. The added functionalities were the possibility to generate a PDF for a CGA session, which later could be archived on the patient's physical profile, and the ability to keep a list of drugs prescribed for each patient.

Its evaluation is underway, by clinicians, the end-users (pilot user group), and is mainly being focused on the functionalities themselves, since the most prominent usability issues were solved in the first two prototypes.

3.5   Security Issues

GeriatricHelper deals with personal clinical data, which must remain confidential and inaccessible to third parties. Implementing this may not be straight-forward, which may explain why most the apps mentioned do not make it available. The security enforcement for this system is based on the separation of demographic and clinical data, i.e., data which may lead to identifying a person, such as name, address and birthdate, is ciphered before being stored on a backend, while the other data, such as sessions and scales, are not ciphered on the backend, since they point out to the ID of a patient, not its personal data.

4   Conclusion

GeriatricHelper development followed a User Centered Design approach and aims at providing a valuable "pocket" application for the Portuguese geriatric community. Its functionalities were designed considering the Portuguese reality, with the active participation of domain professionals. The application is an improvement to the paper-only existing support, making it more practical to calculate scales and browse clinical recommendations.

As future work, the application that is already multilingual, needs to obtain the clinical validation for other health care context, to be used by an international community of practitioners.

Acknowledgements. The authors would like to thank the fruitful collaboration of SPMI-GERMI, especially Paulo Almeida, MD. This research is partially funded by Portuguese National Funds through the FCT - Foundation for Science and Technology, in the context of the project UID/CEC/00127/2013 and Marie Curie IAPP project IRIS (ref. 610986). Samuel Silva is funded by FCT grant SFRH/BPD/108151/2015.

References

1. Bassem Elsawy, M.D., Higgins, K.E.: The geriatric assessment. Am. Fam. Physician **83**, 48–56 (2011)
2. Tsaousides, T., Gordon, W.A.: Geriatric assessment tools. Mt. Sinai J. Med. **76**, 173–181 (2009)
3. Gallagher, P., Ryan, C., Byrne, S., Kennedy, J., Mahony, O.D.: STOPP START toolkit supporting medication review. Eur. J. Clin. Pharmacol. **46**, 1–12 (2008)
4. American Geriatrics Society (AGS), Geriatrics Society Beers Criteria for Potentially Inappropriate Medication Use in Older Adults: AGS Beers Criteria. Most, 2–5 (2012)

5. PT-Measures - Android Apps on Google Play. https://play.google.com/store/apps/details?id=com.sensingfuture.ptmeasures
6. Indicators of dependence - Android Apps on Google Play. https://play.google.com/store/apps/details?id=gt.app.dep
7. iGeriatrics - Android Apps on Google Play. https://play.google.com/store/apps/details?id=com.usbmis.reader.dwtf1
8. OncoScale - Android Apps on Google Play. https://play.google.com/store/apps/details?id=com.agmmultimedia.oncoscale
9. Wilkinson, C.R., De Angeli, A.: Applying user centred and participatory design approaches to commercial product development. Des. Stud. **35**, 614–631 (2014)
10. Sociedade Portuguesa de medicina interna. http://www.spmi.pt/nucleos_estudo_conteudos.php?id_nucleo=17
11. Alertbox: current issues in Web usability. Nielsen Norman Group
12. Brown, W., Yen, P.-Y., Rojas, M., Schnall, R.: Assessment of the health IT usability evaluation model (Health-ITUEM) for evaluating mobile health (mHealth) technology. J. Biomed. Inform. **46**, 1080–1087 (2013)
13. Yáñez Gómez, R., Cascado Caballero, D., Sevillano, J.-L.: Heuristic evaluation on mobile interfaces: a new checklist. Sci. World J. **2014**, 434326 (2014)
14. Martins, A.I., Rosa, A.F., Queirós, A., Silva, A., Rocha, N.P.: European Portuguese validation of the system usability scale (SUS). Procedia Comput. Sci. **67**, 293–300 (2015)
15. MeasuringU: Measuring Usability with the System Usability Scale (SUS). https://measuringu.com/sus/

A mHealth Patient Passport for Adult Cystic Fibrosis Patients

Tamara Vagg[1(✉)], Cathy Shortt[2], Claire Hickey[2], Joseph A. Eustace[3], Barry J. Plant[2], and Sabin Tabirca[1]

[1] Department of Computer Science, University College Cork, Cork, Ireland
{tv3,tabirca}@cs.ucc.ie
[2] Cork CF Centre, Cork University Hospital, University College Cork, Cork, Ireland
{cathy.shortt,claire.hickey1}@hse.ie, b.plant@ucc.ie
[3] HRB CRF, University College Cork, Cork, Ireland
j.eustace@ucc.ie

Abstract. Life expectancy for some Cystic Fibrosis (CF) patients is rising and new complications and procedures are predicted. Subsequently there is need for education and management interventions that can benefit CF adults. This paper proposes a CF patient passport to record basic medical information through a smartphone application (app), giving the patient access to their own data. It is anticipated that such an app will be beneficial to patients when travelling abroad and between CF centres. This app is designed by a CF multidisciplinary team to be a lightweight reflection of a current patient file. The passport app is created using PhoneGap so that is can be deployed for both Android and iOS devices. The app is introduced to seven participants as part of a stress test. The app is found to be usable and accessible. The app is now being prepared for a pilot study with adult CF patients.

Keywords: Cystic Fibrosis · mHealth · Patient passport

1 Introduction

Cystic Fibrosis (CF) is the most common life limiting genetic disease affecting Caucasians. Ireland has the highest occurrence of this disease in the world. Patient education is considered to be an integral part of care and can often improve quality of life [1]. Adult Cystic Fibrosis patients are often considered to be a well-educated cohort, however previous studies have identified knowledge gaps with this population [2, 3]. Life expectancy of this population is predicted to rise, with some patients expected to live to retirement age and as such further disease complications and or medical procedures may arise [4, 5]. With these medical obstacles, CF patients will be given new information and educated respectively. From a study conducted by Kessels it was found that between 40% and 80% of the medical information provided to patients by practitioners is forgotten immediately [6]. With this comes the need for education strategies and interventions which can be of benefit to the care of these patients and to overcoming

© ICST Institute for Computer Sciences, Social Informatics and Telecommunications Engineering 2018
P. Perego et al. (Eds.): MobiHealth 2017, LNICST 247, pp. 155–162, 2018.
https://doi.org/10.1007/978-3-319-98551-0_18

education barriers. It is also imperative that such interventions do not impede on their daily lifestyles.

Self-management often falls under the umbrella of patient education. An intervention such as a patient passport may aid in the delivery of such care and education materials [7]. A patient passport is a paper based intervention which allows the user to collect pertinent medical data to aid in the management and care of their condition. This is often used for those with long term illnesses or learning difficulties. One such passport was developed by Newell et al. [8] for asthma management. The passport is paper based and can be folded so that it fits into a wallet. The agenda of this passport is to store the information needed for an asthmatic to receive care on arrival to an emergency unit. By storing the information in a passport, it lessens the onus on the patient to repeat this information to various medical professionals and allows the care professionals more time with the patient rather than sourcing the information [8]. Similarly, a medication aid passport was developed by Barber et al. [9] which allowed patients to record details of their medicines. This study found that the passport had a positive effect on those patients and that it can aid in the dialogue of medications between patients and healthcare team members [9].

Life expectancy for some CF adults is rising, and considering the benefits of a patient passport, it can be stipulated that such a tool would be beneficial to adult CF patients. This paper proposes a patient passport targeted at adults with cystic fibrosis. However, unlike the aforementioned passports, the proposed passport will be developed as a mobile application (app). To the authors knowledge, this is the first passport app created for CF. The agenda for this app is to provide CF adults with their basic medical information and also to allow them to record their medications. By doing so, adult CF patients may become more educated to their condition which may improve therapy compliance. Additionally, three scenarios have been identified in which the proposed app may be of significance to a CF adult. Firstly, it can allow a patient to receive immediate care when traveling abroad. Secondly, to receive care if travelling between adult CF centres. Lastly, to bridge the gap between health care team members. These scenarios and the design of the passport app will be discussed further in the following section.

2 Design

This section will discuss the three outlined usage scenarios for the proposed app. It will then move on to discuss other design consideration such as the intended data to be recorded, potential pitfalls, solutions implemented, and additional features.

2.1 Usage Scenarios

Providing a tool for adult CF patients to record their basic medical information may prove beneficial, however it is pertinent to highlight scenarios that may require the use of the passport so that such a tool can be incorporated into the current care system. The scenarios in which this passport is considered to be of use are outlined in the following subsections.

Travel Between Centres: There are currently 5 adult CF centres in Ireland. As such patients may transfer between hospitals to receive care, depending on medical/personal reasons. CF patient files are hard copies only and it is not always possible to gain access to this file. As such scenarios where patients will move from one hospital to another, or are transferred, involves a patient arriving to a unit with limited information. This is resolved by frequent phone calls or requests for information. However, with this proposed app, a patient can arrive with their basic care information such as genotype, medications, recent history of lung function results, allergies and other medical conditions.

Travel Outside of the Country: Similarly, if a patient is to travel abroad and is then in need of care, the patient will have access to their most basic information necessary to receive care. The app also records contact details of their health care team members in case further information is required.

Bridging Gaps for the Health Care Team: It is pertinent that all antibiotics that are prescribed to a patient are recorded. Generally, it can be two months between standard clinical visits. In this time, it is possible for a patient to begin a new antibiotic as prescribed by a General Practitioner (GP). During the next clinical visit, CF nurses will ask patients if they have been on any new medications, which can be either forgotten or only partial information is remembered. With the use of this app, a patient can record any interaction with any member of their health care team from phone calls to clinic visits in order to provide a broader view of their care.

2.2   Recorded Medical Data

Members of the CF multidisciplinary team discussed which data is of importance to a patient in the scenarios as outlined previously. It is agreed upon that this mobile application should follow the same structure as that of a patient file, wherein there is data that is recorded only once, such as profile information. There is also data that is recorded rarely and can be edited and amended, such as medical conditions and procedures. Lastly, there is data that will be recorded at each clinic appointment such as weight, height, FEV1 and FVC. To note, although the app follows the same structure as a patient file, it does not record all information that is stored in a patient file, only the basic information required for treatment.

The app is then divided into three sections to reflect the structure above. These sections are named "My CF Information", "My Medical History", and "My Clinic Appointments"; this can be seen in Fig. 1B. The data stored in these sections are discussed below:

My CF Information: Data in this section is recorded once and can be amended by the user if required. Information that can be recorded includes: date of birth, date of diagnosis, sweat test, genotype, blood group, allergies, medications, medical team contact numbers, and physiotherapy techniques. This can be seen in Fig. 1C.

My Medical History: The data in this section will be filled out once initially and amended over time. This section is broken down into two sub sections. The first is

"My Medical Procedures" which records data such as the insertion and removal of a Portacath. The second section, "My Medical Conditions" records other diseases which can affect CF patients such as Diabetes.

My Clinic Appointments: This section is intended to record data for each meeting with a member of the health care team, which can occur every two to four months. The types of data that can be recorded here include Date, BMI, Weight, Health, blood Pressure, FVC Liters, FVC %, FEV1 Liters, FEV1 %, Bugs in Mucus, Treatment, and Comments. This section can also be used for annual assessments, phone calls to the health care team and General Practitioner visits. This can be seen in Fig. 1D.

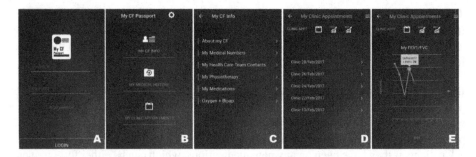

Fig. 1. Images showing: (A) Login Screen. (B) Main Menu. (C) My CF Info Screen. (D) My Clinic Appointments Screen. (E) Graph with FEV1 % and FVC % data.

2.3 Potential Pitfalls

Paper based patient passports have, in the past, been developed for diabetes patients, asthmatics and also for older adults, with each related study reporting a positive response from the patient. In a study conducted by Dijkstra et al. [10] it was found from interviewing patients that while these various patient passports have shown beneficial results, there continues to be issues which may result in a poor adaptation of the passport or negative effects. Such issues include: (1) Security, if the passport was to become lost or stolen there is potential for identity theft, (2) forgetting to bring the passport to appointments with various members of the health care team, (3) size and space, some patient passports can be the size of a small booklet and due to this can be unwieldy for patients to carry on the person, and (4) patients felt they had no time to enter information into their passport and did not want to waste valuable consultation time [10]. Dijkstra et al. [10] also found while interviewing members of the diabetes healthcare team that there are issues that affect using a patient passport as a patient intervention. One such issue is that of a clearly defined agenda for this intervention. As without clearly stating this agenda it is unclear as to how the passport should implemented into the patient's care and at which point of care it should be introduced [10]. Other discrepancies found in this study include: (1) If the passport is of any use to the health care team, (2) clearly stating who is responsible for filling out the passport, and (3) a sufficient introduction to the passport by the health care team so that the patient knows how to use the passport [10].

2.4   Solutions and App Implementation

The issues as outlined above were focused on diabetes passports only, however these problems are transferable. As such the above has been considered in the design of the adult cystic fibrosis passport this paper proposes. From issues outlined by patients, a digital platform has been incorporated as a solution. The CF passport is intended for use as an app for a smartphone device. By doing this, the passport app can be password protected and all data encrypted to avoid security issues in the event the phone is lost or stolen. An image of the login screen can be seen in Fig. 1A. Physical size and space will no longer be an issue as no additional space will be used to carry the app. Subsequently space in memory is now formed as a new consideration, however the data recorded through this app will be for basic information only, resulting in a minimal amount of memory being used on the smartphone device. Lastly, the issue of forgetting the passport is also reduced due to the popularity of smartphones. There has been a growth in smartphone users from 39% of the Irish population owning a smartphone in 2012 to 70% in 2015 [11]. It is also predicted that there are 2.32 billion smartphone users worldwide as of 2017 [12].

The remaining issues as highlighted by members of the diabetes team were discussed with the Cystic Fibrosis nurses, and the corresponding solutions were agreed upon by consensus. The app is intended to be introduced when CF pediatric patients transfer to the adult ward, however it can also be implemented for existing adult CF patients. For those patients who are interested in the app, they will be given a short workshop by the CF nurses who will explain the potential benefit of the app, what can be recorded and why this can of benefit, where to record the data, and how this app can be implemented into their care. During this workshop, the nurses will also assist the patient in inserting data that needs only be recorded once. The nurses will also advise that it is the responsibility of the patient to enter and record data and all data recorded is voluntary and will not be viewed by any other persons. A standard adult CF clinic appointment in Ireland can take up to 1 h and 15 min. In this time, the patient will meet with the CF nurse, the physiotherapist, the dietician and a CF registrar or consultant. The patient will be encouraged to fill in data with the CF nurses and time will be designated for this. However, if they would prefer not to fill it in with the nurses, there is approximately 15 min of non-contact time in between meeting the multidisciplinary team where the patient can record this information.

2.5   Additional Features

Other features are also incorporated into the app to aid patients with self-management. One feature which was added to visualise the recorded data to the patient are interactive graphs. There are two plot graphs currently. The first displays Weight and the second displays FVC % and FEV1 %. An example of this graph can be seen in Fig. 1E. Here the user can tap on the graph for more details on the data points, and hide/reveal values in the x and y axis. The app also provides access to the default device calendar. By doing this the user can save reminders for clinical and other related medical appointments.

3   Methodologies

The app is developed using Cordova Phonegap [13] which utilises web technologies such as HTML, JavaScript and CSS. The web technologies are then compiled so that the app can be deployed to both Android and iOS. The app also utilises the Framework 7 [14] framework for app navigation, style, and layouts for the appearance of a native app. The language used in the app is simple so that it can be understood by non-medically trained persons. All data recorded through this app is encrypted using the Advanced Encryption Standard (AES) algorithm and stored in a local SQLite database. Initially, the data is loaded from the database only after the user has successfully logged in. New data is entered into the local database once the user presses the submit button, and is reloaded each time the user enters new data. Once the user leaves or exits the app, this database is then closed. If the app deleted from the device, the databases will also be deleted. All graphs are developed using the Highcharts.js framework [15]. During the development process, the app was continuously reviewed and validated by members of the CF multidisciplinary team. The current app can be seen in Fig. 1.

3.1   Stress Testing

The purpose of this test is to evaluate the performance of this app and its design. Seven participants were enlisted who all had Android devices. To note, the participants did not have CF. The decision to recruit non-CF participants was so that performance and design issues could be remedied before clinical testing. The participants included three females and four males. The youngest participant was 19 years old and the oldest was 51, this age range is similar to that of the CF adults that the app is intended for. The participants varied in technical background. Some participants were actively working in the technology industry and were familiar with stress testing devices, while others would be considered novices.

The participants were given the app for three months and asked to add, edit and delete information to the "My CF Information" and "My Medical History" sections once a month. Similarly, they were asked to do the same for "My Clinic Appointments" once a week. At the end of every month the participants were asked to report on any performance or usability issues they encountered using the app via email. The participants from technical backgrounds were familiar with stress testing and as such were asked to focus on performance issues. The other users who would be considered novice were asked to focus on usability issues and features of the app that were easy or found difficult.

Overall the app was received positively by the participants. No user reported difficulty using the app or of any serious issues in the apps performance. From the study, some minor cosmetic issues were identified with varying phone screen sizes and resolutions. For example, the button outline would remain stationary on larger screen when the keyboard was visible, as opposed to moving with the button element. All users reported confusion with the format for a date entry. Another common issue reported by the users is that the "Go" Button on their keyboard did not navigate the user through a form as expected. These issues have now been addressed in a newer version of the app in preparation for pilot testing with CF adult patients. The app will be offered to CF adults who will also attend a workshop on how to use the app and its purpose with the Cystic Fibrosis Nurses. The CF adults will then be asked to use the app over a three-month period before answering a short survey. This clinical study is pending ethical approval. It is anticipated that the app will then be made available for all CF adult patients through the app store or other platforms.

4 Conclusion and Future Works

Patient passports have proven to help patients with self-management as it facilitates the ability to closely monitor their own condition, allowing for shared disease management. However as this is a paper based solution, possible issues arise such as the patient forgetting the passport, identity theft if lost, and the patient being over encumbered. These issues could be resolved by translating this intervention to a digital system such as an app. To the authors knowledge, a smartphone patient passport app has not been created for CF adults. This research proposes such a passport application which can allow CF adults to record their medications and basic CF information so that they can receive care. It is anticipated that providing a platform for CF adults to record and observe their CF information and actions may benefit medication compliance. The app is now being prepared to be pilot tested with a small cohort of adult CF patients. This pilot study will aim to evaluate the app and determine if a patient passport app will serve as a solution to the issues discussed with the paper based system. Following the results of this study the app will be subjected to a certification process before deploying to an app store or similar dissemination platform.

Acknowledgements. We would like to acknowledge funding from the European Commission for CFMATTERS, Grant agreement 603038.

References

1. Lycholip, E., Celutkiene, J., Rudys, A., Steponenieni, R., Laucevicius, A.: Patient education significantly improves quality of life, exercise capacity and BNP level in stable heart failure patients. Acta Cardiol. **65**(5), 549–556 (2010)
2. Conway, S.P., Pond, M.N., Watson, A., Hamnett, T.: Knowledge of adult patients with cystic fibrosis about their illness. Thorax **51**(1), 34–38 (1996)
3. Sawicki, G.S., Sellers, D.E., McGuffie, K., Robinson, W.: Adults with cystic fibrosis report important and unmet needs for disease information. J. Cyst. Fibros. **6**(6), 411–416 (2007)
4. Hodson, M.E., et al.: International study of aging in cystic fibrosis, an international/ multicentre report on patients with cystic fibrosis (CF) over the age of 40 years. J. Cyst. Fibros. **7**(6), 537–542 (2008)
5. Edwards, J., Clarke, A., Greenop, D.: Adults with cystic fibrosis–responding to a new ageing population. Chronic Illn. **9**(4), 312–319 (2013)
6. Kessels, R.P.: Patients' memory for medical information. J. R. Soc. Med. **96**(5), 219–222 (2003)
7. 'Patient passports' could help hospitals deliver better care. http://www.healthcarebusiness tech.com/hospital-patient-passport/

8. Newell, K., Basi, T., Hume, S.: Development of a patient passport in asthma management. Nurs. Stand. **29**(7), 37–42 (2014)
9. Barber, S., Thakkar, K., Marvin, V., Franklin, B.D., Bell, D.: Evaluation of my medication passport: a patient-completed aide-memoire designed by patients, for patients, to help towards medicines optimisation. BMJ Open **4**(8), e005608 (2014)
10. Dijkstra, R., Braspenning, J., Grol, R.: Empowering patients: how to implement a diabetes passport in hospital care. Patient Educ. Couns. **47**(2), 173–177 (2002)
11. eir Connected Living Survey. https://www.eir.ie/opencms/export/sites/default/.content/pdf/pressreleases/eir-connected-living-survey.pdf
12. Number of smartphone users worldwide from 2014 to 2020. https://www.statista.com/statistics/330695/number-of-smartphone-users-worldwide/
13. Adobe PhoneGap. http://phonegap.com/
14. Framework 7. https://framework7.io/
15. HighCharts. http://www.highcharts.com/

Suitability of Event-Based Prompts in Experience Sampling Studies Focusing on Location Changes

Anja Exler[(✉)], Sebastian Kramer, Miguel Angel Meza Martínez,
Christian Navolskyi, Michael Vogt, and Michael Beigl

TECO, Karlsruhe Institute of Technology (KIT), Karlsruhe, Germany
exler@teco.edu
https://www.teco.edu

Abstract. Among others, location changes and activity level are indicators for state changes of patients suffering from affective disorders such
as Bipolar disorder, Borderline personality disorder or depression. It is a
common means to assess this information via self-report questionnaires.
Usually, these are sent out either randomly throughout the day or at
fixed points in time. However, this might lead to missing records of location changes. We propose to rely on event-triggers: send out self-report
prompts when a location change is automatically detected. We enhanced
the ESMAC application by a location change detection event. Then, we
created three different study configurations for each trigger type: random, time-based, and event-based. In a three-week within-subject study
we let subjects experience each trigger type in randomized order. We
found statistically significant differences in favor of the event-triggers in
terms of number of prompts, response rate, prompts after detected location changes, and prompts after detected activity changes. We conclude
that event-triggers based on a location change detection shall be used
as trigger type for experience sampling studies focussing on location or
activity changes.

Keywords: Experience sampling method · ESMAC
Location changes · Mobile sensing · User experience

1   Introduction

In clinical psychology the assessment of states and state changes of patients
suffering from affective disorders – e.g. depression, bipolar or borderline personality disorder – is important to perform an appropriate treatment [1,2]. Location
changes and user activity information are relevant as they can provide insights
about motoric activity (lethargically staying at home vs. moving from one place
to another) or avoidance of other people (staying at home vs. changing location) which are symptoms of depression [3]. Such context information relates to
states and state changes [4]. Psychomotoric changes in patients suffering from

© ICST Institute for Computer Sciences, Social Informatics and Telecommunications Engineering 2018
P. Perego et al. (Eds.): MobiHealth 2017, LNICST 247, pp. 163–168, 2018.
https://doi.org/10.1007/978-3-319-98551-0_19

depression is mirrored in the patient's movement behavior and their location changes [5].

The most common method in clinical psychology to assess user behavior information is to apply experience sampling or ecological momentary analysis to monitor the patient by tracking their daily activities with their smartphones and to prompt them to answer self-report questionnaires. These prompts are displayed in form of smartphone notifications. Related work distinguishes three prompting types: random, time-triggered and event-triggered [6]. *Random* means that prompts are sent our randomly over the day, only the number of prompts is fixed. *Time-triggered* means that prompts are sent out at pre-defined points in time such as every full our between 8 a.m. and 10 p.m. *Event-triggered* means that prompts are sent out if a specific event happens such as a location change or when a certain activity is performed.

We investigated the suitability of these three prompting types for assessing information about the location changes and activities within a field-study and present the results.

2   User Study

Study Design. We wanted to oppose three trigger types and assess how user experience each of them and how they quantify against each other in terms of number of prompts and response rate (number of responses/number of prompts) as well as percentage of prompts after actual location or activity changes. We decided to design the study within-subject with randomized order to counteract carry-over effects. Subjects were prompted for self-reports between 8 a.m. and 10 p.m. to allow them to rest over night without being disturbed. 14 prompts were sent out randomly over the day for the *random* condition. *Time*-triggered prompts appeared at each full hour, i.e. also 14 times. *Event*-triggered prompts appeared at each detected location change, i.e. the number varies per day and per subject.

Location Change-Aware Experience Sampling Application. To assess location changes and activities we required an experience sampling application. We enhanced ESMAC, the experience sampling method app configurator [7]. First, we added a location change detection mechanism as a new event-trigger. We defined location changes as a situation in which a user showed movement behavior six times in a row. Movement behavior was defined as moving at least 60 meters in one minute, i.e. moving with at least 1 m/s. Next, we added questions to be displayed to the user. They consisted of questions about the current and last location and about the current and last activity. Last, we had to configure the trigger type for each study condition. In the end, we had three different configuration files: each one for random, time-trigger, and event-trigger, respectively.

Procedure. At the beginning of the study, we met with the subjects, explained the study and asked them to sign a consent form. Afterwards, we installed the app with the first configuration and asked for demographic data. The user study itself lasted three weeks, i.e. one week per trigger type. It took place during lecture time to guarantee fairly similar circumstances for each week. We collected data from Monday to Friday. On the weekend, we exported and pseudonymized all log files and questionnaire answers from the smartphone, handed out feedback questionnaires about the experience with our app during the week and installed the new configuration file. At the end of the user study, we assessed the general experience with our app over all three weeks.

Subjects. Initially, 23 subjects participated the study. However, 4 of them quit during the study and for 2 subjects no data was collected due to technical issues. Three of the remaining 17 subjects were female, 14 were male. They were between 18 and 29 years old. We focused on students as subjects as they are digital natives and used to the usage of smartphones in everyday life. In addition, they have a regular week structure which guarantees comparable circumstances for each experimental condition.

3 Results

We looked into number of prompts, response rates, and the accurate detection of actual location and activity changes. The latter will be presented in form of the relation between the number of questionnaires prompted after an actual location or activity change relative to the total number of prompts. Table 1 gives an overview of the results. It might be surprising that some subjects apparently received less than 70 prompts for random and time-triggered which is the expectancy value (5 days, 14 prompts per day). Apparently, some subjects turned their phone off during the study causing less prompts. What is visible is that event-triggered prompts are fewer but more accurate in terms of prompting after actual location or activity changes. This type also shows a higher response rate that might be caused by a higher user compliance due to fewer prompts.

To evaluate if the differences between different trigger types are statistically significant or caused by coincidence, we ran correlation analyses. As the data is not normally distributed, we decided to perform parameter-free Friedman tests. The results are listed in Tables 2, 3, 4 and 5. Differences between event and time and between event and random triggers show p values below .05 and, thereby, statistical significance. This proofs that location-aware event triggers are most suitable in experience sampling studies focussing on location and activity changes.

Table 1. Overview of number of prompts, response rates, and the accurate detection of actual location and activity changes for each trigger type.

	Time	Event	Random
Number of prompts	62.80 (±39.94)	19.50 (±9.55)	62.70 (±35.11)
Response rate	0.37 (±0.10)	0.43 (±0.09)	0.31 (±0.18)
Percentage of prompts after location change	0.28 (±0.16)	0.71 (±0.23)	0.29 (±0.19)
Percentage of prompts after activity change	0.41 (±0.19)	0.69 (±0.27)	0.37 8 (±0.19)

Table 2. Results of the pairwise comparison of all trigger types for the variable "number of prompts". Significant results are marked: $*p < .05$; $**p < .01$

Number of prompts	Time		Event		Random	
	Mean difference	p value	Mean difference	p value	Mean difference	p value
Time			43.3	.014*	0.1	1
Event	−43.3	.014*			−43.2	.005**
Random	−0.1	1	43.2	.005**		

Table 3. Results of the pairwise comparison of all trigger types for the variable "response rate". Significant results are marked: $*p < .05$

Response rate	Time		Event		Random	
	z value	p value	z value	p value	z value	p value
Time			−1.988	.047*	−1.682	.093
Event	−1.988	.047*			−2.497	.013*
Random	−1.682	.093	−2.497	.013*		

Table 4. Results of the pairwise comparison of all trigger types for the variable "percentage of prompts after detected location change". Significant results are marked: $*p < .05$; $** < 0.01$

Percentage of prompts after detected location change	Time		Event		Random	
	z value	p value	z value	p value	z value	p value
Time			−2.805	.005**	−0.459	.646
Event	−2.805	.005**			−2.701	.007**
Random	−0.459	.646	−2.701	.007**		

Table 5. Results of the pairwise comparison of all trigger types for the variable "percentage of prompts after detected activity change"'. Significant results are marked: $*p < .05$; $**p < .01$

	Time		Event		Random	
Percentage of prompts after detected activity change	Mean difference	p value	Mean difference	p value	Mean difference	p value
Time			0.285	.001**	−0.04	1
Event	−0.285	.001**			−0.326	.048*
Random	0.04	1	0.326	.048*		

4 Conclusion

Within a three-week study we collected location change and activity information from 17 subjects using three different trigger-types for self-report prompts. We opposed all three trigger types in terms of number of prompts, response rate and detection of actual location and activity changes. We found that the event-trigger scored highest in all categories. Statistical tests proof that the scoring differences are significant *between event and time* and *between event and random* triggers. The low number of prompts for event triggers goes together with a high response rate. We assume that this is due to higher user experience: fewer prompts and prompts that relate to the current user context (location and activity change) result in a higher compliance. Hence, we suggest to use event triggers whenever an event trigger is available that relates to items in the questionnaire.

We see a high potential of these findings for context recognition in clinical psychology. Apart from triggering prompts, location changes can reveal regularity, duration, and frequency of location visits. These aspects can give a deeper insight into affective disorder symptoms such as loss of interest to perform usual activities or decreasing motoric activity.

We intend to design and conduct further studies with patients suffering from affective disorders as subjects. Thereby, we want to gain insights about their location change behavior and evaluate the usefulness of our location detection for phase change detection. We might even consider place types[1] [8] or WiFi SSIDs as location [9].

References

1. Trull, T.J., Ebner-Priemer, U.: Ambulatory assessment. Annu. Rev. Clin. Psychol. **9**, 151 (2013)
2. Trull, T.J., Ebner-Priemer, U.W.: Using experience sampling methods/ecological momentary assessment (ESM/EMA) in clinical assessment and clinical research: introduction to the special section (2009)

---

[1] https://developers.google.com/places/supported_types?hl=en.

3. Davidson, G.C., Neale, J.M.: Abnormal Psychology. Wiley Publishing Co., New York (1996)
4. Grunerbl, A., et al.: Smartphone-based recognition of states and state changes in bipolar disorder patients. IEEE J. Biomed. Health Inform. **19**(1), 140–148 (2015)
5. Reichert, M., et al.: Improving motor activity assessment in depression: which sensor placement, analytic strategy and diurnal time frame are most powerful in distinguishing patients from controls and monitoring treatment effects. PLoS ONE **10**(4), e0124231 (2015)
6. Fisher, C.D., To, M.L.: Using experience sampling methodology in organizational behavior. J. Org. Behav. **33**(7), 865–877 (2012)
7. Bachmann, A., et al.: ESMAC: a web-based configurator for context-aware experience sampling apps in ambulatory assessment. In: Proceedings of the 5th EAI International Conference on Wireless Mobile Communication and Healthcare, pp. 15–18. ICST (Institute for Computer Sciences, Social-Informatics and Telecommunications Engineering) (2015)
8. Exler, A., Braith, M., Schankin, A., Beigl, M.: Preliminary investigations about interruptibility of smartphone users at specific place types. In: Proceedings of the 2016 ACM International Joint Conference on Pervasive and Ubiquitous Computing: Adjunct, pp. 1590–1595. ACM (2016)
9. Exler, A., Urschel, M., Schankin, A., Beigl, M.: Smartphone-based detection of location changes using WiFi data. In: Perego, P., Andreoni, G., Rizzo, G. (eds.) MobiHealth 2016. LNICST, vol. 192, pp. 164–167. Springer, Cham (2017). https://doi.org/10.1007/978-3-319-58877-3_22

Advances in Personalized Healthcare Services

Multi-modal User Interface Design for a Face and Voice Recognition Biometric Authentication System

Ilia Adami, Margherita Antona, and Emmanouil G. Spanakis$^{(\boxtimes)}$

Institute of Computer Science, Foundation for Research
and Technology - Hellas, 71110 Heraklion, Crete, Greece
`{iadami,antona,spanakis}@ics.forth.gr`

Abstract. Biometrics refer to unique measurable characteristics and information regarding individual's health, physical or mental condition and can be used to uniquely authenticate or verify a person's identity. They can be sorted in physiological such as fingerprints, palm print, face recognition, iris recognition, retina and DNA and behavioral such as typing rhythm (i.e. signature) and voice and can be described based on the uniqueness, potential change with time (i.e. facial changes), the feasibility to be collected (i.e. fingerprints) and the purposes of usage. In this work we study the use of a biometric technology for eHealth. We present the SpeechXRays project initiative that aims to provide a solution combining the convenience and cost-effectiveness of face and voice biometrics, achieving better accuracies by combining it with video, and bringing superior anti-spoofing capabilities. We explain how a novel user interface biometric platform is designed and adapted, for an eHealth use case, to enable secure access for medical specialists, nurses and patients to a collaborative eHealth platform that provides access to clinical and health related data within and possible outside a hospital. This is the first study, in the field, that gathered all necessary requirements (for a voice/face biometric system) and provides a formative evaluation and implementation of the SpeechXrays system user interface, for both end users and administrators, following a user-centered design approach, based on the holistic consideration of the user experience and the technical implication and functional requirements of the platform.

Keywords: Biometric authentication/verification · Voice · Acoustic
User interface design · Heuristic/guidelines · Smartphone · Mobile
Internet of things · Personal health systems · eHealth/mHealth

1 Introduction

Biometrics refers to the automated recognition of individuals based on biological (i.e., face, fingerprint, iris, voice, DNA, etc.) or behavioural traits (i.e., keyword dynamics, signature, gait, etc.) [13]. Biometric authentication is a natural alternative to traditional authentication systems like password schemes and secure electronic identification cards that promises increased security and user convenience [1]. A typical biometric authentication involves two stages, the enrolment stage and the verification stage.

© ICST Institute for Computer Sciences, Social Informatics and Telecommunications Engineering 2018
P. Perego et al. (Eds.): MobiHealth 2017, LNICST 247, pp. 171–181, 2018.
https://doi.org/10.1007/978-3-319-98551-0_20

During the enrolment, the system acquires a biometric trait of an individual (i.e., iris, fingerprint, face, voice, etc.), extracts a specific feature set from it and stores it in a database as a template. It then assigns an identifier associating the created template with an individual. During the verification stage, the system once again acquires the biometric trait of an individual, extracts a feature set from it, and compares it against the templates that are stored in the database in order to verify the claimed identity [11].

SpeechXRays aims to develop and test, in real-life environments, a user recognition platform based on voice acoustics analysis and audio-visual identity verification. The vision is to combine and pilot two multi-channel biometrics techniques: acoustic driven voice recognition (using acoustic and not statistical only models) and dynamic face recognition. SpeechXRays aims to outperform current state-of-the-art solutions in the areas of *Security*: high accuracy solution, *Privacy*: biometric data stored in the device, *Cost-efficiency*: use of standard embedded microphone and cameras (smartphones, laptops) and most importantly **Usability**: text-independent speaker identification (no pass phrase), low sensitivity to surrounding noise and state of the art **User interface design** for user interaction. Usability evaluation will be performed during the pilot of the two multi-channel biometrics techniques: ***acoustic driven voice recognition*** (using acoustic and not statistical only models) and ***dynamic face recognition*** in the project use cases involving 2000 users in 3 pilots: a *workforce*, an *eHealth* [23, 24] use case and a *consumer use case*. This paper describes the activities concerning the design, formative evaluation and implementation of the SpeechXrays system user interface, for both end users and administrators, following a user-centered design approach, based on the holistic consideration of the user experience and the technical implication and functional requirements of the platform. We present the methodology followed for the design of the user interfaces of the SpeechXRays system based on general usability and user interface requirements, as well as specific use cases requirements [22]. Based on this analysis several UI prototypes were designed and assessed following a formative usability evaluation approach. A mock up system was created to guide user interface development and integration to support UI adaptations as required by the SpeechxRays verification framework. Figure 1 presents the user interaction for the verification of medical personnel, for management of sensitive medial data such as medical information for patients, in the eHealth use case. We present a novel interface design methodology for interactive biometrics applications, taking into consideration all complex functional biometric processes and parameters, such as the scope/goal of the application, the functional and non-functional user requirements, the profile of the targeted end-users, the device type it will be served from, the context of the application (inside a hospital) and the interaction modes (touchscreen vs traditional mouse and keyboard), etc.

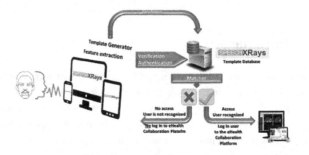

Fig. 1. SpeechXrays workflow for eHealth scenario

2   Design Methodologies and Results

Designing user interfaces for interactive systems in general is a complex process that has to take into consideration many parameters, such as the scope of the end application, its target audience, the functional and non-functional requirements, and the interaction mode (keyboard and mouse, touch, voice, gestures, etc.). In this paper we argue that traditional design guidelines and standards are not adequate, and thus, we focused our work on expanding existing lists with new guidelines to cover emerging interaction requirements for biometric authentication. Similarly, even though we have evidence for the creation of heuristics – for user interface design – in many different domains (robotics, virtual worlds, multimodal mobile applications, Smartphones, etc.), it seems that none of these is biometric related. Quiñones and Rusu [12] presented an extensive literature review conducted from 2006 till 2016 and identified 68 such domains, but none is related to biometric authentication – as described in SpeechXRays project. Even though recent research has shown that usability and reliability play an even more important role than privacy and trust in user acceptance of biometric authentication systems [7] and perceived convenience can be a bigger driver than any increase in security [8], a quick literature review will reveal that the majority of studies in this field concentrate mostly on the technical aspects of various biometric modalities [4, 5] conducting evaluations on their accuracy, reliability and overall performance, such as in the studies presented in [1–3, 9, 10]. As of today, at least to our knowledge, there are no concrete user interface guidelines for biometric authentication systems.

2.1   User Interface Design Methodology

The design of the user interfaces of the SPEECHXRAYS system was based on traditional HCI heuristics applied in the context of biometrics authentication. More specifically, Jacob Nielsen's list of usability heuristics [14] was used as the basis for the application's interface design (Table 1). Nielsen is an internationally known and well-respected usability engineer who along with Rolf Molich in 1990 developed a list of ten design principles for interactive applications [15].

The list was later refined by Nielsen to what is now commonly known as usability heuristics and the evaluation of any interface against these rules is known as heuristics evaluation. This list of guidelines was chosen because it has been validated through many studies over the years in the field of HCI and it has been proven as an effective method for safeguarding usability. In addition, a literature review on biometric authentication systems was performed to gather any design guidelines or principles specific to biometrics applications as they may have been published in recent empirical studies in this field. Lastly, since one of the main requirements of this biometrics, application was for the system to be device independent, common mobile specific design guidelines and principles were used. Table 2 presents with the list of the collected design guidelines that were used for the UI design, along with the suggested design techniques that were used to fulfill them. Finally, Fig. 2 showcases a sample of the user interface prototype along with the respective design guidelines applied.

Table 1. Applying Nielsen's 10 heuristics to a biometric system.

H1. Visibility of system status. The system should always keep users informed about what is going on, through appropriate feedback made available within reasonable time.
The user has to be clear on how long he/she has to speak and look into the camera of the device for the system to take the template sample needed, in order to minimize the risk of premature process quitting and incomplete data processing [1], which can lead to user confusion and frustration.
H2. Match between system and the real world. The system should speak the users' language, with words, phrases and concepts familiar to the user, rather than system-oriented terms. Follow real-world conventions, making information appear in a natural and logical order.
Short textual descriptions should be available to clear out any misunderstandings and the main two processes, enrolment and verification should be presented in a separate way, but also in a way that the user understands that one precedes the other. All structural elements of the application (i.e. navigational menus, action buttons, title bars, etc.) should follow the conventional design guidelines for such systems.
H3. User control and freedom. Users often choose system functions by mistake and will need a clearly marked "emergency exit" to leave the unwanted state without having to go through an extended dialogue. Support undo and redo.
The user of the biometrics authentication system should be able to cancel an already started enrolment or verification process (i.e. provide *CANCEL* button or *BACK* controls). It is also necessary to provide a *REDO* action control – to notify the user to go through the process again – especially for low quality recording, as well as an option to *RETRY* if a verification session is unsuccessful.
H4. Consistency and standards. Users should not have to wonder whether different words, situations, or actions mean the same thing. Follow platform conventions.
In order to achieve uniformity in the way the application is presented and behaves in different operational settings, it is important for the user interfaces to be designed following common design guidelines and standards both for mobile and desktop applications.
H5. Error prevention. Even better than good error messages is a careful design which prevents a problem from occurring in the first place. Either eliminate error-prone conditions or check for them and present users with a confirmation option before they commit to the action.
In the context of biometrics authentication, environmental conditions such as humidity, temperature, and illumination, as well as performance factors such as ability of capturing good quality video and audio samples, may affect significantly the performance and accuracy of the system increasing the likelihood of errors [19]. It is, therefore, essential for the system to be proactive in preventing them from occurring in the first place. In the eHealth use case – where users are mostly occupied with their nursing and treatment work, a proactive system would automatically offered alternative authentication method if certain environmental conditions are not met and cannot be changed, i.e., illumination too low [5].
H6. Recognition rather than recall. Minimize the user's memory load by making objects, actions, and options visible. The user should not have to remember information from one part of the dialogue to another. Instructions for use of the system should be visible or easily retrievable whenever appropriate.

(continued)

Table 1. (*continued*)

User authentication is an interruption in the user's primary task, which may even cause a disruption to the working memory of the user [1]. Multimodal authentication, such as the case of face and voice recognition, is an even more demanding process for the user who is required to perform multiple actions to achieve successful task completion. Thus, the authentication process has to be clear, concise, and able to guide the user seamlessly through the steps.
H7. Flexibility and efficiency of use. Accelerators -- unseen by the novice user -- may often speed up the interaction for the expert user such that the system can cater to both inexperienced and experienced users. Allow users to tailor frequent actions.
The experienced or frequent user of the biometrics authentication system that has already enrolled in the system and wants to access the secured network should be able to do so with just two clicks, one for activating the VERIFICATION mode of the process and one for RECORDING the voice and face sample.
H8. Aesthetic and minimalist design. Dialogues should not contain information, which is irrelevant or rarely needed. Every extra unit of information in a dialogue competes with the relevant units of information and diminishes their relative visibility.
It is very challenging to design complex processes for mobile viewing and careful planning and designing is needed to avoid the risk of overcrowding the interface and creating confusion to the user. This can be achieved by clearly separating the navigational elements from the actual functional elements of the selected process, by providing one main action button for each screen and other types of commonly used mobile patterns.
H9. Help users recognize, diagnose, and recover from errors. Error messages should be expressed in plain language (no codes), precisely indicate the problem, and constructively suggest a solution.
This heuristic deals with what should happen in case an error does actually occurs. When this happens, it is essential for the system to present the error in a meaningful way to the user. This means that it has to be expressed in plain language and be descriptive of what the problem was.
H10. Help and documentation. Even though it is better if the system can be used without documentation, it may be necessary to be provided. Any such information should be easy to search, focused on the user's task, list concrete steps to be carried out, and not be too large.
Educating the user on how the biometrics authentication system works on a higher-level, how and where the biometrics data is stored and used by the application, how the templates are created and accessed, and how the system safeguards their privacy and security from cyber-attacks can eliminate confusion, skepticism, and other negative pre-notions that users that are not familiar with such systems may have formed.

Table 2. List of biometrics design guidelines and their matching techniques

G1: Visibility of system status
• Provide progress bars for all the system processes noted on the screen
• Provide visual/sound feedback after each action
• Visual cues for the status of devices involved in process
G2: Match between system and the real world
• Use familiar to the users wording
• Use design patterns users are familiar with
G3: User control and freedom
• BACK button available at all screens
• EDIT button available for user to change biometrics profile
• TRY AGAIN button in case of failure during the processes of verification and enrollment
• Provide alternative authentication method (i.e., traditional username / password)
G4: Consistency and standards
• Fluid and flexible User Interface (UI) layout and design
• Unified UI look, feel, and experience for all access platforms
G5: Error prevention
• Contextual inline instructions for correct placement of capture objects
• Status of bad operation and status of hardware
• Warning of poor environment conditions during enrollment and verification.
G6: Recognition rather than recall
• All main UI components and navigational elements should be visible at all times
• Follow simple, commonly design patterns for mobile devices
G7: Flexibility and efficiency of use
• Processing time and each process steps should be kept to a minimum
• User should be able to cancel a process and restart it
• Provide instruction section for novice users and immediate action for experienced users
G8: Aesthetic and minimalist design
• UI simple and not overcrowded with navigation elements and information
• Context sensitive information only
• One central action button per screen
• Clear look and feel with discrete graphical elements that are not tiring to the eye
G9: Help users recognize, diagnose, and recover from errors
• Display errors clearly and in descriptive text
• Error messages should not be in code
• Clearly communicate any process errors occurring provide descriptive error messages
G10: Help and documentation
• Provide a dedicated section with instructions / tips on how to create a good quality biometric template
• Provide both textual instructions and instructions in the form of a quick demo video or animated GIF

(*continued*)

Table 2. (*continued*)

G11: Focused content with one clear task
• Provide a goal oriented design by keeping calls-to-action front and center
• All information displayed on each page should be about the function that is provided in the particular page
G12: Provide a clear navigational path
• Use menu and navigation design patterns conducive to mobile interaction
• Keep menus short, one level of option only
• Provide an easy way to get back to the homepage
G13: Develop a single underlying system that allows for a unified experience across platforms and device sizes
• Responsive UI with fluid layouts to accommodate various screen resolutions
• Design the entire site for mobile interaction
G14: Design for Touch
• Design buttons with appropriate touch target size.
• Use appropriate colors & contrast.

2.2 Mobile Application Design Guidelines

There are many sources for mobile application design guidelines, such as articles published by professionals and commercial companies on technology websites and blogs, as well as papers published on scientific magazines and journals. Mobile industry leaders, Apple and Google, have both provided extensive design guidelines to developers of mobile applications for each platform respectively. Many of the published mobile best practices lists are based on Nielsen's traditional heuristics and have been expanded to include guidelines specific to the mobile use context. For the purpose of this project, a selection of four guidelines were extracted from publications [16–18, 20, 21] and used in the design of the user interfaces prototypes. These four were selected because they are complementary to the Nielsen's heuristics.

G1: Focused Content with One Clear Task. Designing with minimalism in mind is even more essential for mobiles than desktop application because in mobile devices the users have to deal with smaller screens and touch interaction. Clutter and competing graphical and interaction elements do not enhance user experience and they should be kept to a minimum. Each page should have one central focus and that should be dedicated to the task at hand [17]. The application should guide the users seamlessly through task completion without disrupting their flow. In the biometrics application context, this applies both for the verification and the enrolment processes which include multiple steps.

G2: Provide a Clear Navigational Path. Again the limitations in the viewing space on mobiles calls for less elaborate menus and navigation mechanisms than those often found in desktop websites. Thus, multi-level menus with sub menus that show on hover

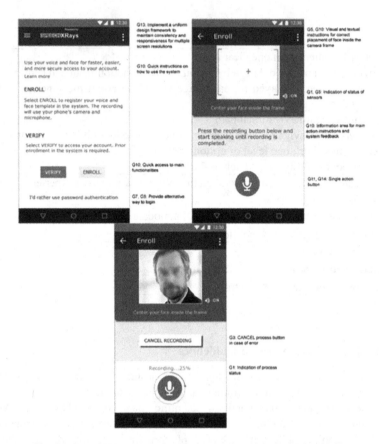

Fig. 2. SpeechXRays user interface samples with applied guidelines

and side navigation bars are not recommended in mobile design. In addition, the navigable path to task completion should be clear so that the users will be able to understand right away how they can interact with the application to achieve task completion [17].

G3: Develop a Single Underlying System that Allows for a Unified Experience Across Platforms and Device Sizes. This guideline is extremely important for all mobile applications and is referred in many studies [16, 17] and especially important for this biometrics authentication system since it addresses one of the main user requirements for the system which is, to be device independent. One of Google's guidelines is to optimize the entire site for mobile use. Participants in their study had a much easier time navigating mobile-optimized sites than trying to navigate desktop sites on mobile devices. Sites that included a mix of desktop and mobile-optimized pages were actually harder for participants to use than all-desktop sites. Thus it is suggested to design the entire site for mobile use.

G4: Design for Touch. Designing for touch requires extra care to account for fingers of all shapes and sizes applying varying kinds of pressure to touch screens that respond differently. All form controls, action buttons, and other interaction elements must measure at least 44 points by 44 points and have adequate space around them, so that they can be accurately tapped with a finger [20, 21].

3   Conclusion and Future Work

Despite the rising issues for the security of the biometric data, biometric technology is used for a number of different types of applications ranging from modest (time and attendance of personnel for a small industry) up to expansive (integrity of a whole population cohort such as voters database). Depending on the applications, the benefits of deploying biometric tools may lead to increased security, increased convenience and increased accountability compared to other authentication methods (PINs, passwords etc.). Prior to opting for a biometric system, one must also consider the existing security solutions and requirement in the specific application domain where the biometric system will be embedded. This is critical especially when dealing with services that would allow access to sensitive medical data. The UI described here along with the presented list of design guidelines, will be evaluated to study insights on how to optimally design a modular biometric platform able to be used in the eHealth domain [25]. Users (i.e. Medical specialists) will use the remote biometrics tool of SpeechX-Rays to access a collaboration platform containing patient's eHealth record and the data for management of patient's chronic conditions. The pilot study will also test the context-dependent feature that allows administrators to modify the false accepting rate or false rejection rate trade-off in order to reduce the risk of false reject for low security data and reduce the risk of false accept for high security data.

Acknowledgement. This work is supported by the research project "SpeechXRays" which receives funding from the European Commission (EC) through Horizon 2020 Grant agreement No. 653586.

References

1. Trewin, S., Swart, C., Koved, L., Martino, J., Singh, K., Ben-David, S.: Biometric authentication on a mobile device: a study of user effort, error and task disruption. In: Proceedings of the 28th Annual Computer Security Applications Conference, pp. 159–168. ACM, December 2012
2. Nandakumar, K., Jain, A.K.: Biometric template protection: bridging the performance gap between theory and practice. IEEE Sig. Process. Mag. **32**(5), 88–100 (2015)
3. Chingovska, I., Dos Anjos, A.R., Marcel, S.: Biometrics evaluation under spoofing attacks. IEEE Trans. Inf. Forensics Secur. **9**(12), 2264–2276 (2014)
4. Toledano, D.T., Pozo, R.F., Trapote, Á.H., Gómez, L.H.: Usability evaluation of multi-modal biometric verification systems. Interact. Comput. **18**(5), 1101–1122 (2006)

5. Bhagavatula, C., Ur, B., Iacovino, K., Kywe, S.M., Cranor, L.F., Savvides, M.: Biometric authentication on iphone and android: usability, perceptions, and influences on adoption. In: Proceedings of USEC, pp. 1–2 (2015)
6. Miltgen, C.L., Popovič, A., Oliveira, T.: Determinants of end-user acceptance of biometrics: integrating the "Big 3" of technology acceptance with privacy context. Decis. Support Syst. **56**, 103–114 (2013)
7. De Luca, A., Hang, A., Von Zezschwitz, E., Hussmann, H.: I feel like I'm taking selfies all day! Towards understanding biometric authentication on smartphones. In: Proceedings of the 33rd Annual ACM Conference on Human Factors in Computing Systems, pp. 1411–1414. ACM, April 2015
8. Patrick, A.S.: Usability and acceptability of biometric security systems. In: Financial Cryptography, p. 105, January 2004
9. De Luca, A., Hang, A., Brudy, F., Lindner, C., Hussmann, H.: Touch me once and I know it's you! Implicit authentication based on touch screen patterns. In: Proceedings of the SIGCHI Conference on Human Factors in Computing Systems, pp. 987–996. ACM, May 2012
10. Blanco-Gonzalo, R., Diaz-Fernandez, L., Miguel-Hurtado, O., Sanchez-Reillo, R.: Usability evaluation of biometrics in mobile environments. In: 2013 6th International Conference on Human System Interaction (HSI), pp. 123–128. IEEE, June 2013
11. Jain, A.K., Nandakumar, K., Ross, A.: 50 years of biometric research: accomplishments, challenges, and opportunities. Pattern Recogn. Lett. **79**, 80–105 (2016)
12. Quiñones, D., Rusu, C.: How to develop usability heuristics: a systematic literature review. Comput. Stand. Interfaces **53**, 89–122 (2017)
13. Jain, A., Ross, A.A., Nandakumar, K.: Introduction to Biometrics. Springer Science & Business Media, Berlin (2011)
14. Nielsen, J.: Usability inspection methods. In: Conference Companion on Human Factors in Computing Systems, pp. 413–414. ACM, April 1994
15. Molich, R., Nielsen, J.: Improving a human-computer dialogue. Commun. ACM **33**(3), 338–348 (1990)
16. Yáñez Gómez, R., Cascado Caballero, D., Sevillano, J.L.: Heuristic evaluation on mobile interfaces: a new checklist. Sci. World J. **2014** (2014)
17. Joyce, G., Lilley, M.: Towards the development of usability heuristics for native smartphone mobile applications. In: Marcus, A. (ed.) DUXU 2014. LNCS, vol. 8517, pp. 465–474. Springer, Cham (2014). https://doi.org/10.1007/978-3-319-07668-3_45
18. Vilar Neto, E., Campos, F.F.: Evaluating the usability on multimodal interfaces: a case study on tablets applications. In: Marcus, A. (ed.) DUXU 2014. LNCS, vol. 8517, pp. 484–495. Springer, Cham (2014). https://doi.org/10.1007/978-3-319-07668-3_47
19. Unar, J.A., Seng, W.C., Abbasi, A.: A review of biometric technology along with trends and prospects. Pattern Recogn. **47**(8), 2673–2688 (2014)
20. Apple Developer: UI design do's and don'ts (2017). https://developer.apple.com/design/tips/
21. Google Developers: Up and running with material design (2017). https://developer.android.com/design/index.html
22. Spanakis, E.G., Spanakis, M., Karantanas, A., Marias, K.: Secure access to patient's health records using SpeechXRays a multi-channel biometrics platform for user authentication. In: 38th Annual International Conference of the IEEE Engineering in Medicine and Biology Society, Orlando, FL, USA, 16–20 August 2016 (2016)

23. Chronaki, C., et al.: An eHealth platform for instant interaction among health professionals. In: Computers in Cardiology 2003, Thessaloniki Chalkidiki, 21–24 September 2003, vol. 30, pp. 101–104 (2003). (02766574)
24. Spat, S., et al.: A mobile android-based application for in-hospital glucose management in compliance with the medical device directive for software. In: 2nd International ICST Conference on Wireless Mobile Communication and Healthcare (MobiHealth 2011), Kos Island, Greece, 5–7 October 2011 (2011)
25. Spanakis, E.G., et al.: Technology-based innovations to foster personalized healthy lifestyles and well-being: a targeted review. J. Med. Internet Res. 18(6), e128 (2016). https://doi.org/10.2196/jmir.4863

Gaze Alignment Techniques for Multipoint Mobile Telemedicine for Ophthalmological Consultations

Ramkumar Narayanan[1(✉)], Uma Gopalakrishnan[1], and Ekanath Rangan[2]

[1] Center for Wireless Networks and Applications (WNA), Amrita University,
Amritapuri, Kollam, India
ramkumar@am.amrita.edu
[2] School of Medicine, Amrita University, Kochi, India

Abstract. Telemedical consultation systems are emerging as a viable medium for patient-doctor interaction in a number of medical specialties. Such systems are already prevalent in fields like cardio diagnosis and it is still very nascent in the field of ophthalmology. But with the emergence of affordable and high quality remote-control cameras, a host of new possibilities have opened up. In this paper, we have developed innovative gaze alignment techniques for ensuring Mutual Gaze, Gaze Awareness and Gaze following. The system is shown to work effectively even for interactions that are as complex as involving multiparty consultations involving remotely located patients through the use of a mobile telemedicine network and general physician/ physician-assistant and specialist ophthalmologist.

Keywords: Ophthalmology · Gaze · Mobile telemedicine

1 Introduction

There are several existing technologies that enable telemedicine consultation in the fields of cardiology [1, 2], neurology etc. However, in the field of ophthalmology, gaze is an important factor that directly impacts the effectiveness of an ophthalmological diagnosis. It is observed that out of the 45 million blind worldwide, 80% is curable. The vast rural populous, particularly in the developing world cannot afford visits to super specialty tertiary hospitals. Mobile Telemedicine Units on vehicles often drive to remote villages and setup camp to provide free checkup.

We have embarked on setting up of a multipoint mobile telemedicine network for ophthalmological consultation, consisting of an (1) ophthalmological *specialist* in a Tertiary Medical Center (TMC) located in an urban area, (2) a *general practitioner* in a Primary Health Care (PHC) center located within the county through which the care for all patients in the neighborhood is usually coordinated, and (3) a Mobile Telemedicine Unit (MTU) that reaches out to remote villages belonging to that county. In such a distributed multipoint telemedicine consultation scenario, targeted to address ophthalmological conditions, there is a need for the patients' gaze to be directed towards either the specialist or the general practitioner periodically during

© ICST Institute for Computer Sciences, Social Informatics and Telecommunications Engineering 2018
P. Perego et al. (Eds.): MobiHealth 2017, LNICST 247, pp. 182–189, 2018.
https://doi.org/10.1007/978-3-319-98551-0_21

the course of the consultation, In fact, there are three major levels of gaze alignment [3, 4] that can be identified viz,.

(1) *Mutual Gaze:* simply refers to eye-contact between interacting patients and doctors.
(2) *Gaze Awareness:* which in this context means knowing where others are looking. The ophthalmological specialist often needs to perceive the gaze direction of the patient while performing the diagnosis.
(3) *Gaze Following:* which reflects an "expectation-based type of orienting in which an individual's attention is cued by another's head turn or eye turn". The ophthalmologist often points his/her fingers at a visual chart asking the patient to look at the object.

In this paper, we develop techniques to dynamically implement the above three levels of gaze alignment so as to transform a mobile telemedicine consultation into an effective medium for ophthalmological diagnosis. Our technique uses a media rich setup that dynamically maps appropriate camera feeds to display units such that gaze directionalities are preserved.

The system is being tested with a tripartite test-bed consisting of a patient at one location, a specialist in another and a general physician in the third location. The system is being tested in our setup consisting of Amrita Institute of Medical Sciences (a 1500 bed super specialty hospital) located in the city of Cochin in Southern India and Amrita Center for Wireless Networks located in Amritapuri, a picturesque rural village on the shores of Arabian Sea 100 km away. Feedback from preliminary experiments is promising.

2   Related Work

There are several telemedicine consultation systems such as MDLIVE, Teladoc, American Well, Doctor on Demand etc. However, they are mostly web portals coupled with peer to peer video conferencing systems. Such systems work fine for direction insensitive consultation systems.

Work done by Blackwell et al. [5], conducted an extensive survey in for ophthalmological telemedicine diagnosis. They conducted their experiments in the remote villages of Australia. This study was conducted as early as 1997 which showed that effectiveness of remote diagnosis did not quite match the face to face interaction.

Work done by Academy of Pediatrics Section on Ophthalmology - Pediatrics, 2015 [6], describes a retinal digital imaging technique for remote detection of retinal impairment.

In the field of head and eye pose detection, Sheela et al. [7], describes an iris based video tracking solution for estimation of gaze directions.

Bai et al. [8], describes tele-ophthalmology system for rural eye care systems such as Aravind Tele ophthalmology Network. These have been proven to be effective.

Ramkumar et al. [9, 10] describes some fundamental techniques in the area of gesture and gaze in an eLearning scenario. This work serves as the motivation for the application described in this paper and includes gesture triggered, gaze switching with the help of rich media devices.

3   Gaze Alignment Architecture in Ophthalmological Telemedicine

Ophthalmology requires a specialist to be able to direct the patient's gaze towards specific targets, such as reading charts or gaze at other objects. For instance, detecting and measuring degree of squint requires a system to provide the doctor with a frontal perspective of the patient. In another example, detecting impairment in peripheral vision in glaucoma patients may require the ophthalmologist to precisely perceive the patients' gaze direction.

Our proposed telemedicine architecture consists of three geographically separated locations viz.,

- Mobile Telemedicine Unit (MTU) hosting the patient - **PA**.
- Primary Healthcare Center (PHC) consisting of a general practitioner – **GP**.
- Tertiary Medical Center (TMC) consisting of a specialist (ophthalmologist) – **SP**.

Let us take a typical consultation interaction pattern i.e., **SP talks to PA**. SP takes the role of the speaker and *PA* takes the role of the listener. In fact, we define three possible roles in any consultation. We define **role** to be a temporary state the users are in depending on their involvement in the consultation interaction. We can observe three different roles in any consultation interaction namely,

(1) **Speaker:** is one of *SP*, *GP*, *PA* who is doing the talking in the consultation at that moment.
(2) **Listener**: is the one to whom the speaker is mainly talking to.
(3) **Observer:** others who are passively witnessing the interaction.

As the consultation interaction proceeds, *PA*, *GP* and *SP* can take on different roles. An interaction is represented by *speaker* → *listener*.

For this particular interaction in which *SP* talks to *PA*, represented by $SP \rightarrow PA$, let us derive the gaze directionalities. We notice the following in TMC (speaker's location), MTU (listener's location) and PHC (observer's location).

- At TMC, since *SP* is talking to *PA*, *SP* will gaze at the display that shows *PA* (denoted by D_{PA}) and this is represented by a vector called the **entity gaze vector**, $\overrightarrow{SP \rightarrow D_{PA}}$ (shown using green arrow in Fig. 1a).

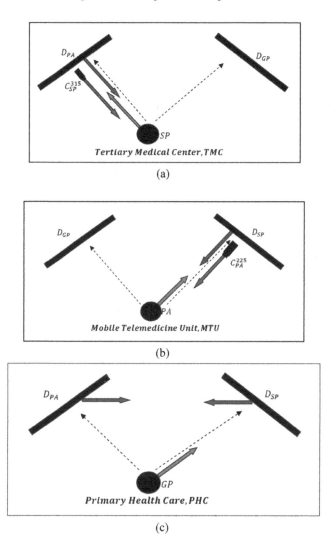

Fig. 1. Ophthalmological consultation consisting of *SP* talking to *PA*. Gaze alignment in (a) TMC, (b) MTU and (c) PHC. (Color figure online)

- At MTU, *PA* will look at the display showing *SP* (denoted by D'_{SP}) and his/her entity gaze vector is given by $\overrightarrow{PA \rightarrow D_{SP}}$ (shown using green arrow in Fig. 1b).
- At TMC, to ensure eye contact, we require *PA's* gaze direction as displayed on D_{PA} to be towards *SP*. This is given by the **display gaze vector**, $\overrightarrow{D_{PA} \rightarrow SP}$ (shown by a blue arrow in Fig. 1a).
- Angle between $\overrightarrow{D_{PA} \rightarrow SP}$ and $\overrightarrow{SP \rightarrow D_{PA}}$ in TMC should be 180° to enable mutual gaze. Now go into MTU, take the reverse of this angle (−180°) from the entity gaze

vector, $\overrightarrow{PA \to D_{SP}}$. This yields the ***camera gaze vector***, $(\overrightarrow{C_{PA}^{225} \to PA})$ which is directed from the camera, C_{PA}^{225} towards PA in Fig. 1b, denoted by a red arrow.

- In order to arrive at the camera gaze vector in TMC, we follow a similar approach with a view to present $SP's$ gaze displayed on D_{SP} in MTU, so as to appear as though directed towards PA. This will yield the camera gaze vector as shown in Fig. 1c, denoted by the red arrow.
- The gaze directionalities of the observer, GP in PHC presents itself with a bit more complexity. The gaze direction of GP is towards the display showing the speaker, D_{SP}. The gazes of D_{SP} and D_{PA} should appear directed towards each other as represented by blue arrows in PHC. How does this translate into camera gaze vectors at PHC? This is derived from the generalized gaze mapping algorithm that we present in the next section.

4 Generalized Gaze Mapping Algorithm

When we generalize the interaction algorithm, there can exist six consultation interaction patterns, viz., $SP \to PA$, $PA \to SP$, $SP \to GP$, $GP \to SP$, $PA \to GP$ and $GP \to PA$, all of which are handled by the generalized gaze mapping algorithm presented below.

Configuration Steps:

Step 1: Map *entities*, $E \in \{SP, GP, PA\}$ to roles, $R \in \{speaker, observer, listener\}$.
Step 2: In each of the three locations, TMC, PHC, MTU, the displays are mapped to distinct remote entities and are called D_{SP}, D_{GP} and D_{PA}. If and when we refer to displays as $D_{speaker}$, $D_{listener}$ and $D_{observer}$ these roles may be substituted by the respective entites.

Entity Gaze Vectors (all drawn in green):

Step 3: The entity gaze vectors of the listener and observer in their respective locations, is directed towards display showing the speaker.
Step 4: In the speaker's location, his/her entity gaze vector is directed towards the display mapped to the listener.

Display Gaze Vectors (all drawn in blue):

Step 5: In the listener's location, a display gaze vector is drawn from the $D_{Speaker}$ towards the *listener*.
Step 6: In the listener's location, a display gaze vector is drawn from the $D_{Observer}$ towards the $D_{Speaker}$.
Step 7: In the observer's location, a display gaze vector is drawn from the $D_{Speaker}$ towards the $D_{Listener}$ and vice versa.
Step 8: In the speaker's location, two display gaze vectors are drawn from the $D_{Listener}$ and $D_{Observer}$ towards the speaker.

Relative Position Vectors, (all drawn in dotted black):

Step 9: Relative position vectors are drawn from an entity to each of the displays in the entity's location.

Computation of Camera Gaze Vectors, (all drawn in red):

Step 10: The camera gaze vector directed towards entity Ei, whose video is presented on a display to entity Ej, where $Ei \neq Ej \in \{SP, GP, PA\}$ is to be computed as follows,

Substep 10.1: calculate θ = angle between

$$relative\ postion\ vector, \overrightarrow{Ej \rightarrow D_{Ei}}$$

and

$$display\ gaze\ vector,\ \overrightarrow{Ei\ in\ Ej's\ room}$$

Substep 10.2: *camera gaze vector* = $Ei's$ *entity gaze vector* $- \theta$

Applying the above algorithm for each of the six interactions, we arrive at the table of angles of camera gaze vectors. Table 1 enumerates them. The notation uses C^φ to indicate a camera positioned at angle φ from the x axis.

Table 1. Angles of camera gaze vectors obtained by applying the generalized gaze vector algorithm for each of the interaction consultations. Camera C^φ indicates a camera oriented at an angle, φ to capture E_i's video in E_i's location and this video is routed to appropriate display at E_j's location so that E_j gets to view a gaze aligned perspective of E_j. Camera locations are highlighted in red whereas display locations are highlighted in blue.

Interactions (Speaker → Listener)	Ei = PA (in MTU) Ej = SP (in TMC)	Ei = PA (in MTU) Ej = GP (in PHC)	Ei = GP (in PHC) Ej = SP (in TMC)	Ei = GP (in PHC) Ej = PA (in MTU)	Ei = SP (in TMC) Ej = PA (in MTU)	Ei = SP (in TMC) Ej = GP (in PHC)
$SP \rightarrow PA$	C^{225}	C^{270}	C^{225}	C^{180}	C^{315}	C^{0}
$PA \rightarrow SP$	C^{225}	C^{270}	C^{270}	C^{315}	C^{315}	C^{0}
$GP \rightarrow SP$	C^{270}	C^{270}	C^{225}	C^{180}	C^{270}	C^{225}
$SP \rightarrow GP$	C^{225}	C^{180}	C^{225}	C^{180}	C^{270}	C^{225}
$GP \rightarrow PA$	C^{270}	C^{315}	C^{0}	C^{315}	C^{270}	C^{225}
$PA \rightarrow GP$	C^{270}	C^{315}	C^{0}	C^{315}	C^{315}	C^{0}

As the consultation moves from one interaction to another the appropriate video switching subsystem chooses the camera corresponding to the appropriate row (determined by the interaction) and column (determined by the camera and display locations - shown in red and blue respectively) in Table 1. A fully equipped telemedicine consultation room with all of the cameras and displays installed is shown in Fig. 2.

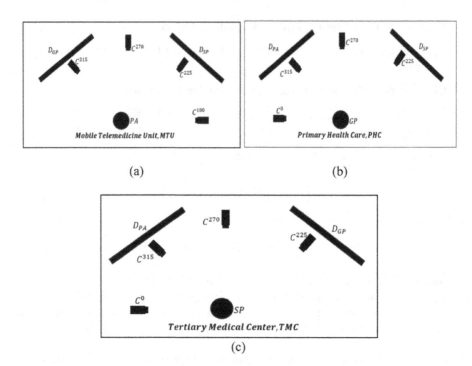

(a)   (b)

(c)

Fig. 2. A fully equipped telemedicine consultation room with gaze alignment for all consultation interaction patterns (a) MTU, (b) PHC and (c) TMC

5   Prototype Implementation

We have implemented a prototype of our system and conducted sample sessions with participants who took on the various roles (see Fig. 3). For instance, the ophthalmologist was asked to detect squint eyes and conduct a basic test for strength of peripheral vision (suspecting glaucoma) by directing the gaze of the patient at certain targets indicated by

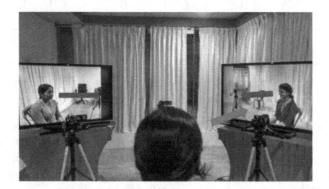

Fig. 3. A prototype system in action for a gaze aligned interactive consultation.

gestures. The ophthalmologist was able to carry out the consultation with much greater ease and naturalness.

6   Conclusion

We have implemented a gaze alignment system for multipoint mobile telemedicine consultation for ophthalmological diagnosis. Since the field of ophthalmology has a direct connectedness to gaze and directionalities in general, this technology is a niche fit. However, it can be extended to other areas of medical diagnosis which are interaction intensive and requires gaze alignment. A prototype implementation shows promising initial results.

References

1. Pathinarupothi, R.K., et al.: RASPRO: rapid summarization for effective prognosis in wireless remote health monitoring. In: Wireless Health (2016)
2. Pathinarupothi, R.K., Rangan, E.: Discovering vital trends for personalized healthcare delivery. In: Proceedings of the 2016 ACM International Joint Conference on Pervasive and Ubiquitous Computing: Adjunct. ACM (2016)
3. Monk, A.F., Gale, C.: A look is worth a thousand words: full gaze awareness in video-mediated conversation. Discourse Process. **33**(3), 257–278 (2002)
4. Flom, R., Lee, K., Muir, D. (eds.): Gaze-Following: Its Development and Significance. Lawrence Erlbaum Associates Publishers, Mahwah (2007)
5. Blackwell, N.A.M., Kelly, G.J., Lenton, L.M.: Telemedicine ophthalmology consultation in remote Queensland. Med. J. Aust. **167**(11), 583–586 (1997)
6. Fierson, W.M., Capone, A., American Academy of Pediatrics Section on Ophthalmology.: Telemedicine for evaluation of retinopathy of prematurity. Pediatrics **135**(1), e238–e254 (2015)
7. Sheela, S.V., Abhinand, P.: Iris detection for gaze tracking using video frames. In: 2015 IEEE International Advance Computing Conference (IACC). IEEE (2015)
8. Bai, V.Thulasi, et al.: Teleophthalmology-based rural eye care in India. Telemedicine e-Health **13**(3), 313–321 (2007)
9. Ramkumar, N., et al.: Gesture triggered, dynamic gaze alignment architecture for intelligent eLearning systems. J. Intell. Fuzzy Syst. **32**(4), 2963–2969 (2017)
10. Narayanankutty, R., et al.: Automatic multi-perspective switching for gaze alignment in e-Learning systems. IJAER **10**(16), 37303–37310 (2015)

Developing a Context-Dependent Tuning Framework of Multi-channel Biometrics that Combine Audio-Visual Characteristics for Secure Access of an eHealth Platform

Marios Spanakis[1], Georgios C. Manikis[1],
Sakshi Porwal[2], and Emmanouil G. Spanakis[1(✉)]

[1] Computational BioMedicine Laboratory, Institute of Computer Science,
Foundation for Research and Technology - Hellas, 71110 Heraklion, Crete, Greece
{marspan,gmanikis,spanakis}@ics.forth.gr
[2] Tech Inspire Ltd., Salford, UK
porwalsakshi@gmail.com

Abstract. The efficiency of a biometric system is identified by the detection error tradeoff (DET) curve, which is a visual characterization of the trade-off between the False Acceptance Rate (FAR) and the False Rejection Rate (FRR). A DET curve is a plot of FAR against FRR for various threshold values, t. FRR refers to the expected probability that two mate samples (samples of the same biometric trait obtained from the same user) will be falsely declared as a non-match whereas FAR is the expected probability that two non-mate samples will be incorrectly recognized as a match. The threshold t defines how much the biometric characteristics must be similar, in order to make a positive comparison, so it measures the correspondence between characteristic to check and template stored in the database. By elevating the threshold, the risk that not authorized users can fool the system diminishes, but, on the other hand, it is more probable that some authorized users can sometimes be refused. In this work, we present the results for SpeechXRays multi-modal biometric system that uses audio-visual characteristics for user authentication in an eHealth platform for osteoarthritis management. Using the privacy and security mechanism provided by SpeechXrays based on audio and video biometrics medical personnel is able to be verified and subsequently identified to the eHealth application for osteoarthritis.

Keywords: Biometrics · Decision threshold · Equal Error Rate (EER)
Detection error tradeoff (DET) · eHealth · Osteoarthritis

1 Introduction

Personal health systems and E-Health platforms aim on improving the interaction among health care professionals with their patients [1–6] and provide the means for secure access to sensitive medical information to people regarding their health status and disease management [7, 8]. To this respect, there is a tremendous need for secure and stratified access to health information [9] by adopting the use of modern ICT technology.

© ICST Institute for Computer Sciences, Social Informatics and Telecommunications Engineering 2018
P. Perego et al. (Eds.): MobiHealth 2017, LNICST 247, pp. 190–198, 2018.
https://doi.org/10.1007/978-3-319-98551-0_22

Today, biometric authentication, is gaining as the leading technological achievement for the verification of a person's identity using a physical trait or behavioral characteristic in order to accept the identity of the person and verify him/her as an authorized user [10, 11]. These systems mainly rely on models derived from pattern recognition, where several characteristics from a person (e.g. voice, facial expression, etc.) are first transformed into one (unimodal) or many features (multimodal) and then are processed to accept or reject the verification and identification of a user [12]. A major prerequisite in this process is the so called training phase of the model composed of a pipeline process in which (a) captured biometric characteristics from specific users are stored in a database, and (b) used for training the model on the basis of that known content. Once training has been performed accurately, the biometric system can be applied for verification and identification.

SpeechXRays[1] is aiming to develop and test in real-life environments (i.e. medical units) a user recognition platform based on voice acoustics analysis and audio-visual identity verification. SpeechXRays provides a state of the art, accurate and user-friendly solution allowing storage and analysis of biometric data for authentication. The e-Health pilot of SpeechXrays will involve more than 400 medical personnel who through SpeechXrays will gain access to hospital's medical image/radiology archiving system as well as a personal health application designed for the management of osteoarthritis (OA) [6]. Recently an evaluation survey and preliminary results regarding acceptability of the approach its functionality, efficiency and user friendly environment were presented along with the acceptance of using the biometric system proposed from SpeechXRays for user authentication [9]. The aim of this work is to present and evaluate the verification rates from various decision thresholds that must be defined and adapted based on the level of security required by the SpeechXRays platform and the confidentiality of the data that the user is attempting to access.

1.1 Biometric System Errors

A biometric verification system usually makes two types of errors: (i) mistaking biometric measurements from two different persons to be from the same person (false match), and (ii) mistaking two biometric measurements from the same person to be from two different persons (false non-match). These two types of errors are often termed as false accept and false reject, respectively [13] and most commonly are described by *FMR (false match rate)/FAR (false acceptance rate), FNMR (false non-match rate)/FRR (false rejection rate, Failure to capture (FTC) and Failure to enroll (FTE).* It is possible to reduce the errors by trying to record more biometric characteristics for every user so that, in case of variations on a template, the other can be used. On the other hand, there are natural variations to biometric characteristics which may not be erased but that could be minimized through the appropriate equipment. Another possibility is to act on the threshold of the system. This threshold defines how much the biometric characteristics must be similar, in order to make a positive comparison, so it measures the correspondence between the characteristic to check and the template stored in database. By

---

[1] http://www.speechxrays.com/.

elevating the threshold, the risk that not authorized users can fool the system drops (FAR is reduced), but, on the other hand, it is more probable that some authorized users can sometimes be refused (FRR increases). Biometric system errors can occur due to various reasons such as: Sampling (imperfect imaging conditions); Changes in characteristics (i.e. bruises or voice changes due to illness); Ambient conditions (temperature humidity); User interaction with the sensor (i.e. distance) and Sensors (different smartphones).

1.2 Efficiency of Biometric System and Application in SpeechXRays Data

The efficiency of any biometric system can be described by a visual characterization of the trade-off between the FAR and the FRR. The most basic and robust method is the calculation of the receiver operating characteristic (ROC) curve. To assess a biometric system performance, detection error tradeoff (DET) curve which is similar to the ROC curve analysis is followed to discriminate between two states that usually overlap such as genuine and impostor users. A DET curve is a plotted as FMR against FNMR for various **thresholds**, *t*. Similarly, EER can be also estimated by the Receiver Operator Characteristic (ROC) curve. A specific threshold *t* can be calculated automatically based on the Error Rate curve of the FAR and FRR. This threshold is the value where FAR and FRR are equal (i.e., where FAR = FRR), and is called Equal Error Rate (EER) (intersection point of FAR & FRR) [10, 13, 14]. Additionally, the more the EER is near to 0% better is the performance of the target system.. In this light, EER is a performance metric with FAR and FRR used as performance criteria simultaneously, since EER is defined by both metrics with the constraint that they are equal.

2   Methodology

The performance of the SpeechXRays biometric system in its implementation will be assessed using experimental protocols based on both unimodal and multimodal data. Data will be randomly separated into enrolment data and data used at the verification level in order to simulate a real case scenario. However, the estimation of the system performance can be influenced by the selection of data used for enrolment and verification, affecting a good generalization in performance. SpeechXRays biometric system will be applied to health domain applications [18, 19], thus such model needs to demonstrate at first adequate verification capability on the data used for designing the system.

In SpeechXRays audio and voice data will be first partitioned into k equally (or nearly equally) sized folds following a k-fold cross-validation method for assessing the generalization performance of the system. Subsequently k iterations of enrolment and verification will be performed such that, within iterations, a different fold of the data is held-out for verification purposes while the remaining k-1 folds will be used as data for the enrolment phase. Finally, k-fold cross-validation will run several times, increasing the number of estimates, where data from the experimental protocol will be reshuffled and re-stratified before each run.

Security requirements such as confidentiality, integrity, authenticity, non-repudiation and availability are essential for computer and network based systems. Following steps were performed by the SpeechXRays biometric system to enrol the person by acquiring and storing the appropriate data, verify by comparing the captured data against the database, and authenticating or revoking access based on the comparison/classification of the biometric trait.

In the context of SpeechXRays, the following phases are studied in a pipeline process for enrolment, verification, authentication, and revocation through the biometric context dependent detection system. **Enrolment Phase:** Medical personnel will provide speech and facial imaging data under different times, environment conditions (i.e. noisy background, low light, etc.), and facial expressions. This multimodal information will be extracted using feature extraction techniques for voice and face data, and stored individually as a biometric template to a database. This template will be linked to a specific token (i.e. ID, name, etc.) related to each medical personnel. Once the information gathering is finished, two separate unimodal biometric systems will be applied to the data in order to construct SpeechXRays biometric system. Through enrolment of the system, appropriate thresholds will be estimated and assigned specifically to the medical data with different levels of security/sensitivity. **Verification Phase:** At the verification level, a medical specialist requires access to medical data classified with a specific security level degree. The user presents a token, facial and speech data, and the biometric feature template associated with the user is retrieved from the database. The system processes the given data, extracts the facial and speech features and compares them with the features stored at the database at the enrolment phase. **Authentication Phase:** if matching, secure session is opened between two parties and if not, the access is denied and **Revocation Phases** – revoke access based on security risk such as template leakage, spoofing attempts, etc. The user can then proceed again to the verification process and depending on the security levels assigned to the medical data a number of attempts can be made.

2.1 Demonstration of the Context Dependent Tuning Framework of SpeechXRays

SpeechXRays unimodal system - Experimental Protocol
According to the SpeechXRays developing procedure, individual unimodal biometric systems will be first applied to both speech and face data. The derived matching scores will be afterwards fused to conclude to the final decision at the verification phase. For that reason, a unimodal biometric system was implemented first using publicly available data from the ORL database[2], composed of 400 facial images of size 112x92. Ten different images of each of 40 distinct subjects-persons were captured in different times, lightning, facial expressions (i.e. open/closed eyes, smiling/not smiling) and details (i.e. glasses/no glasses). All images were acquired against a dark homogeneous background with faces in an upright position in frontal view, with a tolerance for some side movement. Facial features were exported using the methodology described in [15]. Following

---

[2] www.cl.cam.ac.uk/research/dtg/attarchive/facedatabase.html.

an iterative process to assess the verification accuracy of the SpeechXRays biometric system, the entire data of each of the 40 distinct subjects was randomly partitioned into subsets act as enrolment and verification data respectively. Particularly, 80% of the images of each subject contributed to the enrolment phase of the biometric system, while the remaining 20% served as the set for verification. A 5-fold cross-validation was applied to the subset simulating the enrolment phase, to estimate the generalization performance of the system. Linear Discriminant Analysis (LDA) was applied during the enrolment phase to reduce feature dimensionality and construct linear combinations of the available features. Matching score calculations were performed using a nearest neighbour classifier and impostor and genuine distributions were calculated using the Euclidean distance measure.

SpeechXRays bimodal system - Experimental Protocol

Face and speech information in SpeechXRays were integrated according to the matching score fusion process from the post-classification techniques. To follow this approach, matching scores from face and speech were first calculated from individual unimodal systems and then normalized using min-max normalization to produce scores varying from 0 to 1. The data used for building the bimodal biometric system relied on the MOBIO database composed of 152 people with speech and facial data [16]. At last, fusion was achieved using linear regression techniques [17]. Genuine and impostor distributions were calculated and presented in the results.

3   Results

3.1   SpeechXRays Unimodal System

The resulted distributions at the training phase and for each fold are presented in Fig. 1. At the cross-validation phase, verification accept rates were plotted against the associated false accept rates (Fig. 2A). DET curve analysis based on the relationship between the FAR and FRR measurements is shown in Fig. 2B.

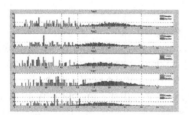
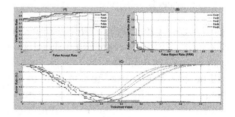

Fig. 1. Genuine and impostor distributions for each fold

Fig. 2. Curves based on: (A) verification accept rate vs FAR and (B) relationship between FAR and FRR. (C) Error rates of FAR and FRR for different folds used

The error graphs of FAR and FRR are shown in Fig. 2C. In any given subset through the cross-validation procedure, the intersection point of these two graphs resulted to the

EER. The calculated value for EER was used to give automatically the threshold of the biometric system. Lower EER results to better system's performance, as the total error rate (sum of the FAR and the FRR at the point of the EER) decreases. A quantitative representation of the identification accuracy of the biometric system is given in the following table for indicative points in the DET curves (Table 1). All folds at the cross-validation process contributed equivalently to the estimation of the performance and an average value was calculated. The measures presented in Table 1 correspond to verification rate of 1%, 0.1, and 0.01 FAR to 82.60%, 72.27%, and 0.25% respectively.

Table 1. Verification rates based on different EER representing different levels of security for ORL dataset in SpeechXRays

Threshold	0% success	50% success	100% success
EER	13/40 subjects	14/40 subjects	13/40 subjects
EER – 10% EER (more strict)	18/40 subjects	11/40 subjects	11/40 subjects
EER – 20% EER (more strict)	19/40 subjects	13/40 subjects	8/40 subjects
EER + 10% EER (less strict)	11/40 subjects	13/40 subjects	16/40 subjects
EER + 20% EER (less strict)	9/40 subjects	11/40 subjects	20/40 subjects
Threshold	0% success	50% success	100% success

3.2 SpeechXRays Bimodal System

The data used for building the bimodal biometric system relied on the MOBIO database [16] and fusion was achieved using linear regression techniques and genuine and impostor distributions were calculated and presented in the Fig. 3. The evaluation of the bimodal SpeechXRays biometric system is also displayed in a quantitative way using specific points at the DET curve according to the Table 2.

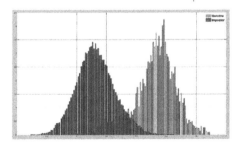

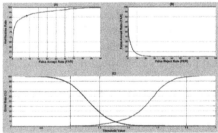

Fig. 3. Genuine and impostor distributions for MOBIO dataset

Fig. 4. Curves based on: (A) verification Rate vs FAR and (B) relationship between FAR and FRR. (C) Error rates of FAR and FRR using MOBIO bimodal data

Table 2. FAR and FRR rates based on different thresholds for bimodal operation in SpeechXRays for MOBIO dataset

Threshold	FAR	FRR
EER	8.33%	8.33%
EER – 10% EER	32.56%	1.98%
EER – 20% EER	73.12%	0.07%
EER + 10% EER	0.87%	22.18%
EER + 20% EER	0.03%	59.68%
EER	8.33%	8.33%

DET curve analysis were performed at the enrolment phase in which: (a) verification accept rates were plotted against the associated FAR, and (b) FAR against FRR are given in Fig. 4. The error graphs of FAR and FRR, (Fig. 4C) were also defined as the probability that an unauthorized user is accepted as authorized, and that an authorized user is rejected as unauthorized. According to the normalized integrated data, the calculated EER was measured with a threshold of **1.3109** and provided as an indicative threshold in the system. Access to the medical data will be given related to the sensitivity of the data in terms of their security levels. For high security the EER will be increased thus making a more secure environment for the user but inconvenient at the same time. On the contrary, medical data that are assigned, as "less secure" information can be accessed using SpeechXRays system with a threshold equal to the EER or less (Table 2). The measures presented in Table 2 correspond to verification rate of 1%, 0.1, and 0.01 FAR to 78.73%, 55.63%, and 29.44% respectively.

4   Discussion

Detection error trade off (DET) curves are used to assess the performance of a biometric system as a trade-off between the False Acceptance Rate (FAR) and the False Rejection Rate (FRR). A DET curve is a plot of FAR against FRR for various threshold values, t. In this work the evaluation on verifying medical personnel's authentication through DET curve analysis for the multimodal biometric system of SpeechXRays was presented. Based on unimodal and multimodal datasets a demonstration of the context dependent tuning framework through DET curve analysis was described in order to test the verification rates based on different thresholds. Through this approach it was evaluated the user acceptance and the various matching thresholds that must be defined and adapted based on the level of security required by the service and the sensitivity of the medical data that the user is attempting to access. SpeexhRays' scope is to bring superior anti-spoofing capabilities and integrate them into an existing healthcare service. Upcoming updates of the SpeechXRays biometric system will include more advanced pattern recognition models for calculating the matching scores (i.e. Support Vector Machines).

Acknowledgement. This work is supported by the research project "SpeechXRays" which receives funding from the European Commission (EC) through Horizon 2020 Grant agreement No 653586.

References

1. Chiarugi, F., Spanakis, M., Lees, P.J., Chronaki, C.E., Tsiknakis, M., Orphanoudakis, S.C.: ECG in your hands: a multi-vendor ECG viewer for personal digital assistants. In: Computers in Cardiology 2003, 21–24 September 2003, pp. 359–362 (2003). https://doi.org/10.1109/cic. 2003.1291166

2. Chiarugi, F., et al.: Real-time cardiac monitoring over a regional health network: preliminary results from initial field testing. In: Computers in Cardiology, 22–25 September 2002, pp. 347–350 (2002). https://doi.org/10.1109/cic.2002.1166780

3. Chronaki, C.E., et al.: An eHealth platform for instant interaction among health professionals. In: Computers in Cardiology 2003, 21–24 September 2003, pp. 101–104 (2003). https:// doi.org/10.1109/cic.2003.1291100

4. Spat, S., et al.: A mobile android-based application for in-hospital glucose management in compliance with the medical device directive for software. In: Nikita, K.S., Lin, J.C., Fotiadis, D.I., Arredondo Waldmeyer, M.-T. (eds.) MobiHealth 2011. LNICST, vol. 83, pp. 211–216. Springer, Heidelberg (2012). https://doi.org/10.1007/978-3-642-29734-2_29

5. Tsiknakis, M., Spanakis, M.: Adoption of innovative eHealth services in prehospital emergency management: a case study. In: Proceedings of the 10th IEEE International Conference on Information Technology and Applications in Biomedicine, 3–5 November 2010, pp. 1–5 (2010). https://doi.org/10.1109/itab.2010.5687752

6. Maniadi, E., Spanakis, E.G., Karantanas, A., Marias, K.: A supportive environment for the long term management of knee osteoarthritis condition. In: Proceedings of the 5th EAI International Conference on Wireless Mobile Communication and Healthcare, London, Great Britain (2015)

7. Kondylakis, H., et al.: Digital patient: personalized and translational data management through the MyHealthAvatar EU project. In: Annual International Conference of the IEEE Engineering in Medicine and Biology Society IEEE Engineering in Medicine and Biology Society Annual Conference 2015, pp. 1397–1400 (2015). https://doi.org/10.1109/embc. 2015.7318630

8. Maniadi, E., et al.: Designing a digital patient avatar in the context of the MyHealthAvatar project initiative. In: 13th IEEE International Conference on BioInformatics and BioEngineering, 10–13 November 2013 pp. 1–4 (2013). https://doi.org/10.1109/bibe. 2013.6701560

9. Spanakis, E.G., Spanakis, M., Karantanas, A., Marias, K.: Secure access to patient's health records using SpeechXRays a mutli-channel biometrics platform for user authentication. In: Annual International Conference of the IEEE Engineering in Medicine and Biology Society IEEE Engineering in Medicine and Biology Society Annual Conference 2016, pp. 2541-2544 (2016). https://doi.org/10.1109/embc.2016.7591248

10. Jain, A.K., Flynn, P., Ross, A.A.: Handbook of Biometrics. Springer, New York (2007). https://doi.org/10.1007/978-0-387-71041-9

11. Li, S.Z., Jain, A.K.: Encyclopedia of Biometrics: I-Z, vol. 1. Springer, US (2009)

12. Ross, A.A., Nandakumar, K., Jain, A.: Handbook of Multibiometrics. Springer, US (2006)

13. Jain, A.K., Ross, A., Prabhakar, S.: An introduction to biometric recognition. IEEE Trans. Cir. Sys. Video Technol. **14**(1), 4–20 (2004). https://doi.org/10.1109/tcsvt.2003.818349

14. Jain, A.K., Ross, A.A., Nandakumar, K.: Introduction to Biometrics. Springer, US (2011)

15. Shen, L., Bai, L., Fairhurst, M.: Gabor wavelets and general discriminant analysis for face identification and verification. Image Vis. Comput. **25**(5), 553–563 (2007). https://doi.org/ 10.1016/j.imavis.2006.05.002

16. McCool, C., et al.: Bi-modal person recognition on a mobile phone: using mobile phone data. In: 2012 IEEE International Conference on Multimedia and Expo Workshops, 9–13 July 2012, pp. 635–640 (2012). https://doi.org/10.1109/icmew.2012.116

17. Ghayoumi, M.: A review of multimodal biometric systems: fusion methods and their applications. In: 2015 IEEE/ACIS 14th International Conference on Computer and Information Science (ICIS), 28 June–1 July 2015, pp. 131–136 (2015). https://doi.org/10.1109/icis.2015.7166582

18. Chiarugi, F., Trypakis, D., Spanakis, E.G.: Problems and solutions for storing and sharing data from medical devices in eHealth applications. In: 2nd OpenECG Workshop, 1–3 April 2004, Berlin (2004)

19. Spanakis, E.G., et al.: Technology-based innovations to foster personalized healthy lifestyles and well-being: a targeted review. J. Med. Internet Res. **18**(6), e128 (2016). https://doi.org/10.2196/jmir.4863, PMID: 27342137

QuantifyMe: An Automated Single-Case Experimental Design Platform

Akane Sano[(⊠)], Sara Taylor, Craig Ferguson, Akshay Mohan,
and Rosalind W. Picard

Massachusetts Institute of Technology, Media Lab, Cambridge 02139, USA
{akanes,sataylor}@media.mit.edu

Abstract. We designed, developed, and evaluated a novel system, QuantifyMe, for novice self-experimenters to conduct proper-methodology single-case self-experiments in an automated and scientific manner using their smartphones. In this work we evaluate its use with four different kinds of personalized investigations, examining how variables such as sleep duration and regularity, activity, and leisure time affect personal happiness, stress, productivity, and sleep efficiency. We describe lessons learned developing the system, and recommendations for its improvement, as well as its potential for enabling personalized insights to be scientifically evaluated in many individuals.

Keywords: Single-case experimental design · Mobile health
Self-experiment · Self-tracking

1 Introduction

Mobile devices today have become nearly ubiquitous full-time extensions of an individual, enabling unprecedented data collection through a combination of mobile and wearable sensors. The collected data can provide an individual with a unique opportunity to determine behavioral patterns and habits about themselves [7]. A common way for individuals to use these data is to compare the logged values of a variable of interest with its recommended values (e.g., sleep, physical activity, and calorie intake), and then adjust daily behavior accordingly. However, these recommendations made by agencies like Center for Disease Control, are averages and ideal values may vary significantly in individuals. Although average values are useful, they do not provide the personalized insights that are best suited for an individual to make optimal behavioral choices.

Our system, QuantifyMe, creates a framework that allows people to find their personal optimal behavioral variables (e.g., bed time or physical activity) to achieve their goals (e.g., productivity or happiness) based on evidence-based experimentation. This is done through a single-case experiment design methodology — a methodology that allows for comparison within an individual instead of between groups. In achieving these aims we are closer to including the general public in dramatically scaling and personalizing the study of daily behaviors.

A. Sano and S. Taylor – Contributed equally to this work.

© ICST Institute for Computer Sciences, Social Informatics and Telecommunications Engineering 2018
P. Perego et al. (Eds.): MobiHealth 2017, LNICST 247, pp. 199–206, 2018.
https://doi.org/10.1007/978-3-319-98551-0_23

2   Related Work

2.1   Quantified Self

Mobile applications and wearable sensors have enabled individuals to collect personal real-time behavioral and physiological data such as physical activity, sleep [10], and diet [11] and use these data to infer their daily activity patterns. This also allows for self-experimentation to make better choices related to their lifestyle, health, and productivity goals. However, using these data to understand optimal values of variables and causal relationships in behaviors like sleep, physical activity, and caloric intake often lacks scientific rigor [3]. Recent mobile applications have provided great tools supporting more systematic and personalized self-experimentation [5,8,13,14]. However, many of these tools do not provide a structured methodology to aid non-scientist quantified selfers, and/or they have not been validated on usability and effectiveness.

2.2   Single-Case Experimental Design

Randomized Control Trials (RCTs) are considered a gold standard in determining whether a causal relationship exists between a specific intervention and observed outcome [16]. However, traditional RCTs operate only across groups, and are unable to provide individual insights [1]. First proposed by Neuringer [17], single-case experimental design provides a methodology that allows researchers to evaluate the effectiveness of an intervention on an individual. An individual serves as his or her own control and is subjected to different experimental conditions at different time periods [1,15]. This contrasts with a group-based design in which outcomes are compared between groups, with each group receiving a specific experimental condition.

3   Survey Study for Understanding Users' Interest in Self-experimentation

Before developing our smartphone app and system, we conducted an online survey study to gauge users' interest in self experimentation and to find which of 32 self-experiments they are interested in. The possible output variables of these proposed experiments (happiness, stress, productivity, sleep efficiency) were chosen from common indicators of wellbeing. The possible independent variables (active time, steps, sleep duration, bed time, meditation duration, outdoor time, fun time, attending a religious service) were chosen based on the ability to be measured with the Jawbone wearable sensor or because they are relatively easily controllable and actionable [14].

A total of 233 individuals completed the survey (90%: 18–24 years old, 5%: 25–29 years old, 5%: over 30 years old). Based on the results of the survey, we decided to focus on four self-experiments — one for each outcome variable: (1) How does my leisure time affect my happiness? (2) How does my activity level affect my sleep efficiency? (3) How does my nightly sleep affect my productivity? (4) How do inconsistent bedtimes affect my stress level? While we selected these four experiments for their popularity for use in the first version of the app, the QuantifyMe system was designed to be flexible to accommodate many different kinds of self-experiments, not just these four.

4 QuantifyMe System for Self-experimentation

The QuantifyMe system consists of three parts: a backend Django application, an Android App, and a Jawbone UpMove fitness tracker. The system could be expanded to other fitness trackers and smartphone platforms.

4.1 Single-Case Experimental Design on QuantifyMe

A traditional suggested design for single-case experiments is an $ABAB$ design, where the A phase corresponds to the baseline, and the B phase corresponds to the intervention period. This design can be modified as a non-terminated sequential intervention $AB_1B_2B_3$ design to see the relationship between different magnitudes of the intervention and their outcomes [18]. This is best suited to our system as we are looking to determine the optimum magnitude of the independent variable. Therefore, we implemented a four-stage design (1 baseline stage and 3 intervention stages) in order to help users determine optimal behaviors with each stage including 4–7 days of data points as suggested by [1].

We quantized behaviors into five zones for each experiment (see Table 1). These target behaviors were predetermined by examining common behaviors based on another study [19].

The "randomized" ordering of target goals was chosen as follows: Stage 1 was a baseline measure. Because a choice needed to be made, we settled on having the middle stage (O2) be the last stage. We also decided to include at least one increase in the target behavior and one decrease in the behavior.

As an example of intervention order, if a user's average sleep duration during Stage 1 (baseline period) is 6.75 h (i.e., within O1), the user would be instructed to sleep 8.5 hr, 6.5 hr, and 7.5 hr during stages 2, 3, and 4, respectively. However, if the mean of the user's sleep duration during Stage 1 was 8.75 h

Table 1. Definitions of target zones of behaviors for each experiment

Zone	Number of steps	Bed time variability	Sleep duration	Leisure time
Under	< 6,500 steps	< ±15 min	< 6 hr	< 15 min
O1	8,000 (6,500–9,500)	±30 min (±15–±45)	6.5 hr (6–7)	30 min (15–45)
O2	11,000 (9,500–12,500)	±60 min (±45–±75)	7.5 hr (7–8)	60 min (45–75)
O3	14,000 (12,500–15,500)	±90 min (±75–±105)	8.5 hr (8–9)	90 min (75–105)
Over	> 15,500 steps	> ±105 min	> 9 hr	> 105 min

(i.e., within O3), the user would be instructed to sleep 6.5 h, 8.5 h, and 7.5 h during stages 2, 3, and 4, respectively. The methodology of imposing sleep targets adds more structure and validity to determining a causal relationship than does simply correlating how long a user chooses to sleep each night with how they feel the next day.

4.2   QuantifyMe Android App

The Android app was designed with the goal of letting the user easily enter data for daily check-ins, while also allowing the user to check on the status of their current experiment. When the user first opens the app after installation, it prompts them for demographic data and asks them to select an experiment. The app connects their Jawbone account to our system's account.

Every morning during the experiment, the user is reminded to check-in on the app and fill out a short daily survey. This survey asks about the amount of leisure time in the past 24 h, along with happiness, stress and productivity levels using 7-point likert scales (not at all — extremely). Finally, the app reminds the user to sync their Jawbone wearable sensor to Jawbone's Up App (syncing takes a few seconds).

After the user has checked-in for the day, the app presents the user with a screen that lets them view their daily goal and experiment progress during that stage (see Figs. 1b and c). In particular, the user is able to see her recorded behavior for all of the days she has been in that stage.

If a user has failed a stage in the experiment, they are shown a message prompting them to restart the stage (see Fig. 1d). Once an experiment has been completed successfully, the user is shown a success screen with their end results, and the experiment's results are added to their history, which they can view from the daily goals screen at any time.

5   App Evaluation Study

After the protocol was approved by the Institute Review Board, we conducted a 6-week pilot study to evaluate the new QuantifyMe application with 13 participants (4 male, 9 female age: 18–27). All participants filled out a Big Five Personality Inventory [12] (not analyzed in this paper) and then chose a self-experiment they liked, which was continued for the 6 weeks. At the end of the study, the participants filled out a post-study survey including a System Usability Scale [2] and questions about their favorite/least favorite parts of the app.

5.1   Results

Self-Experiment Selection. Among the four experiments on the app, 5 people chose "effect of sleep duration on productivity," 4 people chose "effect of leisure on happiness," 2 people selected "effect of sleep variability on stress," and 2 selected "effect of steps on sleep efficiency". This distribution matches that of the survey we conducted before designing QuantifyMe (see Sect. 3).

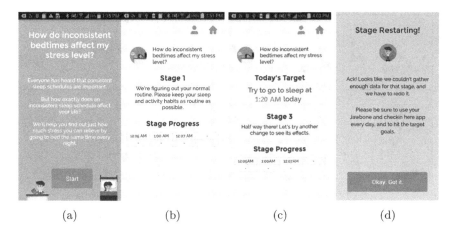

Fig. 1. Screenshots of the QuantifyMe Android App: (a) information provided before starting an experiment, (b) example of instructions during stage 1 (baseline period), (c) example of instructions during stage 3, and (d) example of stage restart notification

Adherence. During the 6-week study, three participants dropped out for various reasons including phone malfunction, side-effects of an un-related medication, and the self-experiment (inconsistent bedtimes and stress) being too difficult to complete. Thus, 10 participants completed the study (i.e., used the QuantifyMe app for 6 weeks); however, only one participant successfully completed a full four-stage scientific self-experiment during the 6-week study.

The average adherence rate for checking-in (i.e., *check-in adherence*) to the QuantifyMe app was 75.8%. *check-in adherence* remained stable throughout the study, and decreased rapidly after the study ended. *Check-in adherence* rates varied widely with four participants checking-in on less than 65% of the days and 3 participants checking-in on more than 90% of the study days. In comparison, we found that on average participants adapted their behaviors to be in the target range on 22.5% of the study days (i.e., *objective adherence*). This lack of adherence to self-experiment instructions was the main reason why only one participant completed a self-experiment in the 6-week period. In other words, many participants had trouble adjusting their behaviors to match the self-experiment instructions (Fig. 2). This resulted in many stage restarts because we required participants to check-in at least 5 out of 7 days and be within the target behavior range for at least 4 of the 7 days.

Post-study Survey. The System Usability Scale (SUS) results presented are from 10 study participants and excludes three who had technical difficulties with use of the app on their phone. The SUS showed a mean of 71 (out of 100) with a standard deviation of 17 (Fig. 3). A SUS score of 68 is considered average [20]. Therefore, our system scored slightly above the average system for usability.

Post-study comments were analyzed from all 13 participants. Seven out of 13 study participants indicated that the daily survey and stage progress allowed

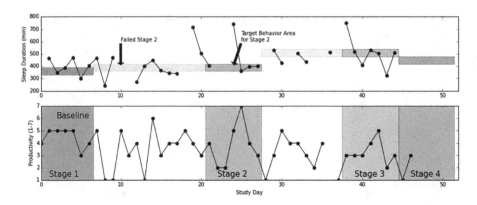

Fig. 2. Example of a participant's self-experiment. The top panel shows their behavior manipulating the independent variable: sleep duration. The bottom panel shows the outcome variable: self-reported productivity. The shaded areas (blue, red, green, and purple) mark each of the 4 stages of the study. In the top panel, we can see that these shaded areas also display the bounds of target behavior. The lighter shaded areas serve as a reference for the target behaviors when the experiment stages had to be restarted.

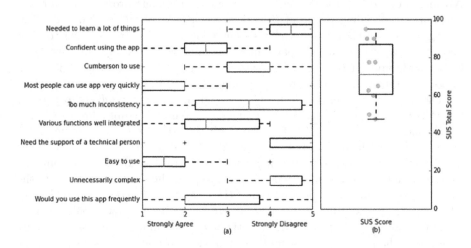

Fig. 3. Results of the system usability scale. Figure (a) shows the distribution of responses for each question and (b) shows the distribution of the SUS total score.

them to be more aware of their behavioral patterns and prompted introspection of their lifestyle. Most study participants indicated their disappointment in not being able to complete the full-four-stage self-experiment during the 6-week study. We also asked about the least favorite aspects of the app. One participant said, "It was hard to follow the instruction about sleep schedule because it was more than I am used to and I wasn't able to plan my schedule around that". Another participant said, "Worrying about when I wasn't able to complete the app instructions" was their least favorite aspect. These comments were consistent with the behavioral lack of success in changing their independent variable.

6   Discussion

This work has several limitations. We assumed that self-experimenters would have enough motivation to maintain the different behaviors being tested. Clearly, better mechanisms to encourage behavioral compliance are needed. Participants suggested it would be valuable to have additional information and motivation about the single-case design methodology such as the number of stages and notifications of why a particular experimental stage would need to be restarted if they didn't reach the target for the independent variable. In the future we recommend that providing study participants with the upcoming targets multiple days ahead and clarifying what flexibility is and is not going to be a set back in the study may allow them to plan for the interventions in advance and increase adherence.

Our population was a set of busy healthy individuals who think they may be interested in trying to find optimal behaviors; they are not likely to be as motivated as an unhealthy population who seeks treatment. We also designed multiple targets they had to meet (instead of sticking with one intervention), adding additional challenges to engaging our healthy population.

Because most participants in our studies were university students who are savvy about technology, experimental design and statistics, these results might not generalize to other populations. Also the participants may have been fairly homogeneous in terms of experiments they may be interested in. One sign supporting this was that the most popular experiment related to the amount of sleep needed. However, all of the participants in the pilot study were novice self-experimenters, which suggests that other tech-savvy novice self-experimenters may encounter similar challenges.

7   Conclusions

In this work, we designed, developed, and evaluated a novel system for users to conduct single case self-experiments in a scientific and automated manner. The QuantifyMe system was designed to create a framework for novice self-experimenters to find their personal optimal behavioral variables to achieve their goals by automating the single-case experimental design process within a mobile application. In a pilot study, we found that although target-behavior compliance was low, our participants still expressed interest in having such an system to determine how to personalize optimal behaviors. Future versions of the QuantifyMe system should include methods of increasing compliance via maintaining motivation on a daily basis and better preparing participants to be able to hit the target behaviors.

References

1. Barlow, D.H., Hersen, M.: Single Case Experimental Designs. Pergamon Press, New York (1984)
2. Brooke, J.: SUS - A quick and dirty usability scale. Usability Eval. Ind. **189**, 4–7 (1996)
3. Choe, E.K., et al.: Understanding quantified-selfers' practices in collecting and exploring personal data. In: CHI 2014, pp. 1143–1152 (2014)
4. Cordeiro, F., et al.: Rethinking the mobile food journal. In: CHI 2015, pp. 3207–3216 (2015)
5. Daskalova, N., et al.: SleepCoacher: a personalized automated self-experimentation system for sleep recommendations. In: Proceedings of 29th Annual Symposium User Interface Software Technology, pp. 347–358 (2016)
6. Dugard, P.: Randomization tests: a new gold standard? J. Context Behav. Sci. **3**, 65–68 (2014)
7. Epstein, D.: Personal informatics in everyday life. In: UbiComp 2015, pp. 429–434 (2015)
8. Evans, B.: PACO Personal Analytics Companion (2017). https://quantifiedself. appspot.com/
9. Halko, S., Kientz, J.A.: Personality and persuasive technology: an exploratory study on health-promoting mobile applications. In: Ploug, T., Hasle, P., Oinas-Kukkonen, H. (eds.) PERSUASIVE 2010. LNCS, vol. 6137, pp. 150–161. Springer, Heidelberg (2010). https://doi.org/10.1007/978-3-642-13226-1_16
10. Jawbone Inc., Jawbone Up App (2017). https://jawbone.com/
11. MyFitnessPal Inc., MyFitnessPal Inc. (2017). https://www.mytnesspal.com/
12. John, O.P., Srivastava, S.: The Big Five trait taxonomy: history, measurement, and theoretical perspectives. Handb. Personal Theory Res. **2**, 102–138 (1999)
13. Karkar, R., et al.: TummyTrials: a feasibility study of using self-experimentation to detect individualized food triggers. In: CHI 2017 (2017)
14. Karkar, R.: A framework for self-experimentation in personalized health. J. Am. Med. Informatics Assoc. **23**, 440–448 (2016)
15. Lillie, E.O.: The n-of-1 clinical trial: the ultimate strategy for individualizing medicine? Per. Med. **8**, 161–173 (2011)
16. Meldrum, M.L.: A brief history of hte randomized controlled trial: from oranges and lemons to gold standard. Hematol. Oncol. Clin. North. Am. **14**, 745–760 (2000)
17. Neuringer, A.: Self-experimentation: a call for change. Behaviorism **9**(1), 79–94 (1981)
18. Newman, F.L., Wong, S.E.: Progress and outcomes assessment of individual patient data: selecting single-subject design and statistical procedures. In: Use of Psychological Tests for Assessing Treatment Outcomes, vol. 1 General considerations, pp. 273–289, 3rd edn. (2004)
19. Sano, A.: Measuring college students' sleep, stress, mental health and wellbeing with wearable sensors and mobile phones. Ph.D. Dissertation. Massachusetts Institute of Technology (2016)
20. Sauro, J.: SUStisfied? Little-known system usability scale facts. User Exp. 14–15 (2011)

Discriminant Analysis Based EMG Pattern Recognition for Hand Function Rehabilitation

Jia Deng[1], Jian Niu[2], Kun Wang[3], Li Xie[4], and Geng Yang[1(✉)]

[1] State Key Laboratory of Fluid Power and Mechatronic Systems, Zhejiang University,
Hangzhou, China
yanggeng@zju.edu.cn
[2] School of Information Science and Technology, Fudan University, Shanghai, China
[3] School of Mechanical Engineering, Jiangnan University, Wuxi, China
[4] Thin Film Electronics ASA, Linköping, Sweden

Abstract. Electromyographic (EMG) signal is playing an important role on hand function training as a neuromuscular rehabilitation tool. Various pattern recognition algorithms (PRAs) have been compared and evaluated in previous research, and Linear Discriminant Analysis (LDA) showed the higher offline accuracy for motion classification. However, it is rarely of comparison for different types of Discriminant Analysis (DA), and the surface electrodes are common methods for signal acquisition. This paper proposes to evaluate the offline performance of LDA and other types of DA, and using Myo armband for recording signals. The offline data was acquired by Myo armband, processing recognizing the data in BioPatRec, an open source platform for motion classification and hand prosthetics control. From the results of average offline accuracy, training time, and testing time of the five types, LDA and Quadratic Discriminant Analysis (QDA) have the better performance than others, and LDA is the fastest algorithm with simple computing.

Keywords: Electromyographic (EMG) signal
Linear Discriminant Analysis (LDA) · Myo armband
Hand function rehabilitation

1 Introduction

Electromyographic (EMG) signal is produced by skeletal muscles, and be displayed with action potentials by recording electrodes, like surface or intramuscular electrodes [1, 2]. The EMG signal which includes a large of neural information could be applied to motion classification, hand control or hand function rehabilitation for amputees. Stroke is a chronic disease, and the hand function by post-stroke is very difficult to recover, and the rehabilitation robots are the most common method to train hand function [3]. Furthermore, EMG-driven systems are more effective than the continuous passive mode [4].

There are many algorithms for pattern recognition such as Linear Discriminant Analysis (LDA) [5], Multi-Layer Perception (MLP) [6], Artificial Neural Networks

© ICST Institute for Computer Sciences, Social Informatics and Telecommunications Engineering 2018
P. Perego et al. (Eds.): MobiHealth 2017, LNICST 247, pp. 207–214, 2018.
https://doi.org/10.1007/978-3-319-98551-0_24

(ANN) [7, 8], and Support Vector Machine (SVM) [9]. The performance of motion classification depends on the classification accuracy, misclassification rate and the time, etc. LDA, a statistical classification method, is the fastest algorithm with low complexity and quick training than other types of the algorithms [5, 10]. The procedures of pattern recognition consist of signal recordings, signal treatment, feature extraction, and pattern recognition. BioPatRec [11] is a modular open source research platform based on MATLAB for prosthetic control.

In BioPatRec, there are friendly GUIs for users to make experiments, and the implementation of algorithms consist of recording signal, signal treatment, feature extraction, motion classification and hand control. LDA has the higher offline accuracy, and most of researches had evaluated the performance of LDA and other PRAs. However, it is rarely used for the evaluation of different types of DA. The surface and intramuscular electrodes are considered as the common tools for acquiring signals [12]. In this study, Myo armband was used to collect EMG signals. Myo armband is a wearable gesture control and motion control device for you to control your mobile phone, computer, and so much more, touch-free by Thalmic Labs [13].

The aim of this work was to evaluate the offline performance of LDA and other types of DA from accuracy, training and testing time of them, especially with QDA, and using Myo armband to acquire the EMG signals.

2   Method

2.1   Signal Acquisition and Processing

BioPatRec provides the offline data from the data repository, which was acquired by the disposable Ag/AgCl bipolar electrodes and NI acquisition hardware board. In this paper, Myo armband was used to acquiring EMG signals. The Myo armband is composed of 8 parts connected together with the expandable flex inside the electrical sensors (Fig. 1 [13]) (e.g. medical grade stainless EMG sensors, highly sensitive nine-axis IMU containing three-axis gyroscope, three-axis accelerometer, and three-axis magneto-meter) for every part, and could recognize 20 motions. The armband is connected to a device (e.g. phone, computer or tablet and supported for most of systems) through Bluetooth 4.0 Low Energy.

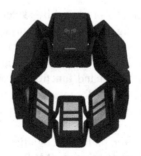

Fig. 1. Myo armband [13]

The placement of the Myo armband was around the forearm proximal third of the forearm, and the part with status LED was placed along the extensor carpi ulnaris. Then a program was developed under Microsoft Visual Studio 2012 environment to read the EMG data saved in csv file, and a creat_recS.m file was developed to save the row data in the structure array recSession which can be later loaded and displayed in BioPatRec GUI. Ten non-amputee subjects participated in this study (six men and four women) with the age of (23 ± 1.25). The sampling rate was set at 200 Hz.

The subjects performed the motion for 3 s, and the relax time was 3 s between each contraction. Repeat each movement for 3 times of 10 movements, including agree (AG), close hand (CH), open hand (OH), extend hand (EH), flex hand (FH), pointer (PT), supination (SP), pronation (PR), side grip (SG), and fine grip (FG), shown in Fig. 2.

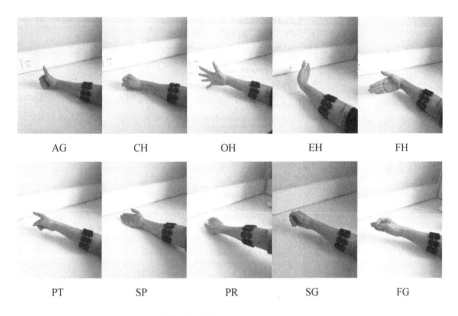

AG   CH   OH   EH   FH

PT   SP   PR   SG   FG

Fig. 2. The ten movements

In order to get the effective information and remain the isotonic contraction, we removed the 15% of the contraction time at the beginning and end of the recording data, which means the contraction percentage (cTp) was 0.7. The acquired data was segmented into 121 time windows of 200 ms with a 50 ms increment. In BioPatRec, there are 4 groups of feature vectors, and we chose the Top 4: mean absolute value, zero crossings, slope sign changes, and wave length time-domain features.

2.2 Offline Pattern Recognition Procedures

Processing the data through applying filters (frequency or spatial), configuring time windows, and selecting the proportion of data sets, mostly is 40%, 20%, and 40% for training, validation and test. Normalization is necessary to unite the weight of standard deviations, otherwise, the learning algorithms would not get the accurate results. Different classifier topologies were applied in different types of classes, including Single, Ago/Antagonist-Mixed, One-Vs-All, One-Vs-One, and All-And-One. Single classifier is the simplest and usually used. In this paper, we chose DA as the pattern recognition algorithm, and training the data with five types of DA. The offline pattern recognition procedures are shown in Fig. 3.

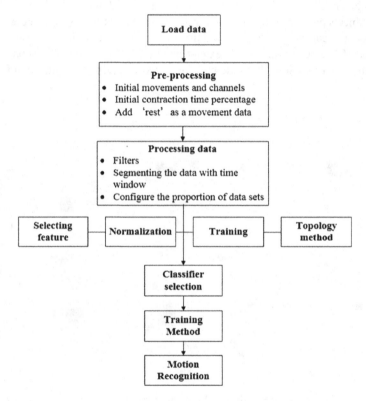

Fig. 3. Offline pattern recognition in BioPatRec

2.3   Pattern Recognition Algorithms

This paper aims to compare the Linear Discriminant Analysis (LDA) and Quadratic Discriminant Analysis (QDA) performance for offline performance.

LDA and QDA are both statistic methods Gaussian Maximum-likelihood based on Bayes' rule [14, 15]. LDA is build a linear function to separate the data by minimizing the inter-class distance with linear boundaries and maximizing the intra-class distance, and the all groups have the equal covariance matrices. QDA could learn the quadratic boundaries, and has different covariance matrices with different classes, which is more complicated than LDA.

3   Results

The offline accuracy and training time are shown in the box plots where the central line represents the median value; the edges of the box are the 25th and 75th percentiles; the whiskers give the range of data values; the diamond markers represent the mean values; and there were no outliers located within ±2.7σ in the data.

The average offline accuracy of Linear, Diaglinear, Quadratic, Diaquadratic, and Mahalanobis was 94.4 (±1.0%), 86.5 (±1.6%), and 96.5 (±0.7%), 89.87 (±1.3), and 95.3 (±0.6), respectively, which is illustrated in Fig. 4. The average training time was 0.100 s (±0.006 s), 0.123 s (±0.008 s), 0.115 s (±0.004 s), 0.112 s (±0.013 s), and 0.119 s (±0.011 s) for Linear, Diaglinear, Quadratic, Diaquadratic and Mahalanobis, respectively, shown in Fig. 5.

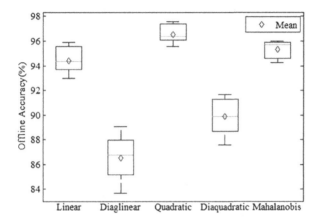

Fig. 4. Offline accuracy for five types of DA

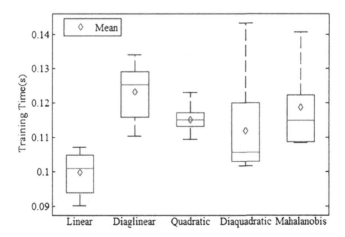

Fig. 5. Training time for five types of DA

The average testing time was 0.629 ms (±0.029 ms), 0.598 ms (±0.005 ms), 1.038 ms (±0.048 ms), 1.007 ms (±0.004 ms), and 1.032 ms (±0.045 ms) for Linear, Diaglinear, Quadratic, Diaquadratic, and Mahalanobis, respectively. The results are illustrated in Fig. 6. The average testing time of LDA is approximately half of the QDA.

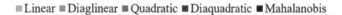

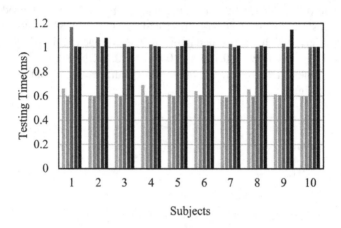

Fig. 6. Testing time for five types of DA

The average accuracy of every movement for the LDA and QDA is shown in Fig. 7. For LDA, the average accuracy was 100%, 100%, 99.8%, 86.5%, 99,8%, 95.7%, 87.3%, 73,7%, 98.2%, and 99.4% for AG, CH, OH, EH, PT, SP, PR, SG, and FG, respectively. For QDA, the average accuracy was 100%, 100%, 99.6%, 98.2%, 99.1%, 98.0%, 86.7%, 100%, and 99.0% for AG, CH, OH, EH, PT, SP, PR, SG, and FG, respectively. The

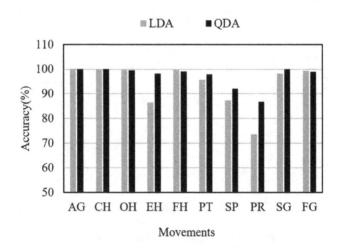

Fig. 7. Offline accuracy of 10 movements for LDA and QDA

lowest accuracy movement of LDA and QDA was both pronation, and the AG, CH, OH, FH, SG, and FG had the extremely high accuracy.

4   Conclusions

The offline results show that LDA and QDA have a better performance for motion classification. The offline average accuracy of them can be higher than 90%, and without statistic difference of the training/validation time between them, but LDA is more stable and lower than QDA. The testing time of LDA is approximately half of the QDA, because the QDA's quadratic boundaries and complicated computing algorithm. LDA finds a linear function, which is more popular and simpler with the fastest training and testing time and used extensively in previous research. QDA could be applied in more complicated classes and massive data. The pronation had the lowest accuracy among the movements for both LDA and QDA. It is likely to be influenced by many factors, such as the placement of the Myo armband, and the subjects' attention and motivation would influence the results. When the amount of training data is relatively small, the LDA is better than QDA. It is necessary to reduce the variance of the QDA model. If the training data contains a large amount of observation data, it will be more likely to use QDA, and the variance of the classifier is no longer a major issue.

In summary, this work aims contribute to the recovery of the post-stroke patients' hand functions. Comparing with motormechanical systems, EMG signals should be seen as the more effective and interactive approach in this aspect. In the future, we could evaluate the real-time classification by the motion test or the Target Achievement Control (TAC) test with Myo armband.

Acknowledgments. The authors would like to thank all of the participants in this study and the open source research platform BioPatRec. The research work was supported by Fundamental Research Funds for the Central Universities, the Science Fund for Creative Research Groups of the National Natural Science Foundation of China (Grant No. 51521064), and National Natural Science Foundation of China (Grant No. 51505190).

References

1. Jiang, N., Falla, D., D'Avella, A.: Myoelectric control in neurorehabilitation. J. Crit. Rev. Biomed. Eng. **38**(4), 381 (2010)
2. Hargrove, L., Englehart, K., Hudgins, B.: A comparison of surface and intramuscular myoelectric signal classification. J. IEEE Trans. Biomed. Eng. **54**, 847–853 (2007)
3. Chen, M., Ho, S.K., Zhou, H.F., Pang, P.M.K., Hu, X.L.: Interactive rehabilitation robot for hand function training. In: IEEE International Conference on Rehabilitation Robotics, pp. 777–780 (2009)
4. Fasoli, S.E., Krebs, H.I., Hogan, N.: Robotic technology and stroke rehabilitation: translating research into practice. J. Top. Stroke Rehabil. **11**, 11–19 (2004)
5. Huang, Y., Englehart, K.B., Hudgins, B.: A Gaussian mixture model based classification scheme for myoelectric control of powered upper limb prostheses. J. IEEE Trans. Biomed. Eng. **52**(11), 1801 (2005)

6. Le, M.D.K., Gale, T.J., Jiang, D., Olivier, J.C., Ortiz-Catalan, M.: Multi-layer perceptron training algorithms for pattern recognition of myoelectric signals. In: Biomedical Engineering International Conference, pp. 1–5 (2013)

7. Hudgins, B., Parker, P., Scott, R.N.: A new strategy for multifunction myoelectric control. J. IEEE Trans. Biomed. Eng. **40**(1), 82–94 (1993)

8. Amsüss, S., Paredes, L.P., Rudigkeit, N., Graimann, B., Herrmann, M.J., Farina, D.: Long term stability of surface EMG pattern classification for prosthetic control. In: 35th Annual International Conference of the IEEE Engineering in Medicine and Biology Society (EMBC), pp. 3622–3625 (2013)

9. Oskoei, M.A., Hu, H.: Support vector machine-based classification scheme for myoelectric control applied to upper limb. J. IEEE Trans. Biomed. Eng. **55**(8), 1956–1965 (2008)

10. Zhang, H., Zhao, Y., Yao, F., Xu, L., Shang, P., Li, G.: An adaptation strategy of using LDA classifier for EMG pattern recognition. In: 35th Annual International Conference of the IEEE Engineering in Medicine and Biology Society (EMBC), pp. 4267–4270 (2013)

11. Ortiz-Catalan, M., Brånemark, R., Håkansson, B.: BioPatRec: a modular research platform for the control of artificial limbs based on pattern recognition algorithms. J. Source Code for Biol. Med. **8**(1), 11 (2013)

12. Hargrove, L.J., Englehart, K., Hudgins, B.: A comparison of surface and intramuscular myoelectric signal classification. J. IEEE Trans. Biomed. Eng. **54**(5), 847–853 (2007)

13. Myo. https://www.myo.com/

14. Srivastava, S., Gupta, M.R., Frigyik, B.A.: Bayesian quadratic discriminant analysis. J. Mach. Learn. Res. **8**(8), 1277–1305 (2007)

15. Chen, X., Zhang, D., Zhu, X.: Application of a self-enhancing classification method to electromyography pattern recognition for multifunctional prosthesis control. J. Neuroeng. Rehabil. **10**(1), 44 (2013)

Advances in Soft Wearable Technology for Mobile-Health

Presentation of a New Sensor Enabling Reliable Real Time Foot Plantar Pressure Distribution Retrieval

Foued Melakessou[1]([⊠]), Werner Bieck[2], Quentin Lallemant[2],
Guendalina Palmirotta[2], and Baptiste Anti[2]

[1] Luxembourg Institute of Science and Technology, L4362 Belval, Luxembourg
foued.melakessou@list.lu
[2] IEE S.A., 5386 Contern, Luxembourg
https://www.iee.lu/en/products/sports-healthcare/smart-foot-sensor

Abstract. Monitoring plantar load conditions becomes useful in many health care fields, e.g. podiatric and orthopedic applications, rehabilitation tools, sports and fitness training tools, and in-field diagnosis and prevention tools for posture, balance, loading and contact times monitoring. IEE target is to provide a single insole-solution for daily usage in order to acquire information on the plantar load distribution for health prophylaxis in a large range of different shoe configurations. In this paper, we introduce for the first time a new **High-Dynamic** (HD) multi-cell smart insole sensor enabling advanced real-time foot plantar pressure monitoring applications. The in-situ measurement of the dynamic plantar load distribution provides an important new source of information that can be combined with traditional monitoring systems often based on accelerometer and gyroscope sensors. In fact, the new smart insole as presented here, facilitates the discovery in an early phase of any biomechanical mismatch in the walking or running gait of its user. Specific datasets have been recorded from a representative healthy population with different monitoring tools, i.e. force plate, pressure matrix and our new smart insole. The aim was to study the similarity of measurements recorded by each system on a defined measurement protocol. It is shown that the new monitoring device provides a competitive methodology to measure static and dynamic foot plantar pressure distribution. The system flexibility and robustness enable the development of new real-time applications, such as high peak pressure detection for diabetics, activity tracking, etc. The paper is organized as follows: we provide in Sect. 1 an overview of challenges and opportunities around foot pressure monitoring and discuss the sensing capabilities. Then we give a description of the new smart insole designed by IEE in Sect. 2. Next we define in Sect. 3 the measurement protocol based on 3 different systems, followed in Sect. 4 by a comparison of their efficiency and reliability. Finally, Sect. 5 provides related works and Sect. 6 concludes the paper.

Keywords: Foot pressure distribution · Smart insole · Force plate

© ICST Institute for Computer Sciences, Social Informatics and Telecommunications Engineering 2018
P. Perego et al. (Eds.): MobiHealth 2017, LNICST 247, pp. 217–224, 2018.
https://doi.org/10.1007/978-3-319-98551-0_25

1 Introduction and Motivation

IEE's smart insole provides users with in-field dynamic monitoring capabilities of the foot plantar pressure distribution. It covers a wide measurement range of pressure and can thus be applied to walking, running, and jumping activities. Connected to a wearable electronic module, it provides real-time data about the plantar contact pressure from proprietary-designed robust high dynamic pressure sensing cells. Each insole is composed by a discrete number of sensor cells, which supports an easy electronic sensor readout and a high measurement frequency. According to an easy integration, it can support foot practitioners in real-life correction diagnosis. The foot pressure map is actually needed in order to identify special gait patterns and design optimized shoes adapted to each person, so that pain and injury risks can be reduced during physical activities thanks to a dedicated training control. This information can also be retrieved with large fixed pressure detection plates that measure on-line the contact pressure between barefoot and the ground under lab condition. Our new thin sensor belongs to a second type of mobile insole-system solutions. It does not affect the overall shoe comfort felt by the user during daily activities due to its high flexibility and robustness. An **E**lectronic **C**ontrol **U**nit (ECU), connected to the sensor, manages data communication to third-party interface systems such as smart-phone, tablet or laptop where additional processing can be applied. This allows mobile real-time applications, that are not feasible with uncomfortable monitoring equipments such as force plates, due to large electronic devices, connectors, cabling etc.

2 Sensor Description

The smart insole is based on a flexible, foil-type sensing device. It detects sole force loads by providing locally in real-time transient dynamic electrical signals. As a consequence, pressure, strain and dynamic force load can be simultaneously monitored. The smart insole is composed by eight individual cells spatially distributed in the main areas where foot pressure changes statistically occurs, i.e. two cells for the heel, one cell for the mid-foot, three cells for the metatarsal area and finally two cells for the toes (see Fig. 1). Each sensor cell covers a

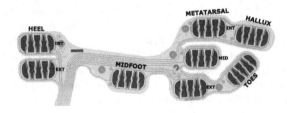

Fig. 1. IEE's smart insole comprising 8-HD pressure cells. The cell design has been elaborated within a comprehensive IEE research project [1,2].

detection area of about $30 \times 15\,\text{mm}^2$ in order to be robust against lateral shifts of the plantar pressure loads that can be due to individual anatomic deviations and relative movements of the foot inside the shoe. The new HD **F**orce-**S**ensing **R**esistor (HD-FSR) multi-cell smart insole sensor enables advanced real-time gait analysis applications. HD-FSR sensors, with their individual triangular cell segmentation, cover a wide pressure range from 250 mbar up to 7 bar. Their robustness enables up to one million actuations under highest humidity conditions. Lifetime variation is smaller than 15%.

3 Measurement Protocol

The goal of the proposed measurement protocol is to show the reliability and repeatability of our sensor in static and dynamic configurations. A calibration process is firstly performed in order to build a unique mapping between each cell response and the applied pressure. An homogeneous pressure from 0 to 6 bar is applied on the complete insole by means of a specific membrane tester system. Then a look up table is generated and links uniquely each sensor **A**nalog to **D**igital **C**onversion (ADC) value to the applied pressure. A spline interpolation model is finally computed in order to convert any ADC value measured by a cell into its pressure load. This calibration process has been applied within IEE's laboratories for each insole in order to provide the same response level to all sensor cells. Each insole has been connected to a Kinematix- ECU enabling data recording at 100 Hz, combined with a 3D accelerometer and gyroscope [3]. Data have been wirelessly exchanged by means of a Bluetooth communication between ECU and a computer.

In order to study the sensor reliability, an alternative monitoring system [5] designed by Lion-Systems S.A. and based on a force plate, has been tested (see Fig. 2). It consists of a walkway of 3.2 m, composed by four blocks ($L80 \times W60 \times H6$ cm). One block includes a force plate from Kistler Instruments that records the ground reaction force exerted by the foot during gait. Four cameras recording 656×490 pixel images at a frame rate of 140 Hz are placed on each corner of the force plate with four metallic arms. Data from the cameras (motion capture based on 3D-coordinates of colored markers located on foot and leg) and force plate are simultaneously recorded. We also used a pressure platform WIN-POD ($L53 \times W60 \times H4.5$ cm) from the French company Medicapteurs [4] in order to retrieve the spatial pressure distribution over time. WIN-POD uses an IEE sensor mat which enables podometry data analysis according to its high sensitivity, its wide dynamic range of measurements, its precision and homogeneity at a frequency rate of 200 Hz. The active surface is about $400 \times 400\,\text{mm}^2$, composed by 2304 individual calibrated resistive cells (48×48 matrix of individual cells of size $8 \times 8\,\text{mm}^2$). The pressure range covers 0.4 N to 100 N.

For this study, five pairs of insoles M (EU-38 for women) and three pairs XL (EU-44 for men) have been used. Twenty three subjects had participated to a predefined measurement protocol for static (standing) and dynamic (walking) activities. The aim of the study was to check the accuracy of the new sensor in

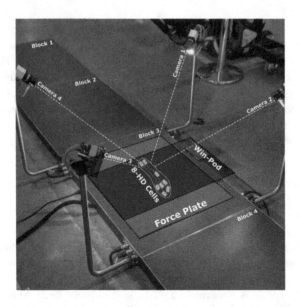

Fig. 2. Measurement set up environment. Three measurement systems (Force Plate, WINPOD and IEE's Smart Insole) have been synchronized in order to record at the same time pressure information of a complete gait cycle.

comparison to more complex systems often used as a reference in gait analysis to monitor plantar pressure distribution under lab conditions. For the static condition, test persons had to keep their neutral position without moving during ten seconds. Users had been also asked to wear flat shoes which can be expected to provide similar plantar load conditions as the barefoot one because any sole effect can be neglected. For the dynamic condition, test persons had been asked to walk at their natural speed on the four blocks. The starting distance from the force plate had been adapted for each person in order to record a specific step without gait modification. Test persons started in a stationary position. Afterwards, they walked forward a few meters with natural pace. Proper time synchronization allows a direct comparison of the pressure signal of the corresponding step reaching the force plate and the data extracted from the smart insole. Each test was composed by three trials in order to study the sensor repeatability.

4   Results

The standard force curve for walking is typically composed by a first peak corresponding to the breaking phase, a drop linked to the support phase and a second peak for the propulsion. If the user touches the ground with a high force, an additional high pressure peak at the heel appears very early during the gait cycle. The peak corresponding to the breaking phase occurs when the pressure is distributed between Heel and Mid-Foot. The force drop can disappear between the breaking and propulsion phases in case of a comparatively large plantar mid-foot surface, for instance for flat feet. For people with a distinct pronounced arch, the drop is more important.

The vertical force measured by the force plate had been correlated with the plantar pressure distribution recorded with the 8-HD sensor cells for each step trial. Both measurements were done simultaneously on the same step. Data had been normalized with the body weight for the force plate, and the sum of all cell responses for the insole, both under static condition. A typical pressure profile obtained with the insole sensor and the corresponding individual cell responses are plotted in Fig. 3(a).

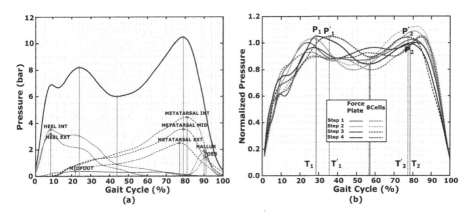

Fig. 3. (a) Typical pressure profile recorded with the new smart insole sensor. (b) Similarity between walking profiles recorded with the insole and the force plate. (Color figure online)

Figure 3(b) compares four steps measured with the insole and the force plate, randomly selected from the global dataset. For each step, the normalized pressure for the complete gait cycle has been plotted as solid (dashed) line for the force plate (insole, respectively). The step duration has been also normalized in order to enable a direct comparison between each walking profile. We can observe a high similarity in the dynamics. For instance, if we consider Step 4 in Fig. 3(b), signals from each system follows the same trends. T_1/T_2 corresponds to the relative timing with respect to the gait cycle duration when the first/second pressure peak occurs of relative amplitude P_1/P_2. The first peak practically occurs at around 25% of the gait cycle. A minimum is reached most of the time at around 60% and the second peak at around 80% of the gait cycle. A similarity metric $S(\delta)$ has been defined as the gait cycle proportion where the ratio between the force plate and 8-HD sensor cells belongs to the range $[1 - \delta, 1 + \delta]$ as can be used to quantify the similarity between the two systems' measurements. If we used an accepted deviation rate of $\delta = 0.2$, a relative difference of 20% is allowed between the two sensors for each time index. The obtained results for S are plotted in Fig. 4 for each step and subject weight. The metric intrinsically

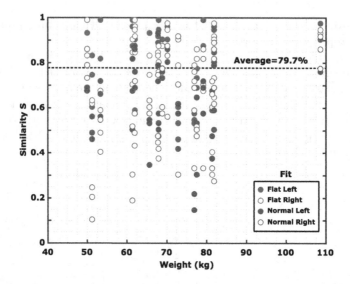

Fig. 4. Similarity metric S comparing force plate vs. insole for the complete dataset plotted versus subject weight. The force plate and the smart insole present similar signals when S is close to 1. (Color figure online)

belongs to $[0, 1]$. $S = 0$ if the difference between the two signals is always greater than 20% during the complete gait cycle. S reaches an average value of 79.7% for the overall experiment. Moreover, S is larger for flat shoes (red symbols) in comparison to normal shoes (blue symbols). This is due to the sole effect mentioned earlier which aims to distribute the pressure over the complete shoe. Thus the data acquisition inside the shoe gives additional information compared with force plate measurements and allow to study the influence and potential differences between different shoe types. As a conclusion, the new insole sensor provides very similar results as the force plate when measuring the total force load.

5   Related Works

Various complex systems have been released on the market enabling detailed gait analysis. They are mainly based on image processing by means of expensive data acquisition systems that need large laboratory environment, floor sensors, and wearables carried directly by the test persons. Researchers often rely on floor sensors, such as so-called sensor matrices or baropodometric mats since they provide a complete overview in real time of the pressure distribution below each patient's foot. Another interesting type of monitoring system comprises force plate sensors. In that case, the main issue is the large set up environment and also the impossibility to monitor the users' gait during their daily activities. Cheap wearables enable to measure different characteristics of the human gait based on pressure sensors directly placed on the patient's insoles and also inertial sensors that are the most widely used monitoring system in gait analysis. Gait data recorded in real conditions outside a laboratory, and also on the long term, become more relevant for an accurate analysis. The main advantage of these systems is that users can wear them in their daily life. Following pre-defined measurement protocols e.g. in case of force plate application is often felt as a heavy constraint by users. This has also an deep impact on data as the recorded gait signals can differ from the natural ones. In fact patients unconscious adapt their gait in order to walk on the right position where the sensor is located. These changes affect the measurement repeatability.

In [6], Herran et al. presented a complete survey on available systems focusing on gait analysis. They referenced a non-exhaustive list of sensors covering a large range of method, application, accuracy, price and ease of use. Force plates and wearables remain the most used candidates. For instance, in [7], Hadopp et al. presented a smart-shoe composed by three pressure sensors mounted on a flexible insole. It can reliably differentiate the most common postures and activities, according to an additional three-axis accelerometer. In [8], Sanghan et al. used the Pedar-x system, composed by an array of 99 capacitive sensors placed on a 2.6 mm thick insole. Da Rocha et al. selected in [9] the pressure mapping system Matscan from Tekscan Inc. In [10], Wafai et al. monitored the dynamic plantar pressure distribution in respect the F-scan in-shoe pressure measurement system composed by 960 sensors from Tekscan. In [11], Ferber et al. presented their smart shoe. They concluded that the pressure recorded by their device is highly correlated with data monitored simultaneously with a gold standard pressure-sensing device.

6   Conclusion and Outlook

In this paper, we introduced a novel smart insole sensor which consists of a flexible carrier foil comprising eight individual pressure cells. This system enables advanced real-time foot plantar pressure monitoring applications. It offers a new research tool in order to monitor in a reliable and accurate way the gait dynamic of its user. We have studied the correlation between the data recorded with the new smart insole, a force plate and a pressure matrix based on a defined measurement protocol. It could be shown that this new sensor device provides in fact a competitive approach to measure static foot plantar distribution and also gate dynamics in daily life. Future works will consist of the design of enhanced algorithms in order to automatically extract gait features. A potential next goal can be the characterization and the classification of individual walking profiles into healthy and non-healthy categories. Warning notifications can be provided in case of walking profile anomalies that can be caused by an illness evolution. For that, sophisticated mathematical models will be used to generate the complete pressure distribution on each foot based on spatial interpolation schemes.

Acknowledgments. We are grateful to the Ministry of Economy & Commerce in Luxembourg who funded the research project [2] prior to this study and to Kinematix for providing the data acquisition electronics [3].

References

1. Steier, A.: Film-type pressure sensor e.g. for article of footwear. Patent US 20140144251 A1 (2014)
2. Bieck, W.: In-situ stress detection of human foot soles using multiple integrated sensing techniques. Founded by Ministry of Economy & Commerce, Luxembourg, MECO Research Project 12942, Ref. CUN10/12/RED Technical Reports I-VI (2012–2015)
3. De Castro, M., et al.: Accuracy and repeatability of the gait analysis by the Walkin-Sense system. BioMed Res. Int. **2014** (2014). https://doi.org/10.1155/2014/348659
4. http://www.medicapteurs.fr/
5. Samson, W.: A portable system for foot biomechanical analysis during gait. Gait Posture **40**(3), 420–428 (2014). https://doi.org/10.1016/j.gaitpost.2014.05.010
6. Herran, A., Zapirain, B., Zorilla, A.: Gait analysis methods: an overview of wearable and non-wearable systems, highlighting clinical applications. Sensors **2014**(14), 3362–3394 (2014). https://doi.org/10.3390/s140203362
7. Hodapp, C., Edgar, R., Fulk, G., Sazonov, E.: Real-time posture and activity recognition by SmartShoe. In: 2012 International Conference on Environment Science and Engineering, IPCBEE, vol. 32. IACSIT Press, Singapore (2012)
8. Sanghan, S., Leelasamran, W., Chatpun, S.: Imbalanced gait characteristics based on plantar pressure assessment in patients with hemiplegia. Walailak J. Sci. Technol. (WJST) **12**(7) (2015). https://doi.org/10.14456/WJST.2015.69
9. da Rocha, E., Bratz, D., Goubert, L., Machado, A., de David, A., Carpes, F.: Influence of obesity on plantar pressure and foot sensitivity of children. In: ISB 2013, Congress of the International Society of Biomechanics (2013)
10. Wafai, L., Zayegh, A., Woulfe, J., Aziz, S., Begg, R.: Identification of foot pathologies based on plantar pressure asymmetry. Sensors **15**, 20392–20408 (2015). https://doi.org/10.3390/s150820392
11. Ferber, R., Webber, T., Kin, B., Everett, B., Groenland, M.: Validation of plantar pressure measurements for a novel in-shoe plantar sensory replacement unit. J. Diabetes Sci. Technol. **7**(5), 1167–1175 (2013)

Humans Sensitivity Distribution in Perceptual Space by a Wearable Haptic Sleeve

Daniel Goodman, Atulya Nagar, Emanuele Lindo Secco,
and Anuradha Ranasinghe$^{(\boxtimes)}$

Liverpool Hope University, Liverpool, UK
{14008961,nagara,seccoe,dissana}@hope.ac.uk

Abstract. Haptic perception plays a major role when vision and audition are partially or fully impaired. Therefore, this paper tries to give a brief overview on humans' sensitivity distribution in perceptual space. During our experiments, a wearable sleeve with 7 vibro-actuators was used to stimulate subjects arm to convey haptic feedback. The basic research questions in this study are: (1) whether humans' perception linearly correlated with the actuation frequency, haptic feedback in our scenario (2) humans' ability to generalise templates via the wearable haptic sleeve. Those findings would be useful to increase humans' perception when humans have to work with fully or partially impaired perception in their day-to-day life.

Keywords: Wearable devices · Haptics · Human-robot interactions
Humans' perceptual space

1 Introduction

According to the Statistical bulletin of national population projection in 2014, the UK population will be increased by 9.7 million over the next 25 years [1]. As the projected population and ageing over the coming years, it is very important think of how to uplift elderly people on daily life, perhaps to become more independent as well. Perception, cognition, and movement control are some of the main concerns of the age related issues when the aged population is grown [2]. When it comes to perceptions, haptics would be the best alternative to enhance their abilities in communication when visual and auditory are impaired fully or partially with ageing. Moreover, there are some situations people have to work in impaired perceptions like indoor fire-fighting, search and rescue, or noisy environments like a factory. In this scenario, having haptic feedback is important. Therefore, it is very important to understand humans' perception in haptic feedback. Haptics would be used to convey messages in some tasks to convey some spatial information when people are partially or fully impaired [3]. There have been some efforts that have been taken to enhance the elderly people daily activities. Some studies focused on effect of haptic supplementation by different methods to support posture stabilization in elderly people [4]. The results of this study concluded that haptic feedback enhances posture control to make them independent. A robotic walker was made to help the elderly people's walking in [5]. In this study, the robotic walker escorts the elderly people. Moreover, previous studies demonstrated that haptic

© ICST Institute for Computer Sciences, Social Informatics and Telecommunications Engineering 2018
P. Perego et al. (Eds.): MobiHealth 2017, LNICST 247, pp. 225–232, 2018.
https://doi.org/10.1007/978-3-319-98551-0_26

perceptions would be the solution to guide humans in unfamiliar/uncertain environments [6–9]. Since haptic feedback has been widely used to convey messages to humans, it is important to understand how humans perceive the haptic feedback.

Vibro-actuators have been widely treated as a good communication equipment in haptic perception in different applications. As an example, the previous study on an active belt with wearable tactile display in [9] can be used to transmit information in multiple direction. In addition to that it can combine with a GPS directional sensor and 7 vibro-actuators. Moreover, there have been some studies on using vibro-tactile displays have showed that it can be used to improve the quality in many ways, for example devices for reading for people with less visual perceptions [10] or to provide haptic feedback of body tilt [11]. Furthermore, haptic feedback has been used in balance control, and postural stability [12, 13] in some studies in the past with some wearable devices. However, our attempt in this paper is to understand humans' arm perception when they wear a haptic sleeve with actuated micro vibrators. The results would give us ideas as to humans' sensitivity and their capabilities in perceptual space.

Amplitude was the most dominant way to convey the messages to humans in most of the haptic-based stimulation in the past [14–17]. However, our argument is that the frequency would be better for persistent perception in order to the nature of mechanoreceptors of the human skin.

This paper focuses on two different experiments. The experiment 1 was de- signed to understand humans' sensitivity distribution in perceptual space by using the wearable haptic sleeve. The experiment 2 was designed to understand humans ability to generalize haptic-based templates when they are trained.

The organization of this paper as follows. Section 2 discusses the experimental methodology to collect data of human participants while they wear the haptic sleeve and the different intensity patterns were played to understand humans' sensitivity and their ability to generalize templates. Section 3 shows the results of experiment 1 and 2. Finally, Sect. 4 presents a conclusion and future works.

2 Materials and Methods

In order to produce wearable haptic based pattern feedback the use of (Precision Microdrives) Pico Vibe 10 mm vibration motor – 3 mm type were used in order to produce a wearable haptic sleeve. In total the Haptic Sleeve consists 7 Pico Vibe 10 mm vibroactuators arranged in equal distance as shown in Fig. 1. In order for the device to be made wearable, the 7 Pico Vibe 10 mm vibroactuators are attached to seven velcro belts allowing the device to be adjusted in order to fit the arm size of the participant as shown in Fig. 1. The different intensities for the vibrations are generated by Genuino Mega 2560 motherboard, However in order to reach the desired and frequency needed to complete the experiment the amplitude is modulated using simple power amplifier circuit as shown in Fig. 1 [18].

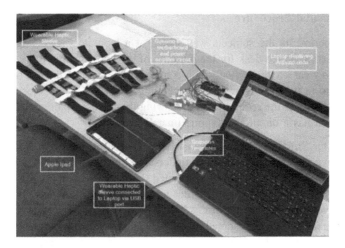

Fig. 1. Experimental Setup: A wearable vibro-tactile actuator arrays, here 7 Pico Vibe 10 mm vibro-actuator motors were attached to the belt. Arduino Mega motherboard was used to different amplitudes. The power amplifier circuit has been used to amplify the signal (amplitudes in here) [18].

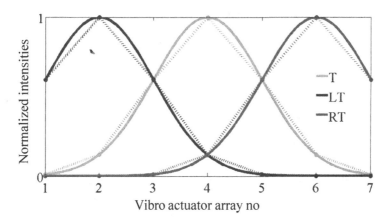

Fig. 2. The templates: The Gaussian Template (T), Gaussian shifted Left (LT), and Gaussian shifted Right (RT) are shown. The standard function $y = gaussmf\ (x,\ [sig,\ c]))$ was used to generate the three different templates. the dashed lines shows the real intensities in experiment 2.

2.1 Haptic Primitives (Templates)

To generate templates, the standard Gaussian function was used. The templates were generated by standard MATLAB function called gaussmf ($y = gaussmf\ (x,\ [sig,\ c])$). The MATLAB programming language (The MATLAB Inc, MATLAB 2014b) was used during the analysis, where $sig = std$, and c is the centre of the distribution. The sig for pattern T, LT, and RT is 1.

2.2 Experimental Procedure

During all experiments the subjects was seated at a laboratory desk, with their arm outstretched resting on the desk for the duration of the experimental trails. The subject was required to wear a vibro-actuator belt containing the seven Vibro- actuators this is then adjusted to fit the arm using Velcro strapping. They are then subjected to Vibro-tactile stimulation with the requirement of drawing the intensity pattern after each trial. Each experiment has a duration of approximately one hour.

Experiment 1: Study Humans' Sensitivity Distribution. Eight subjects were recruited for experiment one in order to understand humans sensitivity distribution in perceptual space. The recruitment criteria stated that potential subject must be healthy and between the ages 18–50 years in order to participate in the study. Subjects were required to give their informed consent before any participation. Within those eight subjects both genders are represented equally. All subjects were required to wear the haptic sleeve containing 7 Vibro-actuators for the duration of the experiment. During the experiment, each subject was subjected to vibro tactile stimulation, in the form of a flat frequency pattern played across all seven Vibro-actuators. During each trial, all vibro-actuators vibrate simultaneously, with each trials lasting roughly ten to fifteen seconds. At the end of each trial the subjects were required to draw intensity pattern across using a drawing app on the Apple ipad (Draw free app (Apple Inc)). Raw data each subjects were then digitized using Getdata Graph Digitizer, all processing of Data and all statistical analysis was analysed by MATLAB 2014a.

Experiment 2: Study on How Humans Generalize Haptic-Based Patterns. Using the same experimental set up from Experiment 1, Experiment 2 was carried out to understand how humans generalize haptic-based patterns. Participants again were required to wear the haptic based pattern feedback sleeve. Throughout the duration of the experiment participants were asked to keep the arm stretched and resting on the desk. Three different intensity patterns were selected Standard Gaussian pattern (T), Gaussian pattern shifted to the left (LT), Gaussian pattern shifted to the right (RT), as shown in Fig. 2. The studies in humans' learning in movements showed that humans learnt through flexible combination of primitives that can be modelled using Gaussian like functions [19]. In this study focuses to explore whether human brain has primitive patterns that can be modelled using Gaussian like functions to represent haptic perceptions as well.

Since the experiment 2 independent from experiment 1, it was conducted with a different group ((4 - male, 4 - female), age between 24 to 26) from experiment 1. During the first fifteen trials, participants were shown the templates and the stimulation was given. Participants were only required to draw a smooth curve in order to represent their perception of each image, using an ipad drawing app. The three Gaussian patterns were played pseudo randomly. The drawing area participants was demarcated to match the size of the printed pattern template so that they would not try to scale the image. This was explained to all participants at the start of each experiment.

3 Results

3.1 Experiment 1

The raw data from experiment 1 for the flat frequency distribution is shown in Fig. 3A for a selected subject. In general, subjects were able to draw the played intensities as shown in Fig. 3A. Subjects were able to distinguish between the 200 Hz and 300 stimulus Hz as shown in Fig. 3A. Interesting, perception frequency is linearly increased with the actuation frequency as shown in Fig. 3B. It would be nice to study a wider range of actuation frequencies. However, due to the technical limitation of the vibro-actuators and humans' most desirable perception frequencies, the perception frequencies was limited to 200 Hz and 300 Hz.

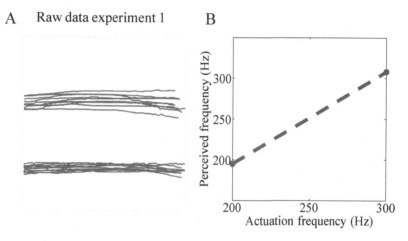

Fig. 3. The experiment 1 was designed to understand human sensitivity distribution: (A) Raw data representation: one of the subjects' sketch data, the total number of trails are 20 for experiment 1, (B) actuation frequency and perceived frequency are shown. Average perceived frequency are shown, 8 subjects participated 10 trials for 200 Hz, and 300 Hz actuation frequencies during the experiment 1.

3.2 Experiment 2

The raw data from experiment 2 for the pattern T, RT, and LT in experiment 2 are shown in Fig. 4A. Here, the black dashed line was used to show templates. The raw data in Fig. 4A were regressed against respective templates in Fig. 2. The average regression coefficients values are shown in Fig. 4B. In Fig. 4, all regression coefficients have increased in the last one third of the experimental trials except for the template T as shown in Fig. 4B. The average regression coefficients of template T are higher during the first and second third of experimental trials compared to LT and RT as shown in Fig. 4B. It implies that subjects have a better ability to generalize scaled template after reasonable number of experimental trials when stimulations are different. However, higher variability in last third of the trials could come due to fatigue. We assume that possible causes for variability could come from physiological factors like muscle tension and psychological factors like attention.

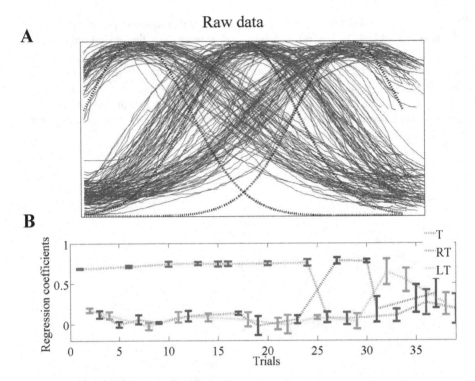

Fig. 4. Sketched data and regression coefficients: (A) The raw data of Experiment 2, and (B) Average regression coefficients when data regressed with templates in Fig. 2. The variability of the regression coefficients are shown by error bars.

4   Discussion

This paper presents experimental evidence of humans perceptions in perceptual space and their abilities to distinguish and generalize a class of primitive haptic feedback patterns after training. The results of the experiments show how humans recognize trained cutaneous feedback patterns as well as their scales. Those results provide us to understand capabilities and limitations of the humans in somatosensory system. Therefore, those preliminary findings could be used to continue our studies to understand humans' sensitivity distribution in perceptual space by using different parts of the body.

In future, we will do more training session to train the templates with human participants. The results of humans' perceptions will give us some degree of freedom to bring humans with less impairments (visual and auditory) more independent: for example, an elderly person living in a house alone with visual and auditory perceptions are impaired due to ageing. Moreover, we can we can use those to enhance the humans' perceptions when they are in noisy environments like in a factory, and search and rescue scenario.

Even though the regression coefficient were improved last one third of the trials in Fig. 4B, the low regression coefficients in first and second half of trials in Fig. 4B suggest that even if recognition of the tactile patterns were high, performance would still be poor if there was a drawing difficulty. Therefore, we deliver some psychophysical experiments to understand the degree of drawing difficulties. This would be the best way to quantify degree of drawing difficulties of the humans. This would be tested on naive and trained participants in the future.

Acknowledgments. The authors would like to thank UK Engineering and Physical Sciences Research Council (EPSRC) grant no. EP/I028765/1 and grant no. EP/NO3211X/1, the Guy's and St Thomas' Charity grant on developing clinician-scientific interfaces in robotic assisted surgery: translating technical in- novation into improved clinical care (grant no. R090705), and Higher Education Innovation Fund (HEIF).

References

1. Statistical bulletin of national population projection, 19 June 2017 https://www.ons.gov.uk/peoplepopulationandcommunity/populationandmigration/populationprojections/bulletins/
2. Fisk, A.D., Czaja, S.J., Rogers, W.A., Charness, N., Sharit, J.: Designing for Older Adults: Principles and Creative Human Factors Approaches. CRC Press, Boca Raton (2009)
3. Hale, K.S., Stanney, K.M.: Deriving haptic design guidelines from human physiological, psychophysical, and neurological foundations. Comput. Graph. App. **24**(2), 33–39 (2004)
4. Albertsen, I.M., Temprado, J.J., Berton, E.: Effect of haptic supplementation provided by a fixed or mobile stick on postural stabilization in elderly people. Gerontology **58**(5), 419–429 (2012)
5. Morris, A., et al.: A robotic walker that provides guidance. In: IEEE International Conference on Robotics and Automation, Proceedings, vol. 1, pp. 25–30 (2003)
6. Gilson, R.D., Redden, E.S., Elliott, L.R.: Remote tactile displays for future soldiers, Technical report, DTIC Document (2007)
7. Jones, L.A., Lederman, S.J.: Human Hand Function. Oxford University Press, Oxford (2006)
8. Gilson, R.D., Redden, E.S., Elliott, L.R.: Remote tactile displays for future soldiers. University of Central Florida, Orlando (2007)
9. Tsukada, K., Yasumura, M.: ActiveBelt: belt-type wearable tactile display for directional navigation. In: Davies, N., Mynatt, E.D., Siio, I. (eds.) UbiComp 2004. LNCS, vol. 3205, pp. 384–399. Springer, Heidelberg (2004). https://doi.org/10.1007/978-3-540-30119-6_23
10. Bliss, J.C., Katcher, M.H., Rogers, C.H., Shepard, R.P.: Optical-to-tactile image conversion for the blind. IEEE Trans. Man-Mach. Syst. **11**(1), 58–65 (1970)
11. Wall III, C., Weinberg, M.S., Schmidt, P.B., Krebs, D.E.: Balance prosthesis based on micromechanical sensors using vibrotactile feedback of tilt. IEEE Trans. Biomed. Eng. **48**(10), 1153–1161 (2001)

12. Maereg, A.T., Secco, A.L., Agidew, T.F., Diaz-Nieto, R., Nagar, A.: Wearable haptics for VR stiffness discrimination. In: International Workshop on Haptics, Pushing the Boundaries of Haptic Research for Health: Current Challenges. European Robotics Forum, Edinburgh (2017)

13. Priplata, A.A., Niemi, J.B., Harry, J.D., Lipsitz, L.A., Collins, J.J.: Vibrating insoles and balance control in elderly people. Lancet 362(9390), 1123–1124 (2003)

14. Van Erp, J.B.: Guidelines for the use of vibro-tactile displays in human computer interaction. In: Proceedings of Eurohaptics, pp. 18–22. IEEE (2002)

15. Stepanenko, Y., Sankar, T.S.: Vibro-impact analysis of control systems with mechanical clearance and its application to robotic actuators. J. dyn. Sys. Meas. Control 108(1), 9–16 (1986)

16. Benali-Khoudja, M., Hafez, M., Alexandre, J.M., Khedda, A., Moreau, V.: VITAL: a new low-cost vibro-tactile display system. In: IEEE International Conference on In Robotics and Automation, vol. 1, pp. 721–726 (2004)

17. Zaitsev, V., Sas, P.: Nonlinear response of a weakly damaged metal sample: a dissipative modulation mechanism of vibro-acoustic interaction. J. Vib. Control 6(6), 803–822 (2000)

18. Goodman, D.: Distributed Haptic feedback via Vibro-Actuator arrays. Undergraduate thesis, Hope University, Liverpool (2017)

19. Thoroughman, K.A., Shadmehr, R.: Learning of action through adaptive combination of motor primitives. Nature 407(6805), 742 (2000)

Daily Life Self-management and Self-treatment of Musculoskeletal Disorders Through SHOULPHY

I. Lucchesi[1,2], F. Lorussi[1,2], M. Bellizzi[1,3], N. Carbonaro[1,3], S. Casarosa[4], L. Trotta[4], and A. Tognetti[1,3(✉)]

[1] Center "E.Piaggio", University of Pisa, Pisa, Italy
a.tognetti@centropiaggio.unipi.it
[2] University of Pisa, Pisa, Italy
[3] Information Engineering Department, University of Pisa, Pisa, Italy
[4] Fisiokinetic, Rehabilitation Centre, Pisa, Italy

Abstract. The aim of the present work is to introduce SHOULPHY: a digital application, which includes a rehabilitation protocol for the treatment of Shoulder Impingement Syndrome (SIS). SHOULPHY, short for Shoulder Physiotherapy, represents a valid contribute for physicians allowing for the creation of a patient-centred physiotherapic program and remote monitoring patient's adherence to it, both in clinics and daily life. The application permits quantitative and effective evaluation of the therapeutic activity and functional level, through the use of wearable devices. The final purpose is to facilitate the functional recovery and maintenance of the physical level gained through the rehabilitation program, allowing for a complete return to sport and ordinary activities.

Keywords: Self-management and self-treatment of musculoskeletal disorders · Sensor wearable systems
Intelligent system for rehabilitation · Daily-life monitoring
Digital application · Virtual reality · Gamification

1 Introduction

Musculoskeletal disorders (MSDs) of the shoulder are common, with as many as 30.3% of adults experiencing shoulder pain annually, with significant economic impact [1]. The most common shoulder disorder regarding the shoulder girdle is Shoulder Impingement Syndrome (SIS), which is caused by a compression of some of the rotator cuff tendons, most prominently the supraspinatus tendon, along with the other soft structures, such as the long head of the biceps, the bursa and the ligaments in the subacromial space. SIS accounts for up to 48% of all consultations for shoulder pain, within primary care [2]. Repetitive activities, involving the use of the upper arm at or above the shoulder level, represent the primary risk factor for SIS; the target population is composed by a wide variety of workers, from construction employees, to athletes, who are directly exposed to

© ICST Institute for Computer Sciences, Social Informatics and Telecommunications Engineering 2018
P. Perego et al. (Eds.): MobiHealth 2017, LNICST 247, pp. 233–241, 2018.
https://doi.org/10.1007/978-3-319-98551-0_27

overhead work conditions, heavy lifting and forceful work, but may include also other categories, performing recreational activities that can be related to SIS [3]. Shoulder Impingement Syndrome is often caused by an imbalance between the forces involved in the shoulder motion, such as the deltoideus, the rotator cuff muscles and the scapula stabilizers. The incorrect activation of these muscular groups affects the movements of the shoulder, leading to changes in glenohumeral joint, with strong evidence of a reduction of the subacromial space during activities, when arm is elevated closer to an angle of 90° [4]. Differential diagnosis of this condition remains critical, since it can be very difficult to identify shoulder impingement relying on very generic symptoms, like shoulder pain and weakness. A large variety of treatment options are available depending on the stage of the condition, the patient's actual level of activity and the intended goals. However physical rehabilitation represents a key factor in the therapeutic protocol, to restore the functional level of activity, in patients presenting SIS [6,7]. The first aim of SIS therapy should be to restore a suitable balance between the forces involved in the shoulder motion in order to re-establish a correct kinematics and reduce the pain [5]. According to the European Musculoskeletal Conditions Surveillance and Information Network [9], the breakthrough in the management of musculoskeletal disorders, e.g. SIS, consists into asserting that patients affected by this condition can actively take part in the management of their physio-care. The main obstacle in the current therapy for SIS is compliance with and motivation to perform the training protocol; this aspect is quite relevant once the patient is discharged from the clinic. Due to the repetitive nature of the tasks, the exercises protocol may result tedious, not challenging and poorly interactive for the patient at home, thus limiting rehabilitation outcomes and functional recovery. Gamification of therapy in the rehabilitation field could be a good strategy to increase compliance and motivation, thanks to the possibility to self-challenge in a highly interactive digital environment, produced by the combined use of virtual reality and wearable devices [8]. In this context the present work has been focused on the development of a custom digital application for Shoulder Impingement Syndrome Telerehabilitation, which allows for patients evaluation and training in both indoor and outdoor environments. The SHOULPHY app, short for Shoulder Physiotherapy, relying on the use of wearable sensing devices and virtual reality, represents a simple, helpful and effective tool for both patients and physicians, in the management of SIS.

2 Materials and Methods

The SHOULPHY app through a wearable sensor platform, constituted by inertial sensors integrated into commonly used technological devices (e.g. smartband, smartphone, smartwatch) and innovative e-textile sensors (made of knitted piezo-resistive fabrics), allow for a continuous patient's activity monitoring. Inertial Measurement Units (IMU) rely upon microelectronic mechanical systems (MEMS), combining the information of accelerometers, gyroscopes and magnetometers, and are now widely used in wearable motion tracking [11,12].

The use of different IMUs, placed on connected body segments, and the additional information on the kinematic constraints enable most joint angles to be measured [13,14]. Textile-based or e-textile sensors are a key tool for unobtrusive human motion detection, having several advantages: low cost, lightweight, low thickness, flexibility, and the possibility of adapting them to different body structures. The main drawbacks are the reduced accuracy, the non-negligible transient time and the hysteresis. In recent works [15–17] we employed and characterized textile-based sensors based on knitted piezoresistive fabrics (KPF) that shown reliable performances as strain and angular transducers. In our recent study [10] a bi-articular model of the shoulder, combining the widely used socket-ball model with an additional joint, capable of describing both the movement of the scapular-thoracic complex and gleno-humeral joint and taking into account the constraint given by the scapular-humeral rhythm has been developed and validated, hence it has been considered as the reference biomechanical model for the reconstruction of the upper limb motion. The model is substantially based on the following relationship:

$$\begin{pmatrix} X_{Tr} \\ Y_{Tr} \\ Z_{Tr} \end{pmatrix} = \begin{pmatrix} A_{10} + A_{11}\sin(\theta_a)\cos(\psi_a) + D_{ht}\sin(\theta_{arm})\cos(\psi_{arm}) \\ A_{20} + A_{21}\sin(\theta_a)\sin(\psi_a) + D_{ht}\sin(\theta_{arm})\sin(\psi_{arm}) \\ A_{30} + A_{31}\cos(\theta_a) + D_{ht}\cos(\theta_{arm}) \end{pmatrix}$$

where A_{ij} with $i = 1, 2, 3$ and $j = 0, 1$ and D_{ht} are patient specific anatomical parameters, representing respectively the parameters related to the acromion position and the distance of the trochlea from the center of the humeral head. θ_a and ψ_a represent the scapular movements, while θ_{arm} and ψ_{arm} the gleno-humeral ones. The unknown parameters A_{ij} and D_{ht} can be identified by the minimization of the following functional:

$$G = \int_I \left(X_{Tr} - \hat{X}_{Tr} \right)^2 + \left(Y_{Tr} - \hat{Y}_{Tr} \right)^2 + \left(Z_{Tr} - \hat{Z}_{Tr} \right)^2 dI$$

Where $\hat{X}_{Tr}$, $\hat{Y}_{Tr}$ and $\hat{Z}_{Tr}$ are the real coordinates of the trochlea derived by the opto-electronic system (gold standard for motion capture systems), as described in [10].

3   The SHOULPHY App

SHOULPHY app represents a valid contribute for physicians allowing for the creation of a patient-centred physiotherapic program and remote monitoring patient's adherence to it, both in clinics and daily life. A gamified tele-rehabilitation approach is given, to allow the patient wearing a minimal set of sensors, to perform exercises, customely created through the application by clinicians, who can monitor remotely in real-time his activity and check his upgrades, stored in a database, as shown in Fig. 1. A comprehensive telerehabilitation program has been created with SHOULPHY, thanks to the collaboration with the expert physicians of Fisiokinetic, a high-qualified centre for physical rehabilitation, to provide the clinical requirements needed. The exercises of the training

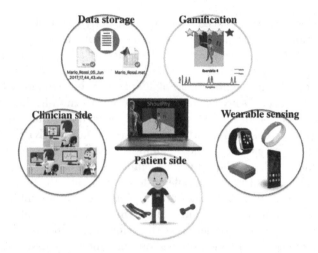

Fig. 1. The components of the SHOULPHY app

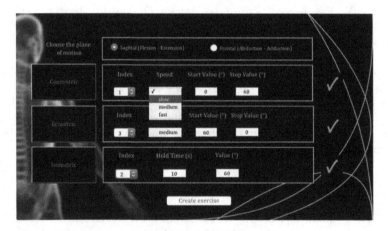

Fig. 2. Exercise creation

protocol can be created, by using different boxes, representing concentric, eccentric and isometric movements, that can be connected in series, thus building the entire exercise; for each box several parameters can be specified, such as the speed of motion, or the holding time, the amplitude and the index referring to the actual position in the training series. Once the exercise has been created, it is saved and loaded to the patient's interface, where it will control the movement of a virtual element, i.e. a ball, whose role is to guide the patient's shoulder motion in real-time. Moreover a video of a 3D avatar performing the exercise correctly is recorded and loaded on the patient's interface, where it acts as a tutorial. The physician should periodically update the training program, taking into account the patient's recovery level, basing on the monitoring of his activity, and checking the results remotely through the access in the progress monitoring section. The application permits quantitative and effective evaluation of the therapeutic activity and functional level, through the use of wearable devices and integrated standard questionnaire. The patient wears two sensors (on the forearm and sternum) that return the shoulder motion in terms of arm position with respect to a trunk coordinate system. With the wearable sensors on, the patient can choose an exercise from a library created ad hoc by physicians. The real-time visualization of the exercise performance is available through the virtual environment in which a 3D humanoid - driven by the sensors - reproduces the actual shoulder and trunk motion. This visualization modality is present on both user and physician interface, with the following advantages (Fig. 2):

1. The patient is alerted about incorrect movement thanks to the implementation of a visual feedback, consisting in tuning the colour of a target virtual object. The colour change depends on the difference between the actual motion and the desired one and permits the patient to adjust the movement during its execution (Fig. 3).
2. The clinician is able to visualize remotely - in real-time or off-line - the actual execution of the patient's motion, thus enabling for an effective monitoring of many rehabilitation sessions at the same time (Fig. 4).

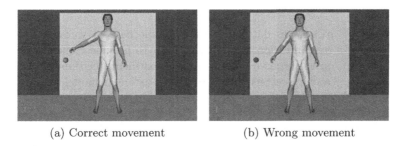

(a) Correct movement   (b) Wrong movement

Fig. 3. Visual feedback: the guide ball color changes when the user does not follow adequately the required movement. (Color figure online)

4   Results and Discussion

A scoring mechanism is implemented to assign virtual awards, in order to increase the patient's awareness about his physical condition. Clinicians rely on standard questionnaires for the functional evaluation of the shoulder. Among many others the Constant Murley test produces a score, ranging from 0 to 100, considering the four patient's domains (pain level, capability to perform ADL, range of motion, total strength). We implemented a modified version of the Constant Murley test by including a quantitative measure of abduction and flexion ROM obtained by sensors data, as in Fig. 5. Furthermore SHOULPHY allows

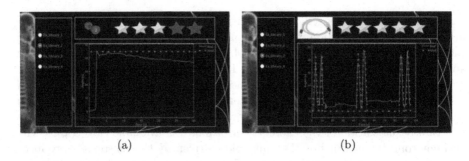

(a)   (b)

Fig. 4. (a) Isometric contraction at 45° on the frontal plane. (b) Concentric and eccentric contraction on the frontal plane.

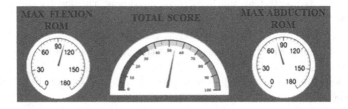

Fig. 5. Constant Murley shoulder test: Traditional score and additional maximum ROM in flexion and abduction

for data storage of sensors data and useful biomechanical variables, to keep track of patient's rehabilitation excursus, in order to provide clinicians a global database to lean on to improve diagnosis and treatment decision-making. The trajectory of the trochlea reconstructed by the bi-articular model, integrated in the SHOULPHY app, follows with high accuracy the real trajectory tracked by the optical system, as shown in Fig. 6. Different subjects have been asked to perform the required exercises created and integrated in SHOULPHY, in order to test the application at Fisiokinetic. The outcome obtained from each rehabilitation session have been delivered to the expert clinicians of Fisiokinetic, who have assessed the feasibility of our approach and the effectiveness to give a quantitative measurement of relevant biomechanical variables, involved in shoulder functional recovery. These data turned out to be helpful for the functional evaluation of the patient's shoulder during his rehabilitation program. The main limitation of our approach is related to the low accuracy of the system to track the upper limb movements at high speed of motion. Nevertheless, the motor tasks involved in a rehabilitation program require speed of motion that are fully compatible with the capability of our system to correctly acquire data from sensors and visualize them in real-time through the virtual humanoid on the user interface.

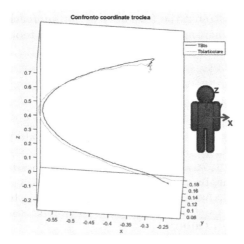

Fig. 6. Trajectory of the trochlea reconstructed by the bi-articular model (green), compared with the optical tracked one (blue) (Color figure online)

5 Conclusions

In our work SHOULPHY app for the evaluation and treatment of Shoulder Impingement Syndrome has been developed and tested. The application includes a standard evaluation test, and a customizable patient-centred rehabilitation program. The clinical specifications required for the development of the physical shoulder treatment have been accomplished thanks to the collaboration with the expert physicians of Fisiokinetic. This collaboration has permitted the creation of a telerehabilitation program through the ShoulPhy clinical interface. The contribute of a personalized virtual reality environment, gamification and a specific data transmission protocol has lead to several advantages, including:

- the opportunity to create a real-time 3D visualization system;
- the remote monitoring of the rehabilitation session by physicians;
- the detection of wrong movements that could potentially turn out to be dangerous;
- the creation of a clinical database, to keep track of the progress or eventually regress obtained through training;
- the increased motivation and adherence of the subjects to a rehabilitation program more involving and interactive, with respect to traditional rehabilitation;

The implemented software provide a digital version of the standard Constant Murley Score, by the addition of a quantitative outcome of ROM reached on frontal and sagittal planes. The training protocol can be adjusted on the specific goals and needs of the patient, moreover it can beuploaded periodically in order to facilitate a more rapid return to work and activities of daily living. As confirmed by the expert clinicians of Fisiokinetic the outcomes achieved by testing the application demonstrated the feasibility of our approach and the effectiveness to give a simple, smart and user-friendly evaluation tool to aid both patient and physician in the treatment of SIS.

References

1. Picavet, H.S.J., Schouten, J.S.A.G.: Musculoskeletal pain in the Netherlands: prevalences, consequences and risk groups, the DMC 3-study. Pain **102**(1), 167–178 (2003)
2. Van der Windt, D.A., et al.: Shoulder disorders in general practice: prognostic indicators of outcome. Br. J. Gen. Pract. **46**(410), 519–523 (1996)
3. Van Rijn, R.M., et al.: Associations between work-related factors and specific disorders of the shoulder-a systematic review of the literature. Scand. J. Work Environ. Health **36**(3), 189–201 (2010)
4. Giphart, J.E., van der Meijden, O.A.J., Millett, P.J.: The effects of arm elevation on the 3-dimensional acromiohumeral distance: a biplane fluoroscopy study with normative data. J. Shoulder Elb. Surg. **21**(11), 1593–1600 (2012)
5. Brent Brotzam, S., Wilk, K.: Clinical Orthopedidic: Rehabilitation. Excerta Medica-Elsevier, pp. 142–161 (2004)
6. Desmeules, F., Côté, C.H., Frémont, P.: Therapeutic exercise and orthopedic manual therapy for impingement syndrome: a systematic review. Clin. J. Sport Med. **13**(3), 176–182 (2003)
7. Hanratty, C.E., et al.: The effectiveness of physiotherapy exercises in subacromial impingement syndrome: a systematic review and meta-analysis. Semin. Arthritis Rheum. **42**(3), 297–316 (2012)
8. Ravenek, K.E., Wolfe, D.L., Hitzig, S.L.: A scoping review of video gaming in rehabilitation. Disabil. Rehabil. Assist. Technol. **11**(6), 445–453 (2016)
9. Report on the impact of musculoskeletal conditions across the Member States - European Musculoskeletal Conditions Surveillance and Information Network - eumusc.net
10. Lorussi, F., et al.: A bi-articular model for scapular-humeral rhythm reconstruction through data from wearable sensors. J. Neuroeng. Rehabil. **13**(1), 40 (2016)
11. Roetenberg, D., et al.: Compensation of magnetic disturbances improves inertial and magnetic sensing of human body segment orientation. IEEE Trans. Neural Syst. Rehabil. Eng. **13**(3), 395–405 (2005)
12. Sabatini, A.M.: Estimating three-dimensional orientation of human body parts by inertial/magnetic sensing. Sensors **11**(2), 1489–1525 (2011)
13. Luinge, H.J., Veltink, P.H., Baten, C.T.M.: Ambulatory measurement of arm orientation. J. Biomech. **40**(1), 78–85 (2007)
14. Roetenberg, D., Slycke, P.J., Veltink, P.H.: Ambulatory position and orientation tracking fusing magnetic and inertial sensing. IEEE Trans. Biomed. Eng. **54**(5), 883–890 (2007)
15. Dalle Mura, G., et al.: Piezoresistive goniometer network for sensing gloves. In: Roa Romero, L. (ed.) XIII Mediterranean Conference on Medical and Biological Engineering and Computing 2013. IFMBE Proceedings, vol. 41, pp. 1547–1550. Springer, Cham (2014). https://doi.org/10.1007/978-3-319-00846-2_382

16. Carbonaro, N., Dalle Mura, G., Lorussi, F., Paradiso, R., De Rossi, D., Tognetti, A.: Exploiting wearable goniometer technology for motion sensing gloves. IEEE J. Biomed. Health Inf. **18**(6), 1788–1795 (2014)

17. Tognetti, A., Lorussi, F., Carbonaro, N., de Rossi, D.: Wearable goniometer and accelerometer sensory fusion for knee joint angle measurement in daily life. Sensors **15**(11), 28435–28455 (2015)

Real-Time Schizophrenia Monitoring Using Wearable Motion Sensitive Devices

Talia Tron[1](✉), Yehezkel S. Resheff[1], Mikhail Bazhmin[2], Abraham Peled[2,3], and Daphna Weinshall[4]

[1] The Edmond and Lily Safra Center (ELSC) for Brain Science, Hebrew University of Jerusalem (HUJI), Jerusalem, Israel
talia.tron@mail.huji.ac.il
[2] Sha'ar Menashe Mental Health Center, Hadera, Israel
[3] Rappaport Faculty of Medicine, Technion Institute of Technology, Haifa, Israel
[4] The Rachel and Selim Benin School of Computer Science and Engineering, HUJI, Jerusalem, Israel

Abstract. Motor peculiarity is an integral part of the schizophrenia disorder, having various manifestations both throughout the phases of the disease, and as a response to treatment. The current subjective non-quantitative evaluation of these traits leads to multiple interpretations of phenomenology, which impairs the reliability and validity of psychiatric diagnosis. Our long-term objective is to quantitatively measure motor behavior in schizophrenia patients, and develop automatic tools and methods for patient monitoring and treatment adjustment. In the present study, wearable devices were distributed among 25 inpatients in the closed wards of a Mental Health Center. Motor activity was measured using embedded accelerometers, as well as light and temperature sensors. The devices were worn continuously by participants throughout the duration of the experiment, approximately one month. During this period participants were also clinically evaluated twice weekly, including patients' mental, motor, and neurological symptom severity. Medication regimes and outstanding events were also recorded by hospital staff. Below we discuss the general framework for monitoring psychiatric patients with wearable devices. We then present results showing correlations between features of activity in various daily time-windows, and measures derived from the psychiatrist's clinical assessment or abnormal events in the patients' routine.

1 Introduction

Clinical literature describes a wide range of motor pattern alternations, manifested in different phases of the schizophrenia disorder. Positive-signs schizophrenia patients are typically psychotic and disorganized, characterized mainly

---

Published in Proc. of 7th EAI International Conference on Wireless Mobile Communication and Healthcare (MobiHealth), Nov 2017, Vienna Austria.
T. Tron and Y.S. Resheff contributed equally to this work.

© ICST Institute for Computer Sciences, Social Informatics and Telecommunications Engineering 2018
P. Perego et al. (Eds.): MobiHealth 2017, LNICST 247, pp. 242–249, 2018.
https://doi.org/10.1007/978-3-319-98551-0_28

by positive symptoms (e.g. auditory hallucinations, delusions and paranoid thoughts). In clinical settings, these patients show involuntary movements, dyskinesia and catatonic symptoms [1]. In negative-signs schizophrenia, there is usually an observed motor retardation, psycho-motor poverty, decreased spontaneous movements, psycho-motor slowing and flattened affect [2,3]. Some patients demonstrate both types simultaneously or during different phases of the illness.

Neurological Soft Symptoms (NSS) can manifest early and during the progression of the disorder, and include deficits in coordination, sensory integration, and sequential motor behaviors [4]. Medical treatment was found to improve some of the motor symptoms, including NSS, involuntary movement and dyskinesia [1]. These medications, however, may also introduce in chronic patients drug-induced movement disorders such as tremor dystonia, Parkinsonism (rigidity and bradykinesia), akathisia and tardive dyskinesia [5].

The diversity and specificity of motor symptoms throughout different phases of the disorder and as a response to drugs, makes them good candidates for patient monitoring and treatment outcome evaluation. Nonetheless, to date, these symptoms are evaluated in a descriptive non etiological manner based on subjective clinical scales such as the Unified Dyskinesia Rating Scale (UDysRS) [6] and the Unified Parkinson's Disease Rating Scale (MDS-UPDRS) [7]. The lack of objective, quantitative methods of measuring these symptoms, and the insufficient conceptual clarity around it, causes multiple interpretations of phenomenology, often entailing low reliability and validity of the diagnosis. In addition, symptom evaluation process requires expert staff and availability of resources, and it is not done frequently enough to capture delicate changes in patients' spontaneous and drug-induced conditions.

The last decade has seen a steep rise in the use of wearable devices in medical fields ranging from human physiology [8] to movement disorders [9,10] and mental health [11]. Accelerometers and gyroscopes, which are commonly embedded in smart-watches and other wearable devices, are now used to assess mobility, recognize activity, and context. In a clinical setting, these sensors may be used in order to detect change in high-level movement parameters, track their dynamics and correlate them with mental state.

The objective of the current study is to develop and evaluate a framework, where wearable devices are used to facilitate continuous motor deficits monitoring in schizophrenia patients in a natural setting. This is an important step towards a detailed automatic evaluation system of symptom severity in schizophrenia. Such a system has a great potential to help understand this illusive disease. An additional goal would be to help with the overwhelming need for detection and characterization of sub-types of the disease towards a better understanding of underlying causes, and the development of better and more personalized treatment.

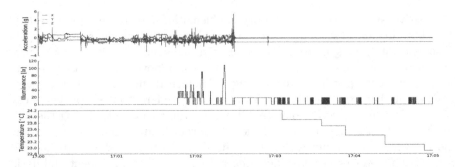

Fig. 1. Raw data as recorded by the smart-watches, including tri-axial accelerometer (top panel), light sensor (middle), and temperature (bottom). This plot shows data from a single patient, recorded on 28 Jan, 2017 at 5:00–5:05pm. Only accelerometer data was used for further analysis.

2   Methods

2.1   Participants and Clinical Evaluation

Twenty seven inpatients from the closed wards at Shaar-Meashe MHC participated in the study after signing appropriate Helsinki legal consents. Most participants (21/27) were diagnosed with schizophrenia according to the DSM-5, 3 with paranoid schizophrenia, 2 with schizoaffective disorder, and one with psychotic state cannabinoids. Participants' age varied from 21 to 58 (mean of 37.48), with course of illness varying from 0 (first hospitalization) up to 37 years (mean of 16.9 years). Two of the patients dropped out of the study after less than a day due to lack of cooperation. The rest (25 patients) were followed for a period of three weeks on average (6–52 days).

The study was conducted in natural settings, where patients were *not* required to change any personal or medical procedure. In addition to routine reports by nurses and physicians, every patient underwent an additional evaluation by a trained psychiatrist twice a week. The procedure included medication monitoring (type, dosage and frequency), as well as clinical evaluation of positive and negative symptom severity (PANSS [12]) and neurological symptoms severity (NES [13]).

All procedures performed in the study were in accordance with the ethical standards of the institutional research committee and with the 1964 Helsinki declaration and its later amendments or comparable ethical standards.

2.2   Data Acquisition

At study onset, each participant was given a smart-watch (GeneActiv[1]). The devices included tri-axial accelerometers, light, and temperature sensors, the high frequency output (50 Hz) of which was stored on memory cards embedded in

---

[1] https://www.geneactiv.org/.

the device (see Fig. 1). Data was collected by the aforementioned smart watches worn continuously by patients throughout the experiment (for a total of 489 days of data from 25 patients). The devices were placed and removed by the medical staff, and the content of the memory card was uploaded to a central storage location upon termination of the experiment for further analysis.

In order to reduce noise introduced by the variability in patient activity due to external circumstances rather than mental state, weekends were excluded from the study; our analysis focused on fixed time windows with regular departmental daily activity: Occupational therapy time slots (10am–11am), lunch (12pm–1pm), and indoor free time (4pm–5pm). In addition, we calculated full day features (6am–10pm) and used night time features (10pm–6am) to evaluate sleep quality.

2.3   Features

Features were computed on the basis of the accelerometer readings, analyzed in 1 min windows (see Table 1 and Fig. 2). Light and temperature data were not used for the analysis. The point-wise sum of values and sum of square values of the tri-axial accelerometer measurements (Energy Square and Energy Sum respectively) were averaged over 1 min intervals. The variance of the sum of squares (Energy Variance) was also computed over the same window. Stepping behavior (Step Detector) was detected as large maxima of the smoothed square norm of the point-wise acceleration. Overall Dynamic Body Acceleration (ODBA), a measure of energy expenditure, was computed as the mean norm of the accelerometer signal after application of a high-pass filter.

Table 1. List of features calculated on the basis of the tri-axial Accelerometers. Average and variance was calculated on a 1 min time window.

Feature	Description
Step Detector	Simple count of the number of steps per minute
Energy Square	Averaged sum of point-wise square acceleration
Energy Sum	Averaged sum of point-wise acceleration
Energy Variance	Variance of point-wise square acceleration
ODBA	Mean norm of a high-passed version of acceleration

2.4   Clinical Assessments

The 30-item scale for positive and negative symptom assessment (PANSS) was reduced to the following 5 literature-based factors: Positive, Negative, Disorganized/Concrete, Excited and Depressed. The dimensionality reduction was done according to the consensus model suggested by Wallwork et al. [14], based on 25 previously published models and refined with confirmatory factor analysis (CFA).

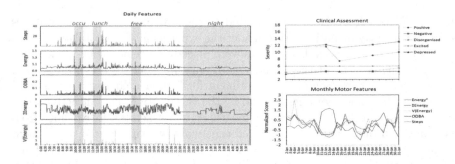

Fig. 2. The daily features of a single subject (left): gray areas indicate the time windows used for aggregated feature calculation. Monthly follow-up of a single patient (right): top panel shows the clinical five-factor PANSS score given by a trained psychiatrist on a bi-weekly basis; bottom panel shows the aggregated features calculated based on the different time windows.

The negative and positive factors had low between-factor correlation ($R = 0.399$), indicating good separation of the symptomatology space. As expected, the positive factor was in high correlation with the mean of all positive PANSS items ($R = .944$), and likewise the negative factor was in high correlation with the mean of all negative PANSS items ($R = .972$).

3   Results

We investigated two distinct ways by which wearable devices can be used for patient monitoring, in order to assist physicians in understanding the state of a patient. The first aspect of monitoring relates to the automatic assessment of a patient's condition, in order to provide automated, continuous, and objective measures of mental state. To this end we investigated the correlation between the computed measures and assessments by physicians, as described in Sect. 3.1. The second aspect of monitoring relates to the detection of change (or anomalous behavior patterns) which warrants additional attention from the medical staff, as described in Sect. 3.2.

3.1   Movement Patterns and Mental State

In order to investigate the correspondence between patterns of movement and mental state, *multiple correlation analysis* was computed between activity related features (described in Sect. 2.2) and PANSS factors. Results (Table 2) indicate the predictive benefit of the computed activity-related features with respect to the PANSS factors. When separately considering features computed in each of the time-windows, it is evident that different time windows provide varying predictive value for the 5 different PANSS factors.

Specifically, the Depressed Factor is described relatively well using features from the *free time* window, with 31.01% explained variance, while all other time-windows are below 10%. Both Positive and Negative factors are described well

Table 2. Percent explained variance based on *Multiple Correlation* between computed features in each of the 5 time-windows and each of the 5 PANSS factors. (See Sect. 2.2 for time-window specifications.)

	free	lunch	occu	day	night	all
Positive Factor	16.30%	11.14%	12.31%	19.80%	5.21%	53.77%
Negative Factor	19.74%	3.15%	2.06%	18.36%	9.77%	55.50%
Disorganized/Concrete Factor	22.73%	0.50%	15.13%	13.42%	5.82%	64.81%
Excited Factor	23.79%	8.75%	15.08%	10.35%	12.70%	57.10%
Depressed Factor	31.01%	9.23%	8.94%	5.78%	6.39%	58.33%

using features from the *free time* as well as *all day* time-windows. The remaining factors are again best described using *free time*. Overall, the *free time* window is the single most effective window, presumably since it imposes less structure on the movement of the subjects, allowing for the manifestation of the underlying mental state. In all cases, combining all time windows (rightmost column in Table 2) leads to substantially higher explained variance, compared to any of the individual windows.

Interestingly, looking at individual variable correlations we see that step count during *free time* was positively correlated with positive, disorganized and exited factor ($R = 0.37, 0.37$ and 0.31 respectively), but not with the negative and depressed factors. In addition, patients who had higher scores in disorganized and exited factors tended to have lower Energy scores during occupational time ($R = -0.28$ for Energy Sum and -0.22 for Energy Variance). This may indicate some motor retardation which is manifested only in non-walking time.

3.2 Continuous Monitoring

Our measures can be used to track changes in the patient's condition as compared to some established normal baseline, and may identify external events which are correlated with the departure from normality. Figure 3 demonstrates such a case: daily *step counts* of a patient dramatically increased 5-fold, at the same time as a significant change in medication dosage was introduced. Whether the

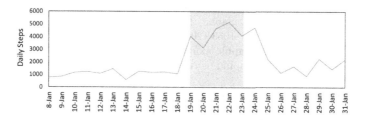

Fig. 3. Mean *daily steps* of a single subject. The gray area corresponds to a short-lasting change in medication regime.

change in medication *caused* the rise in movement propensity or they were both triggered by a change in mental state, this observation points to the relevance of monitoring macro movement patterns as part of routine patient monitoring.

4   Conclusions

We describe a study designed to evaluate the utility of wearable devices fitted with accelerometer, light, and temperature sensors, for the monitoring of schizophrenia patients in a closed ward mental health institution. Initial results show correlations between features of activity in various daily time-windows, and factors derived from the PANSS assessment.

Results indicate that movement features during free time are the most indicative of mental state. This finding is somewhat counter-intuitive, since the more structured activity during occupational therapy or lunch was expected to highlight differences in the state of patients. However, our results clearly show that the behavior of individuals when left to their own devices is better correlated with the PANSS factors.

These findings point to the possibility of automatically and continuously tracking Schizophrenia related symptoms and patient state in a natural setting hospital environment. The benefits of such a tracking system are twofold; first, the continuous tracking will assist physicians in understanding the state of a patient on an on-going basis, as opposed to specific points in time, when assessed by the doctor. Second, long term monitoring of a large number of patients will produce data allowing us to develop objective measures of motor aspects of the illness, and facilitate a more personalized, objective, and data driven approach which is much needed in the field of mental health.

Future work will focus on measuring the utility of this approach as an augmentation tool from a physicians perspective on the one hand, and the ability to predict physician assessments for automation of diagnosis on the other.

References

1. Peralta, V., Cuesta, M.J.: The effect of antipsychotic medication on neuromotor abnormalities in neuroleptic-naive nonaffective psychotic patients: a naturalistic study with haloperidol, risperidone, or olanzapine. Prim Care Companion J. Clin. Psychiatry 12(2), e1-11 (2010)
2. Morrens, M., Hulstijn, W., Sabbe, B.: Psychomotor slowing in schizophrenia. Schizophr. Bull. 33(4), 1038–1053 (2007)
3. Wichniak, A., et al.: Actigraphic monitoring of activity and rest in schizophrenic patients treated with olanzapine or risperidone. J. Psychiatr. Res. 45(10), 1381–1386 (2011)
4. Bombin, I., Arango, C., Buchanan, R.W.: Significance and meaning of neurological signs in schizophrenia: two decades later. Schizophr. Bull. 31(4), 962–977 (2005)
5. Janno, S., Holi, M., Tuisku, K., Wahlbeck, K.: Prevalence of neuroleptic-induced movement disorders in chronic schizophrenia inpatients. Am. J. Psychiatry 161(1), 160–163 (2004)

6. Goetz, C.G., Nutt, J.G., Stebbins, G.T.: The unified dyskinesia rating scale: presentation and clinimetric profile. Mov. Dis. **23**(16), 2398–2403 (2008)
7. Goetz, C.G., et al.: Movement disorder society-sponsored revision of the unified Parkinson's disease rating scale (MDS-UPDRS): scale presentation and clinimetric testing results. Mov. dis. **23**(15), 2129–2170 (2008)
8. Staudenmayer, J., He, S., Hickey, A., Sasaki, J., Freedson, P.: Methods to estimate aspects of physical activity and sedentary behavior from high-frequency wrist accelerometer measurements. J. Appl. Physiol. **119**(4), 396–403 (2015)
9. LeMoyne, R., Mastroianni, T., Cozza, M., Coroian, C., Grundfest, W.: Implementation of an iphone for characterizing Parkinson's disease tremor through a wireless accelerometer application. In: 2010 Annual International Conference of the IEEE Engineering in Medicine and Biology Society (EMBC), pp. 4954–4958. IEEE (2010)
10. Wagner, A., Fixler, N., Resheff, Y.S.: A wavelet-based approach to moniotring Parkinson's disease symptoms. In: International Conference on Acoustics, Speech, and Signal Processing (2017)
11. Wang, R., et al.: StudentLife: assessing mental health, academic performance and behavioral trends of college students using smartphones. In: Proceedings of the 2014 ACM International Joint Conference on Pervasive and Ubiquitous Computing, pp. 3–14. ACM (2014)
12. Kay, S.R., Flszbein, A., Opfer, L.A.: The positive and negative syndrome scale (PANSS) for schizophrenia. Schizo. Bull. **13**(2), 261 (1987)
13. Buchanan, R.W., Heinrichs, D.W.: The neurological evaluation scale (NES): a structured instrument for the assessment of neurological signs in schizophrenia. Psychiatry Res. **27**(3), 335–350 (1989)
14. Wallwork, R.S., Fortgang, R., Hashimoto, R., Weinberger, D.R., Dickinson, D.: Searching for a consensus five-factor model of the positive and negative syndrome scale for schizophrenia. Schizophr. Res. **137**(1), 246–250 (2012)

Smart Shoe-Based Evaluation of Gait Phase Detection Accuracy Using Body-Worn Accelerometers

Marco Avvenuti[1], Nicola Carbonaro[1,2], Mario G. C. A. Cimino[1],
Guglielmo Cola[1(✉)], Alessandro Tognetti[1,2], and Gigliola Vaglini[1]

[1] Dipartimento di Ingegneria dell'Informazione, University of Pisa,
Largo Lucio Lazzarino 1, 56122 Pisa, Italy
{marco.avvenuti,mario.cimino,gigliola.vaglini}@unipi.it,
g.cola@iet.unipi.it
[2] Research Center "E. Piaggio", University of Pisa,
Largo Lucio Lazzarino 1, 56122 Pisa, Italy
{nicola.carbonaro,alessandro.tognetti}@centropiaggio.unipi.it

Abstract. The spatio-temporal parameters of gait can reveal early signs of medical conditions affecting motor ability, including the frailty syndrome and neurodegenerative diseases. This has brought increasing interest into the development of wearable-based systems to automatically estimate the most relevant gait parameters, such as stride time and the duration of gait phases. The aim of this paper is to investigate the use of body-worn accelerometers at different positions as a means to continuously analyze gait. We relied on a smart shoe to provide the ground truth in terms of reliable gait phase measurements, so as to achieve a better understanding of the signal captured by body-worn sensors even during longer walks. A preliminary experiment shows that both trunk and thigh positions achieve accurate results, with a mean absolute error in the estimation of gait phases of ∼12 ms and ∼31 ms, respectively.

Keywords: Accelerometer · Frailty · Gait analysis
Gait phase detection · Smart shoe · Sensorized shoe · Thigh
Trunk · Wearable sensor

1 Introduction and Related Work

A person's manner of walking can reveal important information related to health and well-being. For instance, some studies have shown that abnormal gait is linked with a higher risk of falling, and gait analysis has been proposed for automated fall-risk assessment [13]. Other works have shown that a deviation in gait patterns can be an early indicator of cognitive impairment caused by a neurodegenerative disease [3]. Furthermore, it has been demonstrated that some gait parameters are highly sensitive for the identification of the frailty syndrome, which is characterized by reduced strength and motor ability [10].

© ICST Institute for Computer Sciences, Social Informatics and Telecommunications Engineering 2018
P. Perego et al. (Eds.): MobiHealth 2017, LNICST 247, pp. 250–257, 2018.
https://doi.org/10.1007/978-3-319-98551-0_29

A gait cycle is defined as the interval between two consecutive *heel-strike* (HS) events of the same foot. The duration of a gait interval is known as *stride time*. Gait is further characterized by the instants at which a foot leaves the ground and starts "swinging" forward: this is known as a *toe-off* (TO) event[1]. For each foot, there are two phases: *stance* (ground support) and *swing*. When both feet are in the stance phase, the subject is said to be in the *double support* (DS) phase. The ratio between DS and swing is particularly important, as a relatively longer DS phase has been linked with the frailty syndrome [10].

The typical approach to gait analysis is observational: the patient is required to frequently visit an equipped lab, where a trained clinician visually inspects the patient's gait during predefined tests. In the last years, there has been a significant effort for the development of automated techniques for gait analysis. Particular attention has been devoted to wearable sensor-based systems, as they enable the continuous monitoring of gait and other daily activities in uncontrolled environments [1,2,5]. To foster user acceptance, it is key to obtain an unobtrusive solution, possibly based on just one wearable device.

A commonly adopted trade-off between accuracy and usability is represented by placing a single wearable accelerometer over the lower trunk. In this context, an interesting evaluation of five different methods for the estimation of gait parameters is presented in [12]. Among the considered methods, a particularly relevant work is represented by [14], where the body's center of mass trajectory during walk is modeled as an inverted pendulum. This model is then exploited to estimate some gait parameters, including the detection of HS events based on a simple analysis of antero-posterior acceleration. More recent works, like [7], attempted to also detect TO events by analyzing the vertical component of acceleration.

In this paper, we study the detection of foot contact events (HS and TO) with accelerometers placed at two different body positions: over the lower trunk (approximately near the L3 vertebra) and inside a front trouser pocket. The works described above used an optical system or an instrumented platform with force sensors for their experimental evaluation. Consequently, HS and TO events were measured only for a limited number of consecutive steps. In the experiment proposed in this paper, the ground truth is provided by a sensorized shoe, hence foot contact evaluation becomes possible even during longer and unconstrained walks. A similar approach was proposed by [8], which exploited instrumented insoles to validate gait analysis with an ear-worn sensor.

The technique that we used for gait analysis with the trunk sensor is inspired by the techniques presented in previous works [7,14]. Differently, to the best of our knowledge, this is the first time that a pocket-worn device is used to detect foot contacts. This positioning could be exploited by smartphones, which are often carried in trouser pockets. Indeed some works, like the one recently presented in [9], have already evaluated the use of a smartphone's accelerometer for gait analysis, but the smartphone was placed over the subject's trunk.

---

[1] Some other works refer to heel-strike and toe-off as initial foot contact (IC) and final foot contact (FC) gait events, respectively.

2   Method

The sensor configuration used in this work is shown in Fig. 1. The user wears a single sensorized shoe and two Shimmer3 devices [11], one over the trunk (lower back) and one in a front trouser pocket (thigh). Hereafter, we refer to the two Shimmer devices as *trunk* and *pocket* sensors, respectively. Figure 1 also shows the anatomical directional references (vertical, antero-posterior AP, and medial-lateral directions).

In the following subsections, we first show the algorithm used to detect gait phases (i.e., stance and swing) using the sensorized shoe. Then, we describe the algorithms used to detect gait phases with the trunk and pocket sensors.

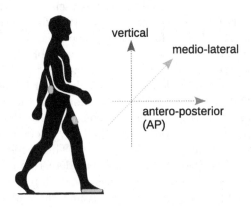

Fig. 1. Sensor placement (trunk, pocket, shoe) and reference anatomical directions.

2.1   Sensorized Shoe

Previous works have shown that gait phases (i.e., stance and swing) can be estimated with high accuracy by means of a sensorized shoe. An example is represented by [4], where acceleration and force sensors were exploited to detect foot contacts. The force sensors recognize heel and toes contact times, whereas the accelerometer is used mainly to avoid wrong detections of steps when the user is not walking.

In this work we used a single sensorized shoe, hence stance and swing times are calculated only with respect to the foot wearing the sensors. The shoe is a FootMoov 2.0, which is a new version of the smart shoe produced by Carlos S.p.A. and described in [4]. As in the first version, sensors and electronics are fully integrated below the insole. However, the full set of sensors has been significantly upgraded. A 9-axis inertial measurement unit (IMU) is positioned under the heel to enable the assessment of foot spatial orientation. Five pressure sensors are available to monitor the mechanical interaction of the foot with the ground. Three of the pressure sensors are positioned under the forefoot, while

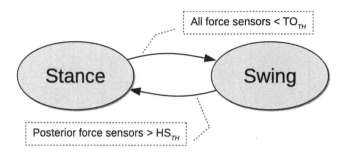

Fig. 2. Detection of gait phases with the sensorized shoe.

the remaining two are under the heel. These sensors are custom-made piezore-sistive transducers produced by using ink-jet printing of a conductive material on a flexible substrate. The Bluetooth 4.0 transmission module, fully integrated with the rest of the electronic unit in the heel of the shoe, enables low energy data transmission to a mobile device (smartphone, tablet).

The algorithm used in this study only required the analysis of four force sensors, two under the heel and two under the forefoot. HS events are detected by using the two sensors in the posterior part of the shoe, whereas the two anterior sensors were used to detect TO events. The detection algorithm is described by the finite state machine in Fig. 2. Initially, the user is in the *stance* state. When all force sensor values are below a threshold (TO_{TH}), a TO event is detected and the user is in the swing state. Swing terminates when both of the posterior sensors measure a force above a threshold (HS_{TH}). As mentioned before, stance time is the interval between HS and TO, whereas swing time is the interval between TO and the following HS.

The foot contact times provided by the shoe are used as ground truth to validate the following methods based on body-worn accelerometers.

2.2 Trunk (Lower Back) Sensor

Shimmer3 devices include an ST Micro LSM303DLHC tri-axial accelerometer, which was set to operate within ±8 g range. The reference frame of the trunk sensor is supposed to be approximately aligned with the anatomical directional references.

Figure 3 shows the acceleration during two consecutive gait cycles. More pre-cisely, the thin line shows the acceleration magnitude signal (Euclidean norm of the three acceleration signals), whereas the thick line shows the acceleration on the AP direction.

The method to detect HS and TO events proceeds as follows. First, gait cycles are identified by using the walking detection algorithm presented in [6], which exploits the groups of acceleration magnitude peaks produced at each step. For each detected step, a region including the group of peaks (gray bands in Fig. 3) is considered to search for HS and TO events. More precisely, foot contacts are found by analyzing the AP signal: HS events correspond to a local

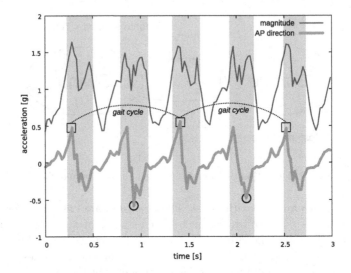

Fig. 3. Detection of gait phases with the trunk sensor.

maximum in the AP signal, as suggested in [14], whereas TO events correspond to a local minimum. The approach used to detect TO events differs from what we found in the literature, as typically vertical acceleration is used to detect TO events [7]. Detected HS and TO events are shown in Fig. 3 using squares and circles, respectively.

2.3 Pocket Sensor

A novel method is proposed to detect HS and TO events with an accelerometer carried in a front trouser pocket. The method enables the detection of the foot contacts produced by the leg that is carrying the sensor.

Figure 4 shows the same gait cycles as in the trunk example, this time measured with the pocket sensor. The thin line is the acceleration magnitude signal, whereas the thick line is the acceleration measured on the axis approximately aligned with the AP direction when the user is standing still. We use the letter z to refer to this axis: this corresponds to the reference frame typically adopted in smartphones (z is the axis orthogonal to the screen, and is approximately aligned with AP when the device is in a front trouser pocket). Differently from the trunk scenario, the pocket sensor "swings" during gait cycles because of leg movements, hence the orientation of the accelerometer with respect to gravity is not fixed.

Despite the significantly different pattern, the walking detection algorithm in [6] can still be used to detect steps and gait cycles by processing the acceleration magnitude signal. All the steps are highlighted with gray vertical bands. The proposed algorithm first needs to discriminate between the steps made with the leg carrying the sensor (*dominant steps*) and the ones made with the contralateral leg. To discriminate between dominant and contralateral steps the average

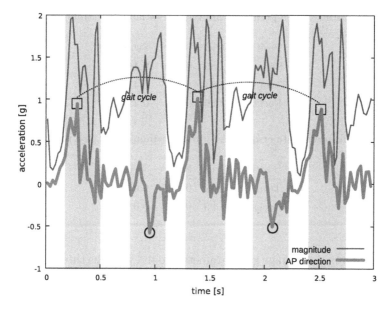

Fig. 4. Detection of gait phases with the pocket sensor.

value on the z axis is used: as shown in Fig. 4, during dominant steps there is a significant positive acceleration. Dominants are used to detect HS events by finding the local maximum value on z. Instead, contralateral steps are used to find TO events, by finding the local minimum on z. Detected HS and TO events are shown in Fig. 4 using squares and circles, respectively.

3 Evaluation and Discussion

For this preliminary experiment we recruited a healthy volunteer, who wore the three devices (sensorized shoe, pocket and trunk sensors) as in Fig. 1. The experiment consisted in walking two times through a straight corridor. In total, 44 gait cycles were performed. The shoe is capable of sampling force sensor data at ∼50 Hz, whereas the Shimmer's accelerometers were sampled at ∼200 Hz and then downsampled to 50 Hz. All the collected samples were stored into persistent memory to ensure repeatable evaluation.

The force sensor signals on the shoe were used to find the following parameters for each gait cycle: stride time (i.e., the duration of a gait cycle), swing and stance time relative to the left foot (the one wearing the instrumented shoe). In our approach, these parameters represent the ground truth. The methods for gait phase detection at trunk and pocket position were applied to the respective acceleration samples. As a result, we obtained estimations of stride, swing, and stance time for each gait cycle, which can be compared with the ground truth provided by the shoe.

Table 1. Temporal gait parameters estimation results [s]

Position	Stride	Stance	Swing
Shoe	1.085	0.670	0.415
Trunk	1.084	0.665	0.419
Pocket	1.086	0.675	0.411

Table 2. Mean absolute error (MAE) in the estimation of gait parameters [s]

Position	Stride	Stance	Swing
Trunk	0.011	0.012	0.014
Pocket	0.029	0.033	0.031

Table 1 shows the average gait parameters found with the three sensors. Interestingly, both trunk and pocket are able to estimate the three parameters with a maximum average error of 5 ms. More detail on the estimation error committed on each gait cycle is provided in Table 2, where it is shown the mean absolute error (MAE). The trunk sensor achieves higher accuracy, with a MAE between 11 and 14 ms. Notably, the error is significantly lower than the sampling period used (20 ms). This result confirms the accuracy reported by [12] for different approaches based on a single sensor placed over the trunk.

The results of the pocket experiment are promising. Despite the more challenging positioning (the orientation of the sensor changes during the swing phase), the average error is similar to the trunk experiment (Table 1), whereas the MAE is slightly higher (between 29 and 33 ms). The proposed technique is based on the assumption that one of the reference axes of the pocket sensor is approximately aligned with the AP direction. This is a reasonable assumption if we consider a smartphone carried in a front trouser pocket: due to the form factor of the device, the axis orthogonal to the screen is typically aligned with AP while the user walks. These results suggest that a smartphone could be used as a novel means to perform continuous gait analysis during everyday activities. In particular, the ratio between stance and swing times could be used to automatically detect early signs of motor ability issues.

In future work we plan to perform extensive experiments to further investigate the use of a pocket-worn device for gait analysis. Future experiments will take advantage of a higher sampling rate, and will include older adults with gait pathologies in the experiments. In fact, the results presented in this work, as well as in most of the works from the literature, have been obtained on healthy subjects. Specific experiments are required to prove that the methods can be used with (or adapted to) pathologic gait. Another important aspect that needs further investigation is the possibility of using a pocket-worn sensor to detect gait parameters relative to the contralateral leg (i.e., the leg that is not carrying the sensor). Finally, we plan to perform similar tests with a wrist-worn device, which could represent a further step towards unobtrusiveness and ease of use.

References

1. Alfeo, A.L., Barsocchi, P., Cimino, M.G.C.A., La Rosa, D., Palumbo, F., Vaglini, G.: Sleep behavior assessment via smartwatch and stigmergic receptive fields. Pers. Ubiquitous Comput. **22**(2), 227–243 (2018)
2. Alfeo, A.L., Cimino, M.G.C.A., Vaglini, G.: Measuring physical activity of older adults via smartwatch and stigmergic receptive fields. In: ICPRAM, pp. 724–730 (2017)
3. Buracchio, T., Dodge, H., Howieson, D., Wasserman, D., Kaye, J.: The trajectory of gait speed preceding mild cognitive impairment. Arch. Neurol. **67**(8), 980–986 (2010)
4. Carbonaro, N., Lorussi, F., Tognetti, A.: Assessment of a smart sensing shoe for gait phase detection in level walking. Electronics **5**(4), 78 (2016)
5. Cola, G., Avvenuti, M., Vecchio, A.: Real-time identification using gait pattern analysis on a standalone wearable accelerometer. Comput. J. **60**(8), 1173–1186 (2017)
6. Cola, G., Vecchio, A., Avvenuti, M.: Improving the performance of fall detection systems through walk recognition. J. Ambient Intell. Humanized Comput. **5**(6), 843–855 (2014)
7. González, R.C., López, A.M., Rodriguez-Uría, J., Álvarez, D., Alvarez, J.C.: Real-time gait event detection for normal subjects from lower trunk accelerations. Gait Posture **31**(3), 322–325 (2010)
8. Jarchi, D., Lo, B., Ieong, E., Nathwani, D., Yang, G.Z.: Validation of the e-AR sensor for gait event detection using the parotec foot insole with application to post-operative recovery monitoring. In: 11th International Conference on Wearable and Implantable Body Sensor Networks, BSN 2014, pp. 127–131 (2014)
9. Pepa, L., Verdini, F., Spalazzi, L.: Gait parameter and event estimation using smartphones. Gait Posture **57**(June), 217–223 (2017)
10. Schwenk, M., Howe, C., Saleh, A., Mohler, J., Grewal, G., Armstrong, D., Najafi, B.: Frailty and technology: a systematic review of gait analysis in those with frailty. Gerontology **60**(1), 79–89 (2014)
11. Shimmer (2017). http://www.shimmersensing.com
12. Trojaniello, D., Cereatti, A., Della Croce, U.: Accuracy, sensitivity and robustness of five different methods for the estimation of gait temporal parameters using a single inertial sensor mounted on the lower trunk. Gait Posture **40**(4), 487–492 (2014)
13. Verghese, J., Holtzer, R., Lipton, R.B., Wang, C.: Quantitative gait markers and incident fall risk in older adults. J. Gerontol. Ser. A Bio. Sci. Med. Sci. **64A**(8), 896–901 (2009)
14. Zijlstra, W., Hof, A.L.: Assessment of spatio-temporal gait parameters from trunk accelerations during human walking. Gait Posture **18**(2), 1–10 (2003)

Work in Progress

Comparison of Predictive Equations for Basal Metabolic Rate

Ardo Allik[✉], Siiri Mägi, Kristjan Pilt, Deniss Karai, Ivo Fridolin,
Mairo Leier, and Gert Jervan

Tallinn University of Technology, Akadeemia Tee 1, 12616 Tallinn, Estonia
ardo.allik@ttu.ee

Abstract. The aim of this study was to compare and evaluate multiple predictive equations for basal metabolic rate in order to choose the most suitable one for energy expenditure models. Eight different predictive equations were compared to each other using regression analysis and with the results of indirect calorimetry tests with 25 participants. Mifflin-St Jeor, Livingston-Kohlstadt and Henry-Rees predictive equations performed better than other formulas with Mifflin-St Jeor having the lowest RMSE of 175 kcal/day compared to the results of indirect calorimetry. The results of this study can be used to develop more accurate energy expenditure models.

Keywords: Energy expenditure · Predictive equations · Basal metabolic rate
Resting metabolic rate · Activity trackers · Physical activity

1 Introduction

Monitoring the physical activity (PA) is moving towards activity specific energy expenditure (EE) models that first recognise the activity and then apply a suitable EE algorithm for the specific activity type [1], which relies on accurate assessment of basal metabolic rate (BMR). For dietetics purposes BMR is commonly estimated using predictive equations, that use simple anthropometric variables such as the weight, height, age and sex of the person [2]. The aim of this study was to assess the BMR predictive equations by comparing different equations and validating their results with IC in order to choose the most suitable one for EE models.

2 Methods

The predictive equations explored in this study for BMR were Harris-Benedict [3], Schofield [4], FAO/WHO/UNU [5], Henry-Rees [6], and Kleiber [7] and for RMR were Mifflin-St Jeor [8], Owen [9, 10], Livingston-Kohlstadt [11]. EE values achieved with different predictive equations were compared to each other and with indirect calorimetry (IC) measurements. IC measurements were done using open-circuit indirect spirometry device "CareFusion MasterScreen CPX", which calculates EE based on Weir equation [12]. System was calibrated before each test subject.

© ICST Institute for Computer Sciences, Social Informatics and Telecommunications Engineering 2018
P. Perego et al. (Eds.): MobiHealth 2017, LNICST 247, pp. 261–264, 2018.
https://doi.org/10.1007/978-3-319-98551-0

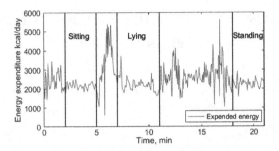

Fig. 1. Energy expenditure of one test subject during indirect calorimetry experiment.

The study group consisted of 25 healthy Caucasian adults, of whom 13 were male and 12 female. During IC measurements, EE was measured during three different positions – sitting on a chair, lying on a bed and standing up. The EE values during the experiment of one test subject are shown on Fig. 1. EE was calculated only based on the last minute of each activity. Even though standing and sitting should have approximately 1.3 times higher EE than lying [13], it was not possible to differentiate between these activities in this study (based on t-test results, $p < 0.05$). EE values from IC were divided by 1.3 and the values achieved with RMR equations were divided by 1.1 in order to compare the results with BMR equations.

3   Results

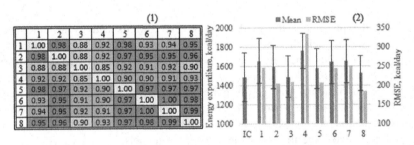

Fig. 2. (1) Coefficient of determination R^2 between different predictive equations. (2) Mean and SD of average BMR with indirect calorimetry (IC) and predictive equations; RMSE of BMR between predictive equations and IC. 1 – Harris-Benedict, 2 – Mifflin-St Jeor, 3 – Owen, 4 – Kleiber, 5 – Livingston-Kohlstadt, 6 – Schofield, 7 – FAO/WHO/UNO, 8 – Henry-Rees

4   Discussion

Based on regression analysis most equations had similar results, with Owen and Kleiber formulas being the outliers, which respectively had the lowest and highest average BMR results (Fig. 2). The average BMR values with Mifflin-St Jeor formula (1447 ± 204 kcal/day) were the closest with IC results (1485 ± 255 kcal/day) and also had the lowest RMSE of 175 kcal/day compared to IC. Based on paired t-test (p < 0.05), the results with Mifflin, Livingston-Kohlstadt and Henry-Rees equations were not statistically distinguishable from IC results.

While the results of this study can be used to compare different predictive equations and for developing different EE models, there are some limitations which can be improved on in future studies. First, the test group in this study was very homogeneous since only healthy adults of same race were included. Secondly, the IC calorimetry tests conducted in this study were part of a larger experiment, which is why each position was held for a minimal amount of time needed to reach an EE plateau.

The research was funded partly by the Estonian Ministry of Education and Research under institutional research financing IUTs 19-1 and 19-2, and by Estonian Centre of Excellence in IT (EXCITE) funded by European Regional Development Fund.

References

1. Altini, M., Penders, J., Amft, O.: Energy expenditure estimation using wearable sensors: a new methodology for activity-specific models. In: Wireless Health 2012, San Diego (2012)
2. Frankenfield, D., Roth-Yousey, L., Compher, C.: Comparison of predictive equations for resting metabolic rate in healthy nonobese and obese adults: a systematic review. J. Am. Diet. Assoc. **105**, 775–789 (2005)
3. Harris, J.A., Benedict, F.G.: A biometric study of human basal metabolism. Proc. Natl. Acad. Sci. USA **4**, 370–373 (1918)
4. Schofield, W.N.: Predicting basal metabolic rate, new standards and review of previous work. Hum. Nutr. Clin. Nutr. **39**, 5–41 (1985)
5. FAO/WHO/UNU: Energy and protein requirements: Report of a joint FAO/WHO/UNU expert consultation. World Health Organ. Technical report. Series 724 (1985)
6. Henry, C.J., Rees, D.G.: New predictive equations for the estimation of basal metabolic rate in tropical peoples. Eur. J. Clin. Nutr. **45**, 177–185 (1991)
7. Kleiber, M.: Body size and metabolism. Hilgardia **6**, 315–351 (1932)
8. Mifflin, M.D., St Jeor, S.T., Hill, L.A., Scott, B.J., Daugherty, S.A., Koh, Y.O.: A new predictive equation for resting energy expenditure in healthy individuals. Am. J. Clin. Nutr. **51**, 241–247 (1990)
9. Owen, O.E., et al.: A reappraisal of caloric requirements in healthy women. Am. J. Clin. Nutr. **44**, 1–19 (1986)
10. Owen, O.E., et al.: A reappraisal of the caloric requirements of men. Am. J. Clin. Nutr. **46**, 875–885 (1987)
11. Livingston, E.H., Kohlstadt, I.: Simplified resting metabolic rate-predicting formulas for normal-sized and obese individuals. Obes. Res. **13**, 1255–1262 (2005)

12. Weir, J. B. de V.: New methods for calculating metabolic rate with special reference to protein metabolism. J. Physiol. **109**, 1–9 (1949)
13. Ainsworth, B.E., et al.: 2011 Compendium of physical activities: a second update of codes and MET values. Med. Sci. Sports Exerc. **43**, 1575–1581 (2011)

Secure Mobile Automation of Ecological Momentary Assessments (EMA) for Structured Querying

Nikhil Yadav[1]([✉]), Mehrdad Aliasgari[2], Christopher Azzara[1], and Fazel Keshtkar[1]

[1] Division of Computer Science, Mathematics and Science, St. John's University, Queens, NY, USA
{yadavn,keshtkaf}@stjohns.edu, christopher.azzara14@my.stjohns.edu
[2] Department of Computer Engineering and Computer Science, California State University, Long Beach, CA, USA
mehrdad.aliasgari@csulb.edu

Abstract. The ubiquitous nature of mobile devices like smartphones and tablets make them ideal platforms for engaging users in Ecological Momentary Assessments (EMA). In EMA, participants are repeatedly assessed frequently (daily or multiple times per day) through a set of questionnaires. In this short paper, we present a secure EMA platform developed using Android mobile devices. The platform is flexible and can scale up to perform data mining tasks for sentiment analysis in patient rehabilitation settings.

Keywords: Mobile health · Data collection · Health surveys

1 Introduction

The ease of developing applications on mobile devices has meant that it is much more easier to create and deploy EMA studies on a large scale, as opposed to traditional paper and pencil methods [1]. Levels of engagement for users on devices such as smartphones are typically very high, meaning that they are ideal platforms for high frequency EMA studies [2]. Recent work has looked at coupling EMA and sensor data to assess physiological states, leading to an abundance of data for the interest of the medical and social science communities. In the rest of this paper we focus on the task of building a secure analytics framework leveraging EMA like surveys on Android tablet devices.

2 Implementation

A simplified EMA like mobile survey was implemented following the techniques and questions of some existing tests like the PHQ-9 (Patient Health Questionnaire) and D.I.R.E. (Diagnosis, Intractability, Risk, Efficacy). Results are stored on an Amazon web server communicating with the mobile application. The mobile survey is shown in Fig. 1.

© ICST Institute for Computer Sciences, Social Informatics and Telecommunications Engineering 2018
P. Perego et al. (Eds.): MobiHealth 2017, LNICST 247, pp. 265–267, 2018.
https://doi.org/10.1007/978-3-319-98551-0

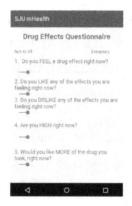

Fig. 1. Ecological Momentary Assessment Administered on Android Device

2.1 Data Flow and Security

The Transport Layer Security (TLS) protocol is used to provide the highest level of protection against outsider adversaries trying to intercept communication channels between the mobile application and server. The data collected on the mobile devices are encrypted prior to being stored. Each record is encrypted with a fresh new AES 256-bit key. In addition, a hash-based message authentication code (HMAC) of each encrypted data is appended to records prior to storage. The keys are themselves encrypted with a master key. In other words, for a record r, the following data structure is stored in the mobile application's database: $< c = \mathsf{Enc}_{k_e}(r),\ t = \mathsf{hmac}_{k_i}(c),\ \mathsf{Enc}_{k_m}(k_e, k_i) >$. Note that the encryption key (k_e) and the message integrity key (k_i) are generated anew for each record. The master key is an AES 256-bit encryption key that is generated when the application is installed. This key is securely stored in a secure storage service provided by the operating system (e.g., Keychain in iOS). The above scheme ensures confidentiality and integrity of user data collected on a mobile device. In order for an insider mobile adversary to compromise the security of user data, it is required to compromise the operating system and access the encryption master key (k_m) along with all encrypted records. With this mechanism, sensitive data is always stored encrypted and access is limited only to those entities that require them.

3 Results

3.1 Structured Data Storage

The format of the survey data collected is shown in Table 1. The *User* column is the MD5 hash of the full name of the user (truncated for display purposes). *EMA1* to *EMA5* correspond to the current five EMA questions on the mobile survey application, scored between 1 and 10. *PHY1* corresponds to a physiological indicator like heart rate. *BSL* in the table indicates whether the data is a baseline reading or not, and *ACT* indicates whether the data has been taken when the subject is in an active state, e.g., after some physical exercise.

Table 1. Structured EMA and Physiological Data

User	EMA1	EMA2	...	EMA5	PHY1	BSL	ACT
baa*	10	9	...	8	5	T	F
Cod*	5	2	...	1	3	T	T
baa*	10	8	...	8	5	F	F
Cod*	7	3	...	1	3	F	T

3.2 Structured Querying of EMA and Physiological Data

Some samples of queries that can run on the system in SQL syntax are shown below:

1. *SELECT User, PHY1 from EMA_PHY_TABLE, where EMA2<5*: Returns the physiological indicator, e.g., heart rate, for all users who do not want more medication drugs.
2. *SELECT EMA* from EMA_PHY_TABLE, where BSL<> 'T'*: Returns the momentary assessment scores which are not baselines.

4 Conclusion and Future Work

Future work will focus on integrating physiological health sensor IoT hardware with the developed platform, and create an API for researchers and health practitioners to modify (or replace) EMA surveys and analyze the data collected over time using data mining techniques.

References

1. Trull, T.J., Ebner-Priemer, U.W.: Using experience sampling methods/ecological momentary assessment (ESM/EMA) in clinical assessment and clinical research: introduction to the special section. Psychol. Assess. **21**(4), 457–462 (2009)
2. Intille, S.S.: Technological innovations enabling automatic, context-sensitive ecological momentary assessment. In: Shiffman, S., Stone, A.A., Atienza, A.A., Nebeling, L. (eds.) The Science of Real-time Data Capture, pp. 308–337. Oxford University Press, New York (2007)

MoodRush: Designing a Language-Free Mobile App for Mood Self-assessment

Sylvia Hach[1(✉)], Nilufar Baghaei[2], Ray Jauny[3], Christian Hayward[4],
and Abdolhossein Sarrafzadeh[5]

[1] Healthcare, Unitec Institute of Technology, Auckland, New Zealand
shach@unitec.ac.nz
[2] Department of Computing, Unitec Institute of Technology,
Auckland, New Zealand
nbaghaei@unitec.ac.nz
[3] Department of Nursing, Unitec Institute of Technology,
Auckland, New Zealand
rjauny@unitec.ac.nz
[4] IBM, Auckland, New Zealand
chayward102@gmail.com
[5] High Tech Transdisciplinary Network, Unitec Institute of Technology,
Auckland, New Zealand
hsarrafzadeh@unitec.ac.nz

Abstract. Depression affects a large percentage of young adults across the globe. The delivery of mental health information and the provision of tools for the self-assessment of mood are important means in addressing this problem. While self-assessment of mood is becoming more common through web resources and mobile applications, existing resources are limited in multiple ways. First, they typically include a significant language component and are therefore not suitable to youth with limited literacy/speakers of other languages. Second, existing tools are not visually engaging, usually constituting questionnaires presented on monochromatic background. Third, existing tools are limited in their clinical validity. This paper presents the background to the creation of a prototype mood self-assessment tool delivered via a mobile app. Based on a clinically validated mood self-assessment measure, the prototype guides the user through 21 pictorial questions and provides overall feedback. The user's level of engagement is assessed using data provided by Google Analytics and compared to their engagement with, and response to, the standard written self-assessment questionnaire.

Keywords: Mobile app · Depression · Young adults

1 Background and Problem

New Zealand has the second highest youth suicide rate of all OECD countries and the most critical age range is 15–24 (Bromet et al. 2011). In addition, international students globally experience high rates of depression (Furnham and Tresize 1981). This is coupled with lower usage rates of mental health support services by the international

© ICST Institute for Computer Sciences, Social Informatics and Telecommunications Engineering 2018
P. Perego et al. (Eds.): MobiHealth 2017, LNICST 247, pp. 268–272, 2018.
https://doi.org/10.1007/978-3-319-98551-0

student body (Ward 2001). Contributing factors include lower service accessibility and increased isolation/decreased social contact (Sam and Eide 1991).

A range of mental health support options including community-based, computer-based and phone depression treatment as well as online mental health information are available to young people in New Zealand. The provision of online offers seems particularly important given that in New Zealand 91% of people aged between 18 and 34 own a smartphone and spend significant amounts of time on their device (Vacaru et al. 2014).

In addition to mental health support, the delivery of online mental health information allowing the individual to identify whether they are affected by a mood disturbance that warrants treatment (Levitt et al. 2007) is crucial. Self-assessment is therapeutically beneficial, contributes to a better defined self-concept, facilitates self-regulation and is a key to goal setting (Sedikides 1993).

Existing online mood self-assessment tools are limited in that they most often include short versions of clinical self-assessment measures with limited clinical validity. Similarly, mood apps, even if carrying official endorsement, often have not undergone testing for clinical validity (Leigh and Flatt 2015) or efficacy (Donker et al. 2013). Existing tools also require a level of language proficiency and (health) literacy that may not be given in young people with English as a second language (Butcher and McGrath 2004). Finally, mood self-assessment questionnaires on monochromatic background arguably are limited in how engaging/attractive they are.

2 Aim and Research Question

The aim of the present project is to design and implement a prototype mood self-assessment mobile application based on a validated clinical assessment tool that is language-free and engaging for youth.

The overarching research question is whether, compared to existing online mood questionnaires, a language-free mood self-assessment tool in the form of a mobile application is; (i) more engaging/attractive to a young population, (ii) more accessible to a young population with English as a second language, and (iii) valid and reliable in identifying young adults who are native speakers of English and those with English as a second language affected by mood disturbance.

3 MoodRush Mobile Interface Design

A prototype mobile app named MoodRush containing pictorial versions of the 21 item Beck Depression Inventory (BDI-II) (Beck et al. 1996) has been created. Pioneered in the work with Latino populations, pictorial information in the form of a fotonovela has previously been shown to be particularly useful in delivering mental health information to young people (Cabassa et al. 2012). In order to increase potential uptake overall and increase uptake across all categories of socio-economic status/minimise selection bias, the prototype app has been designed for the Android Operating System.

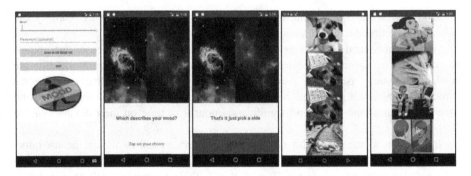

Fig. 1. MoodRush prototype log in/start screen, MoodRush user tutorial, tutorial positive feedback screen and MoodRush prototype sample items exemplifying the choice of image style and content (left to right).

To date, the design for the log on screen (see Fig. 1, far left) and language-free instructions have been completed with reference to the relevant guidelines (Android User Interface Guidelines 2017; Eichner and Dullabh 2007; Nielsen 1994). After the user logs in, they are presented with a tutorial (see Fig. 1, left). In line with Nielsen's (1994) aesthetic and minimalist design guidelines and in order to reduce executive demands (Maalouf et al. 2011), the explanations included as part of the tutorial activity were kept to a minimum. Tapping one of the tutorial pictures gives the user instant positive feedback. Images are presented in a user-timed fashion, meaning they stay on screen for as long or short as the user requires to make their decision. A back button has not been included in the design to allow comparability between users' MoodRush scores and their BDI-II score which includes instructions to not overthink the response.

Since the intended audience for MoodRush is likely to come from a wide range of cultures and backgrounds and, for a proportion of users, English will be a second language, design decisions were not based on Western-centric models where possible. Examples of this can be seen in the more inclusive top to bottom screen design (see Fig. 1, right and far right) and the use of a diverse range of pictorial response choices mostly comprised of cartoons and animals ensuring that not one race or ethnicity is highlighted (Clarkson et al. 2007).

MoodRush tracks user engagement and logs the data using GoogleAnalytics. Specifically, session time, completion rate and time spent interacting with the app in each session will be recorded. The prototype has also been configured to apply a weighting to user responses, to sum the weightings and store these in its internal database. The design of language-free feedback screens based on the sum of the weightings is ongoing.

4   Future Directions

Pilot data will be collected from 20 Unitec students (10 domestic; 10 international students; age range 17–24). An interview will provide accessibility data; number of completed MoodRush items and User Engagement Scale (Wiebe et al. 2014) will assess engagement; and a comparison of participants' MoodRush and BDI-II scores will provide first clinical validity estimates. A large-scale evaluation study will follow and desirability of mood tracking, data sharing and caregiver involvement will be explored.

Acknowledgements. We gratefully acknowledge the 2017 Unitec Strategic Research Fund.

References

Android User Interface Guidelines (2017). https://developer.android.com/guide/practices/ui_guidelines/index.html. Accessed 20 July 2002

Beck, A.T., Steer, R.A., Brown, G.: Manual for the Beck Depression Inventory-II. Psychological Corporation, San Antonio (1996)

Bromet, E., Andrade, L.H., Hwang, I., Sampson, N.A., Alonso, J., de Girolamo, G., Kessler, R.C.: Cross-national epidemiology of DSM-IV major depressive episode. BMC Med. **9**, 90 (2011)

Butcher, A., McGrath, T.: International students in New Zealand: needs and responses. Int. Educ. J. **5**(4), 540–551 (2004)

Cabassa, L.J., Molina, G.B., Baron, M.: Depression fotonovela: development of a depression literacy tool for Latinos with limited English proficiency. Health Promot. Pract. **13**(6), 747–754 (2012). https://doi.org/10.1177/1524839910367578

Clarkson, J., Coleman, J., Keates, S., Lebbon, C.: Inclusive design: design for the whole population. Springer, London (2007)

Donker, T., Petrie, K., Proudfoot, J., Clarke, J., Birch, M.R., Christensen, H.: Smartphones for smarter delivery of mental health programs: a systematic review. J. Med. Internet Res. **15**(11), 1–12 (2013). https://doi.org/10.2196/jmir.2791

Eichner, J., Dullabh, P.: Accessible Health Information Technology (IT) for Populations with Limited Literacy: A Guide for Developers and Purchasers of Health IT (2007)

Furnham, A., Tresize, L.: The mental health of foreign students. Soc. Sci. Med. **17**, 365–370 (1981)

Leigh, S., Flatt, S.: App-based psychological interventions: friend or foe? Evid.-Based Ment. Health **18**(4), 97–99 (2015)

Levitt, J.M., Saka, N., Hunter Romanelli, L., Hoagwood, K.: Early identification of mental health problems in schools: the status of instrumentation. J. Sch. Psychol. **45**(2), 163–191 (2007). https://doi.org/10.1016/j.jsp.2006.11.005

Maalouf, F.T., Brent, D., Clark, L., Tavitian, L., McHugh, R.M., Sahakian, B.J., Phillips, M.L.: Neurocognitive impairment in adolescent major depressive disorder: state vs. trait illness markers. J. Affect. Disord. **133**(3), 625–632 (2011). https://doi.org/10.1016/j.jad.2011.04.041

Nielsen, J.: Enhancing the explanatory power of usability heuristics. In: Proceedings of the ACM CHI 1994 Conference, pp. 152–158, Boston, MA (1994)

Sam, D.L., Eide, R.: Survey of mental health of foreign students. Scand. J. Psychol. **32**(1), 22–30 (1991). https://doi.org/10.1111/j.1467-9450.1991.tb00849.x

Sedikides, C.: Assessment, enhancement, and verification determinants of the self-evaluation process. J. Pers. Soc. Psychol. **65**(2), 317–338 (1993)

Vacaru, M.A., Shepherd, R.M., Sheridan, J.: New Zealand youth and their relationships with mobile phone technology. Int. J. Ment. Health Addict. 1–13 (2014). https://doi.org/10.1007/s11469-014-9488-z

Ward, C.: The impact of international students on domestic students and host institutions. Export education policy project, New Zealand Ministry of Education. Wellington: Ministry of Education (2001)

Wiebe, E.N., Lamb, A., Hardy, M., Sharek, D.: Measuring engagement in video game-based environments: Investigation of the user engagement scale. Comput. Hum. Behav. **32**, 123–132 (2014). https://doi.org/10.1016/j.chb.2013.12.001

Supporting Technologies for Improving Formal Care Management of Senior Patients with Alzheimer's Disease

Adriana Alexandru$^{(\boxtimes)}$, Marilena Ianculescu, Eleonora Tudora, and Dora Coardos

National Institute for Research and Development in Informatics, 8–10 Averescu Avenue, 011455 Bucharest, Romania
adriana_alexandru@yahoo.com,
{manina,gilda,coardos}@ici.ro

Abstract. Senior patients with Alzheimer's disease (AD) have some particularities that bring important challenges for their formal care management inside a health unit. Integrated smart services provided by Internet of Things (IoT)-based applications and Radio frequency identification (RFID) technologies bring a sustainable support to the healthcare providers. This paper puts forward the benefits obtained due to the setting up of these technologies for meeting the specific needs of those with Alzheimer's. A brief presentation of SeniorTrackway software application for the management of institutionalized patients with AD demonstrates the value of embedding the above technologies.

Keywords: Patients with alzheimer's disease · RFID · Internet of things
Real-Time locating system · Patient's tracking · Medication management

1 Introduction

The increasing longevity and the global ageing of the population have brought an expansion of Alzheimer's disease (AD) incidence. Once the disease is diagnosed, a long-term care is expected, together with a continuous deterioration of the senior's quality of life and health having impact not only on the independence and autonomy of the older person, but also on his/her family. That is a main reason for frequent institutionalization of them. A senior with AD in later stages needs almost permanent surveillance, assisted living to daily activities and a personalized management of the disease.

Health informatics, smart devices and IoT-based technologies are increasingly involved in the healthcare of seniors with AD with a proved impact on patients' life.

By attaching radio frequency identification (RFID) tags to different entities (people and objects), identification, tracking, location, security and other capabilities are provided. Any RFID system is composed of a set of discrete components: Tags – passive, semi-passive or active, Readers/Antennas – also known as Interrogators, Application Software & Middleware.

© ICST Institute for Computer Sciences, Social Informatics and Telecommunications Engineering 2018
P. Perego et al. (Eds.): MobiHealth 2017, LNICST 247, pp. 273–275, 2018.
https://doi.org/10.1007/978-3-319-98551-0

In the digital transformation of healthcare towards a patient-centered service delivery, Internet of Things (IoT) applications have as a main core the link between physical and digital environment. RFID, as a fundamental groundwork of IoT, provides data that identifies a particular person/object in a determined location and time.

SeniorTrackway software application for the management of institutionalized patients with AD is an example of how an informatics solution can bridge their specific needs and demands with the requirements of a proper and efficient formal care.

2 SeniorTrackway - a Software Application for the Management of Institutionalized Senior Patients with Alzheimer's Disease

SeniorTrackway is an *under development* Real-Time Locating System (RTLS) that aims to be aligned with IEEE 1847 standard and it is implemented in collaboration with AD Romanian specialists. Each RFID tag periodically transmits its own unique ID that is logged against the person to whom it is attached, thus allowing the system to locate the patient at risk within the building.

The objectives of the software application are:

1. *Protection of vulnerable patients* (institutionalized senior patients with AD) and *insurance of their safety* by offering real-time visibility of their position to the staff.
2. *Increased safety of patient at risk* by generation of local and remote audio/visual alarms and the automatically locking of the access door.
3. *Proving facilities of individual free movement within a defined indoor safe area.*
4. *Helping caregivers to provide the best care by using Active RFID Technology.* The system allows caregivers to keep tabs on all patients under their care and protect them without impeding their freedom of movement or that of their staff.
5. *Deployment of a cost effective solution.*

In SeniorTrackway deployment, each patient at risk of wandering wears a special RFID wristband - with a unique personal ID and some information about him (e.g. blood type, medical allergies, or other health history - which allows the individual free movement within a defined safe area. In addition, the same ID is contained in self-adhesive RFID labels for all patients' paper medical histories and other important documents. The position of each patient is tracked in real time. Any movement of a tagged patient beyond this area will generate an acoustic/light alarm signal or lock an exit door.

RFID readers are placed at strategic places within the hospital:

- RFID gates are mounted at admission and exit doors of the AD special care units.
- Each medical operational room contains minimum one RFID reader.
- RFID sensors are also placed in galleries and important offices (either placed next to the door or under the desks).
- The each staff member (doctors, nurses, caregivers and other employees) has a handheld device (PDA, mobile phone, etc.) equipped with an RFID reader and WiFi connection to the web.

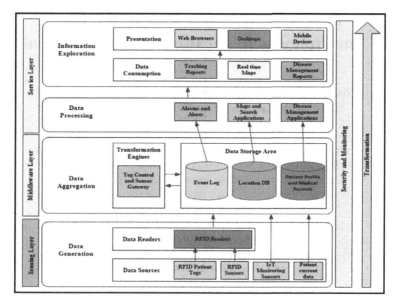

Fig. 1. SeniorTrackway Architecture

The architecture includes three main layers (see Fig. 1):

- *Sensing Layer*: RFID physical components sense the movement and targeted patients and capture the data from the individuals. The layer collects the information from RFID tags or RFID sensors.
- *Middleware Layer*: translates the raw data from the physical layer to the context (position and movement of the person), analyses and processes the data. The software in this layer may combine multiple sensors to analyze a data stream intelligibly.
- *Service Layer:* store the information about the tracked individuals and make it accessible by medical staff and caregivers in queries throughout real time monitoring servers. Notifications or warnings are provided in case of risks to the caregivers through monitoring and assessment consoles.

3   Conclusions

Providing a new approach for the Romanian healthcare domain, SeniorTrackway software application offers: (1) Easy and accurate detection of people within a safe area; (2) Advanced perimeter security performance; (3) High-quantity and high-density tag handling; (4) Reliable tag communications; (5) A holistic approach of specific AD issues as disorientation, abnormal behavior or comorbidities; (6) A particular design targeting directly the disease management of senior in-patients with AD.

Acknowledgments. This work has been developed under the framework of *"Using Big Data Technologies in Government Computer Systems"* and *"ICT in healthcare: A comparative analysis of the eHealth solutions in Member States and successful models in the world"* projects funded by the Romanian Ministry of Communication and Information Society (2015–2017).

Benefits and Limitations of the Use
of Smartphones by Healthy Older Individuals

Blanka Klimova[1(✉)], Petra Maresova[1], Hana Tomaskova[1],
Hana Mohelska[1], Michal Novotny[3], Marek Penhaker[2],
and Kamil Kuca[1]

[1] Faculty of Informatics and Management, University of Hradec Kralove,
Rokitanskeho 62, 500 03 Hradec Kralove, Czech Republic
{blanka.klimova,petra.maresovav,hana.tomaskova,
hana.mohelska,kamil.kuca}@uhk.cz
[2] Faculty of Electrical Engineering and Computer Science,
Technical University of Ostrava, Poruba, Czech Republic
marek.penhaker@vsb.cz
[3] Biomedical Research Centre, University Hospital Hradec Kralove,
Hradec Kralove, Czech Republic
michal.novotny@fnhk.cz

Abstract. Currently, there is a considerable increase in the number of older population groups worldwide. Therefore there is constant effort to prolong the active life of these older individuals as long as possible. And mobile devices such as smartphones seem to offer some benefits for enhancing the quality of life of seniors in the field of healthcare, independent living, socializing, or commerce. The purpose of this work in progress paper is to explore the main issues, benefits and limitations of the use of smartphones by older individuals. The research indicates that the smartphone use is not ubiquitous among the aging population groups, which is a pity since the use of smartphone could contribute to the improvement of quality of life of these older people and could increase seniors contributions to the society. Therefore there is an urgent call for the implementation of training in the smartphone use among the older generation groups in order to enable them to become aware of the benefits of smartphones for the enhancement of their quality of life.

Keywords: Smartphone · Older people · Use · Benefits · Limitations

1 Introduction

At present, there is a considerable increase in the number of older population groups worldwide. For example, in Europe seniors aged 55+ years represent 25% of the whole population [1]. Therefore there is constant effort to prolong the active life of these older individuals as long as possible [2]. And mobile devices such as smartphones seem to offer some benefits for enhancing the quality of life of seniors in the field of healthcare, independent living, socializing, or commerce [3]. In addition, current seniors aged 55+ years are now digitally aware and use smartphones widely. Therefore it might be expected that the use of smartphones among the older generation groups will rise

© ICST Institute for Computer Sciences, Social Informatics and Telecommunications Engineering 2018
P. Perego et al. (Eds.): MobiHealth 2017, LNICST 247, pp. 276–278, 2018.
https://doi.org/10.1007/978-3-319-98551-0

substantially [4]. In fact, the number of smartphone owners increases every year. In 2016 there were 2.1 billion of smartphone users worldwide and this number should reach 2.87 billion by the year of 2020 [5]. Moreover, 80% of the internet users own a smartphone [6].

The purpose of this review study is to explore the main issues, benefits and limitations of the use of smartphones by older individuals.

2   Current Situation in the Use of Smartphones by Older Healthy Individuals

At present, older adults, especially those aged 65+ years resist using smartphones due to their interface complexity, size of the device, anti-ease of use, and cost, as well as due to their physical (impaired visual and motor skills) or cognitive impairments.

On the other hand, Cota et al. [7] indicate that digital games played by the elderly people on their smartphones may delay cognitive decline of the aging population groups. They also show that although these digital games could be played on any mobile device, the elderly people prefer those which could be controlled by touching the screen. In addition, the study by Hong et al. [8] reveals that the use of smartphones considerably influences the internet literacy of its use by older people. Generally, the main benefits of the use of smartphone by the elderly include freedom and social connectedness [9]. Conci et al. [10] point out that older people are willing to accept and adopt a new technology such as a smartphone if it meets their needs and expectations. Zhou et al. [11] list six critical factors influencing older people to accept new functions. These include awareness and attractiveness, soft keys and multi-tap, touch screen, connectivity, concern of learning and social influence. In addition, McGaughey et al. [3] argue that it is especially motivation that makes the elderly people use the smartphone, as well as by proper training in order to let older people discover the benefits the smartphone can bring them since there is very low awareness of its benefits among these older people [12]. Klimova [12] lists several benefits of using the smartphone applications for health purposes, which are as follows: suitable and stimulating intervention and diagnostic tools for elderly; enhanced access to healthcare for elderly living in remote areas; improvement of elderly people's quality of life; cutting potential costs of treatment and care on elderly people; ecological approach.

On the contrary, the key limitations of the use of smartphones by healthy elderly include interface complexity, small size of the device, a lack of training, prize of the device, a lack of confidence, physical and cognitive impairment, or low awareness of the benefits of the smartphone use.

3   Conclusion

Overall, the smartphone use is not ubiquitous among the aging population groups, which is a pity since the use of smartphone could contribute to the improvement of quality of life of these older people and could increase seniors contributions to the society [8]. Therefore there is an urgent call for the implementation of training in the smartphone use among the older generation groups to enable them to become aware of the benefits of smartphones for the enhancement of their quality of life such as freedom, connectedness, health control, or enhancement of feelings of safety. In addition, there is a need for evidence-based studies revealing the effectiveness of smartphone use by these people, as well as showing them the benefits of this use.

Acknowledgments. The paper is supported by the project GAČR 2017 No. 15330/16/AGR Investment evaluation of medical device development run at the Faculty of Informatics and Management of the University of Hradec Kralove, Czech Republic.

References

1. Global AgeWatch index 2015: Insight report (2015). http://www.population.gov.za/index.php/npu-articles/send/22-aging/535-global-agewatch-index-2015-insight-report
2. Klimova, B.: Use of the Internet as a prevention tool against cognitive decline in normal aging. Clin. Interv. Aging **11**, 1231–1237 (2016)
3. McGaughey, R.E., Zeltman, S.M., McMurtrey, M.E.: Motivations and obstacles to smartphone use by the elderly: developing a research framework. Int. J. Electron. Finan. **7** (3–4), 177–195 (2013)
4. Virginia assistive technology system. Assistive technology and aging. A handbook for virginians who are aging and their caregivers (2017). http://www.vda.virginia.gov/pdfdocs/Assistive%20Technology%20&%20Aging%20-%20All.pdf
5. Statista (2017). https://www.statista.com/statistics/330695/number-of-smartphone-users-worldwide/
6. IMPACT (2016). https://www.impactbnd.com/blog/mobile-marketing-statistics-for-2016
7. Cota, T.T., Ishitani, L., Vieira, N.: Mobile game design for the elderly: a study with focus on the motivation to play. Comput. Hum. Behav. **51**, 96–105 (2015)
8. Hong, S.G., Trimi, S., Kim, D.: Smartphone use and internet literacy of senior citizens. J. Assist. Technol. **10**(1), 27–38 (2016)
9. Anderson, M.: For vast majority of seniors who own one, a smartphone equals freedom (2015). http://www.pewresearch.org/fact-tank/2015/04/29/seniors-smartphones/
10. Conci, M., Pianesi, F., Zancanaro, M.: Useful, social and enjoyable: mobile phone adoption by older people. In: Gross, T., et al. (eds.) INTERACT 2009. LNCS, vol. 5726, pp. 63–76. Springer, Heidelberg (2009)
11. Zhou, J., Rau, P.L.P., Salvendy, G.: Older adults' use of smart phones: an investigation of the factors influencing the acceptance of new functions. Behav. Inf. Technol. **33**(6), 552–560 (2014)
12. Klimova, B.: Mobile health devices for aging population groups: a review study. In: Younas, M., Awan, I., Kryvinska, N., Strauss C., van Thanh, D. (eds.) MobiWIS 2016. LNCS, vol. 9847, pp. 295–301. Springer, Cham (2016)

Author Index

Printed in the United States
By Bookmasters